THE FOUNDATION PROGRAMME

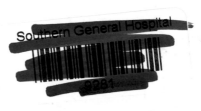

'Due to my poor planning, the rapidly changing situation on the ground and various competing projects, my contribution to this book was written before and after (but thankfully not during) the addition of baby Lucas to our family. I am eternally grateful for Nicky's tolerance and indulgence of my hours at the keyboard during its year long gestation.'

Mark Welfare

'Someone once told me the key to happiness is having a reliable shower and a decent ironing board. Well now I can add two more things to this one-sided equation: continuous inspiration (thanks to my fiancée Alixe), and this book. Thank you to Alan, who, I hope, knows who he is. I would also like to dedicate this to all the unsung docs out there, who never sing out of tune.'

Jonathan Carter

Commissioning Editor: Ellen Green, Pauline Graham
Development Editor: Hannah Kenner
Project Manager: Jess Thompson
Designer: Erik Bigland
Illustrator: Jonathan Haste

THE FOUNDATION PROGRAMME

The Medics' Practical Guide to Thriving and Surviving

Mark Welfare MD FRCP
Senior Lecturer
University of Newcastle;
Consultant Gastroenterologist
Lead for Educational Research
Northumbria Healthcare NHS Trust
Newcastle-upon-Tyne, UK

Jonathan Carter MBBS MRCP
Senior House Officer (Medicine)
University Hospital of North Tees
Stockton-on-Tees, UK

Foreword by
Phil Hammond MB BChir MRCGP
General Practitioner;
Writer and broadcaster;
Honorary Teaching Fellow
Royal United Hospital, Bath, UK

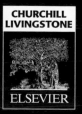

CHURCHILL
LIVINGSTONE

ELSEVIER

Edinburgh   London   New York   Oxford   Philadelphia   St Louis   Sydney   Toronto   2008

CHURCHILL LIVINGSTONE

CHURCHILL LIVINGSTONE
An imprint of Elsevier Limited

First published 2008

ISBN-13: 978-0-443-10334-6

British Library Cataloguing in Publication Data
A catalogue record for this book is available from the British Library

Library of Congress Cataloging in Publication Data
A catalog record for this book is available from the Library of Congress

Notice
Knowledge and best practice in this field are constantly changing. As new research and experience broaden our knowledge, changes in practice, treatment and drug therapy may become necessary or appropriate. Readers are advised to check the most current information provided (i) on procedures featured or (ii) by the manufacturer of each product to be administered, to verify the recommended dose or formula, the method and duration of administration, and contraindications. It is the responsibility of the practitioner, relying on their own experience and knowledge of the patient, to make diagnoses, to determine dosages and the best treatment for each individual patient, and to take all appropriate safety precautions. To the fullest extent of the law, neither the Publisher nor the Authors assume any liability for any injury and/or damage to persons or property arising out of or related to any use of the material contained in this book.

The Publisher

CONTENTS

Contents

Contents

Chapter 9 **When medicine is difficult 215**

Mark Welfare

FOREWORD

Phil Hammond

In the good old pre-Bristol/Harold Shipman days, medicine was a job for life. It was very hard to get kicked out of medical school and, once you qualified, you could be the worst doctor in the world (even a mass murderer) and still have a heaving (though gradually dwindling) waiting room. Clinical freedom was restrained only by cost, and quality control was down to individual conscience. It worked because the vast majority of doctors try to do their jobs well.

But paternalism and blind trust in doctors are no longer fashionable. Medicine is now ruled by criteria, targets and guidelines which masquerade as evidence-based but on closer scrutiny may be anything but. There is some good news. As the journalist who exposed the Bristol heart tragedy and called for surgeons to publish their results, I'm mighty relieved that such openness and scrutiny has not led to heart surgeons cherry picking easier operations. Not only are they taking on harder cases but the act of collecting and sharing their results appears to have driven mortality rates down.

On the downside, we have had the MMC mismanagement. However good the intention – to replace a job application process polluted with nepotism, discrimination and the old boy network with one that is fair, open and objective – the end result appears to have been anything but. Medicine has always been competitive, but the new system seems to combine incompetence (sending people to both ends of the country on the same day for jobs they didn't apply for) with unfairness (excellent candidates not being short-listed at the expense of erudite disaster zones). As an example, the MTAS website allowed confidential information on thousands of applicants, including their sexual orientation and previous convictions, to be publicly accessed. You couldn't make it up.

The upside of this scandal is that it united doctors and galvanized them into action. As a result, heads have rolled, the application process is under review and applicants have been guaranteed an interview for their first-choice job. But there are plenty more battles ahead. The NHS is being destroyed by political and bureaucratic incompetence, huge wastes of public money and the desperate belief that things would be better if we sold it off to large health corporations. Whatever stage you are at in your training, you need to stand up and shout about the errors and iniquities you encounter. This book is an excellent start, for both trainers and trainees. Unlike MTAS, it's independent, objective and funny. And the scope is very impressive, with topics ranging from the genesis of the Foundation programme to sound advice on career options and how to survive in a job that is as stressful as it can be rewarding.

The bottom line is clear. Just as patients no longer wish to be passive recipients of medical care, neither should trainees just take what's handed to them. Get informed, get involved and fight your corner. Heart surgery may be blazing the trail when it comes to accountability, but training programmes are closing because of the dubious belief that statins and stenting will make surgeons redundant. To survive in the NHS you'll need to be flexible and multi-skilled with fewer hours to train. Clearly training will have to get a whole lot better.

Nothing could be more important for patient welfare than the right people getting the right jobs and being given the resources to do them well. When I'm finally dragged kicking and screaming onto an NHS ward, I want to be treated by a doctor with sufficient wisdom, skill and motivation to do the job properly, not a dumbed down generic health worker reading from a guideline. So please – if only for my sake – keep shouting until you get the training you deserve. And when the going gets tough, remember the three Ps; Pace yourself, Pamper yourself and P*ss yourself laughing.

Phil Hammond, GP, writer and broadcaster

PREFACE

We set out to address two unmet needs in this book. First, there is the need for a book that helps new doctors to cope with the pressures of their initial year, which has always been stressful. Second, we offer a map through the radically altered new training system.

As it says on the label, we hope that the book not only helps you survive the Foundation programme, but also thrive and go on to achieve your future career wishes.

For trainers reading this book, we hope that it will help you understand better the reasons behind the changes, the detail of the Foundation programme curriculum and assessment processes, and what you can do to help your trainees survive and thrive.

Perhaps more importantly we want the book to be independent of all the official bodies that have been involved in its development (including the British Medical Association [BMA] and Modernising Medical Careers [MMC]) so that it is seen by its readers to be free from spin and as objective and unbiased as possible.

SURVIVING AND THRIVING IN THE FOUNDATION PROGRAMME

Mark Welfare and Jonathan Carter

'Do not believe something because it is in a book or a sage has told you it is so: go and examine it yourself.'

The last lesson of Buddha

Introduction

Mark Welfare

❝ The trick to forgetting the big picture is to look at everything close up. ❞

Chuck Palahniuk

This book hopes to fill a gap

The transition from student to doctor has always been a rewarding but tricky one. It is exciting and exhilarating and may feel like a relief after your long training. But new responsibilities and pressures can be difficult to deal with, particularly when you are sleep-deprived.

Most books on becoming a doctor have concentrated on the clinical aspects of the job, giving summary guides to clinical problems and prescribing. There has been little on managing your learning or career, or on ways of avoiding problems.

Then, on top of the difficulties of your own transition, a transition in the training of doctors has been thrown in. The changes in medical training are revolutionizing the trainees' experience, but they have been introduced rapidly and have caused much confusion and heartache. The provision of information about the changes has been patchy and often polarised. The views of seniors have been mixed; many do not understand why the changes have been seen as necessary. Lack of familiarity with the new ways of training has meant that some have withdrawn their goodwill and involvement. Much of the preparation (e.g. teaching materials or applications systems) was inadequate or patchy.

The historical context of this book is also important. Chuck Palahniuk in the epigraph to this chapter gives us a pertinent warning. Doctors are not immune to this forgetting disease so a review of the history is important to enable readers to understand the context.

WHY WAS THE FOUNDATION PROGRAMME INTRODUCED?

The Foundation programme is a part of the revision of postgraduate medical training which started with a review of SHO training with the publication of *Unfinished Business* in 2002 and will not be fully realised until the first GP educated under the new system receives the Certificate of Specialist Training in 2009 and the first consultant specialist is appointed in approximately 2013. Such change occurs only once in every two or three generations so it is understandable that the implementation phase has required adjustments and fine-tuning. Many problems were identified in the old training system and efforts have been made to overcome them. A whole new lexicon of abbreviations and education terminology has been invented. Unfortunately, new problems have been discovered or created on the way. There can, however, be little doubt that the new system has the potential to improve the experience of doctors in training and benefit the health service and patients if its potential is fully realised.

Naturally, such extensive change raises antibodies and suspicion in many, particularly those who are caught in its wake. Doctors are like any other group of workers in that respect. The provision of adequate information to so many people, compounded by rumour and counter-rumour, in such a rapidly changing environment has proved challenging. This has led to a feeling of lack of involvement on the part of many trainers, trainees and medical students who feel threatened and worried that the changes are not for their benefit but for the benefit of the government. When they are set in the context of the many other changes in the NHS, which are not always understood or welcomed by doctors, that suspicion deepens. An understanding of how we got here is essential if we are to realise the potential in the programme.

AN EXTENDED METAPHOR

Imagine the system of educating house officers before the MMC as like trying to navigate between Land's End and John o'Groats without a map (Figure 1.1). After an initial struggle through the back lanes of Cornwall, most house officers found their way on to the motorway and sped north. Their educational supervisor guided them remotely from a helicopter and met them at an occasional service station, but could only come part of the way then handed over to someone else around Bristol, who in turn passed them on around Manchester. The house officers picked up what learning they could, but it depended entirely upon which road they found themselves. They really had the choice of only two roads during that part of their career (medicine or surgery), so they missed out on the chance for views of the countryside from other (career) paths. When they got to John o'Groats they were met briefly by their final educational supervisor who signed a form to say that they had arrived; they then achieved full registration. It did not matter how they had got there or what had occurred on the way. A few unfortunate souls with no map were destined to go round and round the Birmingham motorway system repeating their wrong turns in a Kafkaesque nightmare until they were sent back to Land's End to start again, no wiser as to where they had taken a wrong turn. Others remained blissfully unaware of the trail of accidents left behind them in the fog on the M6 and made it to John o'Groats (full registration) despite very poor navigation skills and the carnage behind them.

Continuing the metaphor, once they had reached John o'Groats the trainee set off up a very rocky and uncertain path to scale the career mountain. If they could get a suitable post, they started up the steep mountain path of their choice, carrying a huge burden consisting of exam papers for their chosen college. The paths were wide to begin with and carried many people, but

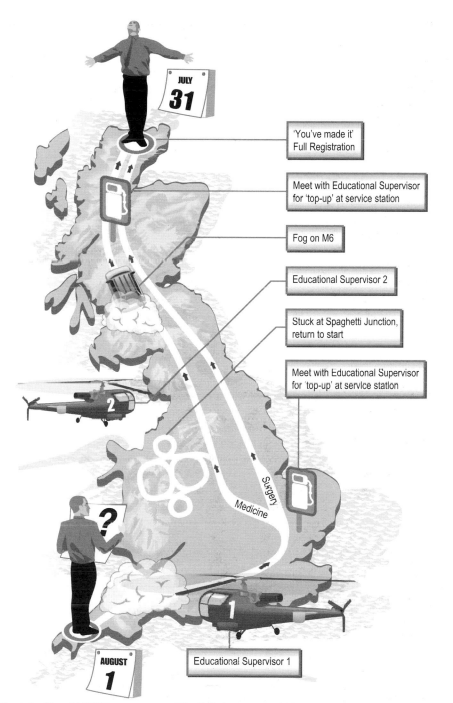

Fig. 1.1 The old PRHO system . . . and the SpR mountain to climb

tapered as they got higher so that many people had to give up. Gates were erected in the way and trainees could only pass through these, and shed part of their burden, when they had passed an exam. Some colleges had three separate gates and it could take some trainees five years to pass through all of them and shed their burden before they entered higher specialist training. Some of the trainees found excellent guides, consultants who could see the way through the fog, offer timely advice and help them over obstacles or rock falls. But many did not find a guide and became exhausted or injured and had to start again at the bottom of the mountain, perhaps this time climbing a road less steep. Many spent time at the bottom of the mountain or halfway up, counting the blades of grass (doing research) or maintaining the path (doing Trust posts), waiting forlornly for the path ahead to clear. Doctors coming from overseas often climbed up seemingly parallel paths, but found that their path never quite reached the final gate.

The victors got into higher specialist training and most went on to complete their training successfully, occupied the mountain peak and proclaimed themselves the world's best qualified doctors. Many were nearly 40 before they could practise independently. Meanwhile, some of the paths became overgrown because so few people travelled along them and as a result at the top of the mountain there was a shortage of certain specialists. Some hospitals could keep open only by employing retired specialists or over-working those in certain specialties (e.g. radiology and psychiatry) because of the shortage of qualified specialists. Even popular specialties such as medicine could only fill two-thirds of advertised consultant posts. Some specialties had so few people reaching the mountain top that they recruited non-medically trained people (e.g. Public Health).

So, the government decided that the route to the top was not working well for all doctors or for the health service and therefore not for the health of the nation. It is fair to say that the BMA was closely involved in the development of the Foundation programme and the post-Foundation system so the profession has a lot of responsibility for the revised scheme. The Foundation programme attempts to replace the rather chaotic pre-registration house officer (PRHO) system with a clear road map, consisting of a curriculum and a better system of assessing the course of the journey which will let trainees know how they are doing on the way, not just at the end. It will also offer more guidance on the way from an expert, who can coach the new doctor through the complexities of the pathway and meet them regularly to review their progress. The Foundation programme will mean a slower route than the chaotic motorway of PRHO jobs, but newly qualified doctors will have an opportunity to travel by different roads and obtain a variety of views of their potential career paths before selecting the one most appropriate for them.

The post-Foundation specialist training will attempt to allocate people to the right path at the bottom of the mountain and it will also make sure that the neglected paths are restored and trainees tread them more frequently. The paths will be shorter and more gently sloping with fewer gates and will not taper. They will only allow the 'right' number of people to enter at any one time. Trainees will have a reduced burden of factual exams to pass, but will have to show that their regular practice is up to scratch to get through the gates. Most hospital doctors could then reach the top of the mountain and

> **Box 1.1   Unresolved questions about the new training system**
> - We may be assessing the pathway that the Foundation trainees take, but do we have good enough methods and are we measuring the right thing?
> - Does the map (curriculum and teaching) include the most important things that a trainee needs to know to get to the right point at the end of the Foundation programme? Is that endpoint John o'Groats or somewhere else?
> - Is the mountain high enough to maintain standards? Will newly qualified consultants have sufficient expertise as opposed to competence?
> - Will the queue at the bottom of the mountain (post-Foundation) to get into specialty training become just as big a problem as that to get into SpR posts previously?
> - After the Foundation programme, how many people will still not have enough information to know which pathway to enter?
> - Why force people onto paths they don't want to follow? Surely it would be better to make the view from the path more attractive so that people want to take it?
> - How many of our graduates will decide they don't like the view and go off to climb career mountains in Australia or the US?

finish their training just 7–8 years after qualifying, although for GPs the minimum length of post-qualification experience is likely to be increased from four to five years.

Of course, there are some unresolved questions from this metaphor (see Box 1.1).

To some, it may sound like a fairy story, but we hope it makes some sense to you and reminds us why the change was thought by many in medical education and NHS circles to be necessary.

UNFINISHED BUSINESS – THE END OF AN ERA

The official start of the new specialty run-through training programme was August 2007. At this point the SHO (senior house officer) grade ceased to be. Existing SHOs and F2s will be able to apply for run-through training programmes. Doctors who have completed the Foundation programme will enter at BST1 level, whereas doctors who have done SHO or non-recognised posts will be able to apply at a level commensurate with their past experience, particularly if they have evidence of the competencies that they have achieved.

The history of the development of the change is interesting. There had already been reforms in the training of PRHOs and registrars. What about the workhorse workforce that made up 50% of all doctors in training? A review of SHO training led to the publication of *Unfinished Business: Proposals for Reform of the Senior House Officer Grade* (Sir Liam Donaldson, London: DoH, 2002) and this provided the catalyst to review the whole structure, from graduation to senior appointment. Its aims include the smoothing out of training so that there are fewer bottlenecks at the mid-way point, reducing the number of people leaving medicine, introducing competency-based training and ensuring that training is 'fit for purpose' in that fully qualified doctors have the appropriate skills for their role in the NHS. Instead of three levels of training – PRHO, SHO and SpR (specialist registrar) – there will now be two – Foundation programme and Specialist run-through training. The organisation of these programmes will pass from individual Trusts to central organisations, mainly the deaneries or newly constructed schools. There will be clearer training paths for future academic doctors, although there will be more training levels to pass through – Foundation programme, Academic Clinical Fellowship (up to three years), Training Fellowship (when you would complete an MD or PhD) and Clinical Lectureship (up to four years).

THE PILLARS ON WHICH THE FOUNDATION PROGRAMME IS BUILT

The design and implementation of Foundation programmes will be guided by seven pillars. Some of these appear to produce potential conflicts between each other and there are certainly some limitations on the extent to which they can be realised at present.

Pillar 1

The Foundation programme is meant to be trainee-centred.

This may imply that you will get the training opportunities that you need or hope for, but obviously that is tempered by what is on offer. Whether you get the post that you want is likely to be dependent on how many points you get in your Foundation application (see Chapter 2). Pillar 1 also produces tensions when working in the NHS, which is generally patient-centred. It can, for example, be particularly difficult to get off the ward and go to Foundation teaching as an F1 and you may get SpRs and consultants questioning the value of the teaching of professionalism in comparison to seeing patients. It can be tough to down tools and leave the ward, considering that you were the only person that was going to take out a patient's chest drain, speak to the relatives of the lady who fractured her hip in a fall on the ward and put the blood forms out for tomorrow. This is where pillars 1 and 4 appear to clash.

Pillar 2

The Foundation programme will be competency assessed.

You must show evidence that you are competent, and not just rely on word of mouth that someone once heard that you had a strong forearm and were quite handy at reaching the desired body cavity with a number 14 needle (see *The House of God*, referenced in Chapter 10). The defined competencies follow the *Duties of a Doctor* and *Good Medical Practice* and range from practical procedures, including simple things like performing ECGs on the ward, to breaking bad news and ethical dilemmas. Every step of the way there will be an opportunity to prove that you are competent at something through observation and feedback. These competencies are assessed using the tools described in Chapter 6. These exist not just for other people to assess you, but to see if you have the ability to reflect on critical incidents or interesting cases. This learning model fits that of life-long learning and professional development. After the Foundation programme the idea is that you take your academic, reflective and practical skills forward into your career and refine them.

Pillar 3

The Foundation programme will be coached.

The idea here is that you will have a personal educational supervisor who will guide you throughout the Foundation programme. They will facilitate your development generally by helping you plan your learning and assessments, offering a degree of pastoral support appropriate to their training and helping you manage your career. The role of the educational supervisor is discussed in detail in Chapters 5 and 7. In many teaching centres there will now be the same educational supervisor for the whole of the Foundation programme. This is a major change and should improve the support offered to trainees, although some Trusts are still offering a new educational supervisor with every post.

Pillar 4

The Foundation programme will be service-based.

This recognises two factors: first, most of your learning will be through your clinical work rather than through classroom teaching; second, it acknowledges that in the current NHS, doctors in training are providing an essential service and are not there just for their own education. Previously it had been popular to describe PRHOs as 'supernumerary', which seemed to imply that if they were not there the NHS could keep running. It would not, and the fact that you get paid reflects this. Pillar 4 covertly acknowledges the tension between service and education that you will undoubtedly encounter.

Pillar 5

The Foundation programme will be structured and streamlined.

This is an interesting pillar. Foundation programmes are definitely structured and the change from six- to mostly four-month jobs is generally to be welcomed as it will give you a broader range of experience. In most posts the learning is maximised within four months and can become repetitive after this. Of course, for service delivery the longer you are in a post the better as you have more experience, so this is one change that has benefited trainees over the service. Whether or not the changes deliver streamlined training and whether this is a good thing remain to be seen. It will actually take longer to qualify as a GP (two years Foundation and three years GP training) than the minimum period possible under the old training scheme (one year PRHO and three years GP training). Maybe that is a good thing. And in theory previously you could become a consultant gastroenterologist in eight years (one year PRHO, two years SHO and five years as an SpR), now it will still take a minimum of eight years (two years Foundation programme, two years general medicine training and four years gastroenterology higher training) but if five years are needed in specialty training it could be even longer. And for the large numbers of people who are not able to enter specialty training immediately but have to undertake an FTSTA (Fixed Term Specialty Training Appointments) post, the notion of 'structured and streamlined' may seem somewhat obscure. The jury is definitely out on this one.

Pillar 6

There will be flexibility in the Foundation programme.

There are some important flexibilities that have been introduced by the new system, in particular the theoretical provision to apply for a transfer to another deanery without having to be interviewed. The reduced number of stages in training will favour women as they are less likely to be between posts when needing maternity leave. (In previous generations many women missed out on their rights to maternity leave because of frequent job changes.) However, truly flexible training, where for reasons of childcare or other dependants, sickness or international-level sport commitments, trainees had the chance to work part-time, has been seriously eroded in the last two years because of apparent reductions in funding. This is a very detrimental step. The flexibility to choose a post-PRHO job to gain more general experience when you are still uncertain about your future career has also been eroded, as has the opportunity to gain valuable experience overseas and have that recognised as part of accredited training. Indeed, the flexibility and opportunity to go to Australia or New Zealand may have been seriously eroded.

Pillar 7

The Foundation programme will be quality assured.

This is potentially where some of the biggest gains from the Foundation programme will come. Clear standards for your teaching and education have been laid down by the MMC. You should know what is expected of the Trust or practice that you are working in. For example, if you are not getting your three hours average teaching per week, ask why. And if your educational supervisor does not find time to meet you as often as stipulated, challenge this. For the quality assurance programme to be effective, however, it requires the active participation of trainees. So, use the opportunities made available to feed back to the Trust and the deanery, whether formally or informally.

SUMMARY

This introduction has set the scene for the changes and the background to them and enabled you to see 'the big picture' as well as to have an awareness of some of the micro-issues that have arisen from the introduction of the Foundation programme.

Chapter 2 will look at the application process and some of the factors that you may use to decide which post to apply for. Chapter 3 is designed to complement your induction process and tells you all you need to know about the NHS and Chapter 4 is designed to help you through the first few days and weeks of your post. Chapter 5 looks at what you need to know from the curriculum and some hints on learning and Chapter 6 looks at how to approach your assessments. Chapter 7 looks at the roles and responsibilities of the trainers. Chapter 8 looks beyond the Foundation programme to the rest of your career. It may seem a long time off, but in order to get on to specialty training you will need to have used your Foundation programme to demonstrate appropriate skills and sustained interest, so don't leave it too late to start. Chapter 9 gives some hints on avoiding becoming a doctor in difficulty, a polite term for someone who is suffering from health or performance problems or is facing disciplinary action, and some issues around other people making your life miserable. Finally, Chapter 10 is a list of resources that you may find helpful.

Choosing and applying for a Foundation programme

Mark Welfare

> ❝ Where before a student was impartially assessed, he is now assessed by his own views of himself and by his ability to enrich his achievements. ❞
> Part of text of online petition October 2006,
> www.ipetitions.com/petition/Thedoctorlottery/

INTRODUCTION

'MDAP Monday (Multiple disasters and problems)'

This was the heading for an article in the *BMJ* Careers Focus section on 11 March 2006 (pp. 98–9) about the multi-deanery application process (MDAP) for Foundation posts beginning in August 2006. The next week, the *BMJ* carried a Personal View article (*BMJ* 2006, 332: 675), which expressed the view that 'the desire to move the applications process away from an "old boys" network had created a completely new set of tribulations'. Many students complained that they had not been able to complete their online application due to excessive traffic. MMC was also unpopular because it sent letters to candidates who scored low on the application form suggesting that they might not be competent and would need further training. MMC has admitted that this was a mistake and has promised to improve the process. But it was not a good start. At the time of writing we await the details of the replacement for the MDAP, which after a lot of thought is called the Medical Training Application Service (MTAS). Spookily similar!

Your application for a Foundation programme will seem like one of the most important decisions of your life so far. You may well feel that the electronic application system has its faults and does not allow all options to be fully explored, but we are stuck with it (and the general principles are being extended to post-Foundation posts). This chapter will help guide you through the process, answer some of the questions that you may have and help you balance your educational, personal and career needs. It should also help you choose which schools or posts to apply for and how to maximise the points you get in the scoring process. If at times you feel frustrated or upset by this process, remember, there is a job for all UK graduates. Although you may not get your first choice, you will get a place somewhere.

Another bit of history

The career market is changing rapidly as a result of the MMC, as outlined in Chapter 1. For SHO and SpR jobs, doctors sometimes made hundreds of applications before getting an appointment. There was a wide-based pyramid with many more SHO posts in some specialties than were needed to fill the number of SpR posts. This meant a lot of attrition (enforced career change) at the transition stages, often after up to five years as an SHO. Appointments were made on the basis of interview and there is no doubt that there was an advantage in being a local candidate; consequently, it was easier to get a job locally. Moving to a specific part of the country could be very hard indeed and there was no provision for moving between deaneries as a PRHO or SHO without going through a repeat application process. Few PRHOs worked outside their medical school's attached Trusts. There were also more stages in an individual's career with a minimum of four job applications, but sometimes many more. This disadvantaged women having a family because they frequently missed out on maternity rights as they were between jobs.

The most significant changes will be the reduction in the number of stages in your career, the narrowing of the base of the pyramid to give approximately the correct number of posts to take you from ST1 through to a Certificate of Completion of Training and the change in application process so that people are essentially appointed on the basis of an application form scored 'objectively' and anonymously. There should also be formal arrangements for transferring between deaneries in either the Foundation programme or specialty training. These measures will act to reduce the pressure on the appointments process. The main pressure in the new system is likely to be in the immediate post-Foundation application because of the narrow pyramid and the fact that appointment to these posts will more or less guarantee that you achieve a senior post. This is discussed in Chapter 8.

The mechanics of the appointments system also needed to change in parallel with the career structure. In the days before the Foundation programme, each medical school or deanery operated its own system, some being based on so-called 'matching' systems, some on competitive interviews with a restricted number of applications along a set time-frame and some a complete free-for-all. Each system had its advocates and strengths and weaknesses. Consultants liked to interview because they felt, rightly or wrongly, that they could choose the most suitable applicants for their jobs, and after all choosing the devil you know is sometimes better than one that you don't. In the view of some, however, interviews allowed consultants to exercise their prejudices, whether this was for the 'rugger buggers', UK graduates, Oxbridge students or any other bias that allowed merit to be ignored. Having taken part in countless interviews, I feel that the choices we made always reflected the candidates' ability as demonstrated in the interview and I was certainly never aware of direct or indirect discrimination against women or candidates from ethnic minorities. Nevertheless, interviews have many weaknesses and most of private industry has developed much more sophisticated means of appointing key employees. General practice training schemes have also developed more structured and diverse means of selecting candidates. This includes more appropriate assessment of the knowledge, skills and behaviours triad matched to the needs of the job.

Anyway, sweeping the brush of newness before it, the MMC decreed that there was to be a new system which would not discriminate against anyone and which would allow the appointments process to be done online and so

> **Box 2.1   Advantages and disadvantages of the single application process**
>
> *Advantages*
>
> - Should reduce the scope for discrimination based on gender, ethnicity or sexuality
> - One single application reduces wasted applications (assuming you get a job in the first round)
> - Opportunity to move deaneries, subject to medical school approval
>
> *Potential disadvantages*
>
> - May not give sufficient weight to academic performance as an undergraduate, thereby not motivating students to work hard
> - Difficult for assessors to weigh equally the differing grading systems from each medical school. Would you know how much weight to give a Merit for a second-year essay at Newcastle?
> - You have to accept the offer if you apply. This is against the previous principle that once offered a post you could think about it and then decide. Your personal circumstances may have changed between application and the offer of the job
> - Bias cannot be totally eliminated. For example, some assessors will value having been captain of the rugby team over playing in an orchestra or organizing a religious retreat, and vice versa

avoid the need for interviews. Students in Nottingham had been responsible for initiating a new system that worked within that one institution, where students had had similar experiences and their assessors were familiar with the local grading system. And so, based on this limited experiment, the electronic application was born. Some of the positives and negatives of the system are detailed in Box 2.1. If you want a humorous critique of the new application process and some left field suggestions of what to put in it, see John Firth's view ('Muddling medical careers – the Foundation appointment process', *BMJ* Careers Focus, 3 December 2005, pp. 237–8). There will also be many participants who question the validity of choosing people for important posts based solely on what they write about themselves, with or without help, in 150 words in answer to six questions, as the quotation at the beginning of this chapter reveals.

HOW DOES ELECTRONIC APPLICATION WORK?

The MMC has changed the supplier for the electronic application system and, as of August 2006, all applications for Foundation programme and specialty training will be made through the Medical Training Application Service (http://www.mtas.nhs.uk/). The information contained in this chapter was accurate at the time of writing, but this is a rapidly changing area and not all details were available. The electronic application is designed to assess your suitability for the post against the person specification for the post. The questions should therefore match the criteria in the person specification. A new draft of both the person specification and the application form is likely to be available by the time you read this chapter, so concentrate on the general messages in this chapter as well as the details.

Applications to the Foundation programmes for all four UK countries are now done through a single process using 27 Foundation schools. The schools vary in size and complexity, with some based loosely on the current deanery boundaries, some quite small, and just one school for the whole of Scotland. Full details of the application process are given on the MMC website (www. mmc.nhs.uk/pages/foundation/application) and you are advised to check up-to-date information from that source. From 2007, all applications will initially be to the schools, and the way in which students are allocated to each post will be decided by the schools at the local level. It is likely that some will use interviews to decide which individual post or rotation you enter, whereas others will rely on the scores obtained from the electronic application system.

The means of application is an electronic form that seeks evidence from two sources:

- your academic achievement in the undergraduate course
- your fit to the job specification, based on your written submission

Academic achievement

Your medical school will give a statement on your placing within the assessment system of the school, probably restricted to which quartile you are in, and details of any prizes you have won. Early guidance suggests that 60% of the marks available will be for your academic achievement.

Your fit to the job specification

On the original system for applications in 2006 this was assessed using six questions, but this may well change for 2007 or subsequent years. The significance of your submission is considerably less than in 2006 and only 40% of your marks will be for this part. In each category you are allowed a set number of words (75 in 2006) to describe the evidence of your performance and skills and its significance to you. Your application is then scored by two trained scorers and a mark of 0–4 is given for each answer, giving a maximum score of 48.

There are more than 5000 applicants for Foundation posts in England and the spread of scores is very limited (0–48), so for popular schools many candidates might achieve identical scores. This means that selection may have to be based partly on random selection within the borderline scores.

You will receive your offer and it seems from the guidance notes that you are pretty much obliged to accept a post that you have applied for if it is offered. The guidance notes for 2006 say that if you do not accept the school offered, you will be deemed to have withdrawn from the system and will have no further part in that round of applications. If, for some reason, such as a change in personal circumstances, you do not wish to work in the school you are offered, you will probably have to turn up on the first day and ask for a transfer to another school or post. This assumes that there are vacant posts in the school to which you wish to transfer. Failure to start a post once accepted without good reason (e.g. health or failing finals) is considered unprofessional and could lead to your being reported to the GMC. Once you have accepted an offer the school will contact you to arrange the appointments into posts/rotations.

The overall implications of these changes for your decision on which Foundation programme to apply to are that the jobs that you do in the Foundation programme should not influence your chances of achieving the post-Foundation job that you want. It's what you do in the job rather than which job you happen to have. The new appointments process should reduce the influence of patronage and should also create a level playing field for all applicants, irrespective of which part of the UK, or indeed the European Economic Area, they come from. This probably means that your choice of Foundation school and the posts within it can reflect more accurately the educational opportunities you wish to pursue and the ethos of the post and your personal preference for a post that matches your lifestyle.

HOW WILL I DECIDE WHERE TO APPLY?

The 2007 system will be a single port of entry for all programmes, but the deaneries/schools will be able to choose their own method for allocating the posts in the Foundation school once candidates have been accepted. You will be asked to rank all 27 schools in your application. Better buy a map of the UK to find some of the more remote ones! Your application will be scored by your first choice.

We will therefore consider the options under three main areas: factors specific to you; factors specific to the school; and factors specific to the post.

Factors specific to you

There will be many students who need to be in a specific area of the country for personal reasons and have little opportunity to move. Historically, the majority of graduates stayed in the area where they graduated if they could obtain a post there. Students put down firm roots in the area in which they have studied and a few may have children or other dependants which makes it necessary to stay locally. Dependants will be seen as a valid reason to stay locally. Equally, having dependants in another part of the country may be a valid reason to move. However, having a property and mortgage will not be seen as a valid reason to be given a job locally. Having a partner or spouse in a particular location may well be a strong motivator for you to stay put or move, but will not score any points in the application. When considering moving to be with a partner, consider the possibility of the relationship not working out. How would you feel if, having moved from Scotland to Penzance, you and your partner split? Hobbies and interests are other factors that will motivate you in your decision about where to live, although unless you are competing at national level, they will not score any points in the application system. One of the authors graduated in Southampton and wished to move to a part of the country where the bird watching was better – hence his migration to the north-east.

Reasons to stay locally

Obviously, there are many reasons why you may wish to work in a specific area. Bear in mind that the first year after qualification is probably the most stressful year of your working life and so having friends around you will help you survive and thrive the year. We know one colleague who moved away from their place of graduation and suffered a severe depressive illness, so if you are prone to stress and depression it may be wise to stay locally. Alternatively, your best support systems may be in another part of the country. Staying in the area of your medical school will also help ensure that the senior doctors that you come across are to some extent familiar and you will be able to seek them out if necessary or even continue your relationship with your undergraduate tutor. Being familiar with the hospitals you will work in will be important at first, but after a few weeks you will be more or less used to a new hospital.

Reasons to move to a different deanery

There are an equal number of reasons to wish to move away from the area of your study. You may wish to move closer to your partner or family. It may be time for a change of view and subculture, or you may want to pursue a sporting interest or hobby. You may wish to move from an urban to a more rural setting, or vice versa. Moving away from the scene of your undergraduate career allows you to re-invent yourself as you move from one stage of life to another. You will after all be moving from being a student to being a health professional, and there may be other changes in your life, such as starting a family. You may have experienced prejudice and wish to move to an area where you will feel more accepted.

You may also wish to consider that the number of moves in your career is likely to be small. You may have only three appointments in your whole career – Foundation programme, specialist training and final GP or consultant position. So, if you do want a move at some point, now may be the time to go.

School-specific reasons

The national implementation of the Foundation programme and the national Quality Assurance scheme that is being introduced mean that there should be few differences between schools in the implementation of the Foundation programme. Nearly all posts will have six four-month rotations, will follow the same curriculum and use the same assessment tools. Some schools will be stronger in certain areas, but the variation between Trusts within a school is likely to be greater than the variation between schools. So there should be little to choose between schools in educational terms.

There may be very specific reasons to choose a particular school. For example, some deaneries have more opportunities for flexible training (part-time working) than others and some may have better educational opportunities than others, particularly if they have been closely involved in the pilot scheme. You may find that only one or two schools offer a choice that you wish to pursue (e.g. diving medicine). However, as you can never be guaranteed a particular post it would be a very long shot to expect to get that particular post.

One of the biggest differences between schools is in the quality of careers advice and management. The Windmills model (www.windmillsonline.co. uk) is being used in some deaneries (e.g. Trent and North Western in 2006) and seems very interesting and worthwhile. It seeks to build your career management skills looking at the whole of your life not just the job part. In time, however, all schools and deaneries will develop better careers advice structures, so this will also become less relevant.

Other reasons to apply to different schools might include the method of choosing F2 posts and the timing at which the F2 choices are made, working conditions and pay and hours, and the amount of travelling required between posts. In these days of environmental awareness, the size of your carbon footprint is important as well as time wasted on travel.

At present there is very little data available to compare deaneries or schools. This information is due to be placed on the MTAS website, including comparisons between numbers of local students and posts, but this information will not be independent. You may like to consider questions such as 'Which have the most efficient administration and get you your contract on time? Which allow the greatest degree of choice in swapping posts or in the choice of your F2 slots? What are the effects of travel and do you get travel expenses if you have to work across many sites in the two years?'

The website for Jobscore (see below) does not currently include school-based data even though this is clearly a need of trainees. Jobscore hopes to include the deaneries and schools in its evaluations at some point soon and be able to provide you with a trainee's view of the schools.

In the end, personal reasons are more likely to influence your decision than deanery-specific factors.

Factors specific to the post or rotation

Once you have been accepted into a school, there will be a process for appointment to a particular Trust and rotation. In some schools the full two-year rotation will be appointed from the beginning; in others you will make choices for F2 during F1. Each rotation will have factors that you will feel are more or less important. You need to consider which of the many variables are most important to you (Box 2.2). The Foundation programme is designed to be generic and give all trainees the experience needed to achieve the competencies required at the end of two years, so the theory is that the posts you do within a rotation will not affect your appointment to future training posts. However, human nature being what it is, if you have a specific career aim at this stage you will probably want to gain some experience of it in your Foundation programme to help confirm your choice and bolster your application.

Box 2.2 Factors to consider in applying for particular posts
- Rural, town or city
- Teaching hospital or district general
- Posts in the rotation
- Posts relevant to your future career or not
- Within your university area or not
- Consultants that you know or not
- Educational opportunities, both formal and on the job
- Work environment – car parking, food, accommodation possibilities, architecture
- Hours and pay
- Distance to travel

You may wish to have a job that gives specific experience to give you a better idea of the implications of that career. For example, if you have an interest in forensic pathology and there is only one rotation that does it, you may well consider it useful to inform your career choice to have that experience in F2. Some posts may have a better reputation for educational opportunities or have consultants who are known to be supportive and positive.

Getting information on individual posts can be difficult. Your own experience will be invaluable here. It is wise to speak to the current crop of F1s as the experience of being a junior doctor may be different from the experience of being a student. Most Trusts publish material on their websites or in glossy magazines listing the educational opportunities and training of their consultants, but this information is not independent. Further information on the quality of jobs can be found at www.jobscore.co.uk which is written by junior doctors. Most big hospitals are included, but the ratings are currently by hospital not Foundation school. The opinions given are sometimes those of a single trainee and so may not be representative, but some hospitals have many reports so the information should be accurate. Jobscore looks at the post from two aspects: the working environment (with subcategories of hospital, job and academic) and quality of life (with subcategories of accommodation, mess and leisure time). You can also email people who have filed reports and get further information. The role of Jobscore is recognised by many authorities and is well worth a look before deciding on which Trust to apply for. The Jobscore website is due to be revised to take into account the new structures recognising the role of Foundation schools and deaneries. We would encourage you to contribute to the site to keep it accurate and up to date.

Trusts and Foundation schools will usually run open days or careers fairs. These are your best opportunity to see what is on offer and talk to the current incumbents. The days of meeting all the consultants before the interviews and being shown round the unit are now past. As a consultant who has done a lot of interviewing in the past, I feel that it is not appropriate to meet the applicants for posts such as Foundation jobs as it could easily lead to bias in the interview stage.

Other questions to consider

Teaching hospital or district general?

There are many preconceptions about different types of post. Traditionally, hospital jobs were viewed as being in 'teaching' or 'district general' hospitals (DGHs). Film and literature characterise teaching hospitals as full of egocentric and insensitive consultants, whereas some view DGH consultants as more benign and forgiving. Teaching hospitals are also regarded as offering incredible experience of rarer disorders and a high level of care and expertise that you would never see in a DGH. Teaching hospitals offer potentially less supervised experience as the academic consultants may be frequently absent and registrars may be more interested in their own research. In contrast, DGH jobs have been characterised as offering experience mainly of common conditions with lower standards of expertise whilst being less stressful, with consultants who are more supportive. There has also been a perception that teaching hospital jobs offered a better chance of progressing your career due to the patronage of senior consultants and academics such as professors. Like most NHS stereotypes, any validity that these views might have had in the distant past has been eroded and bears little resemblance to the reality of the modern NHS.

So what has changed? Today nearly every hospital in the UK is a 'teaching' hospital in that they all play a role in the education of medical students. The increase in the number of medical students and the shorter stay of in-patients have been largely responsible for this, as well as an appreciation of the opportunities available in all hospitals and in primary care. Academic posts (senior lecturers and professors) are found in smaller and medium-sized hospitals throughout the UK. The standards of care in hospitals are increasingly driven by National Service Frameworks and NICE recommendations so differences in care among hospitals of different types are becoming very small. It should always be remembered that any condition that is seen as a tertiary referral was probably seen first in primary care and/or a DGH. On recent 'takes' in a teaching DGH I have seen patients with pneumococcal meningitis, staphylococcal toxic shock syndrome and acute renal failure due to Henoch Schonlein purpura, whilst in four years in a tertiary liver unit I saw only one case of Wilson's disease and one of focal nodular hyperplasia among all the paracetamol overdoses and alcohol-related liver disease.

So, how should you choose what type of hospital to work in? In reality all hospitals will have a mix of consultants who are more or less supportive and more or less interested in education and will offer variable experience. Choose the posts that best suit your educational needs and will help you plan your career most appropriately. Use the rankings in www.jobscore.co.uk to compare the hospitals in your school. You may be surprised at what you find.

In the north-east of England posts are distributed between hospitals over an area of at least 100 miles square. Consultants like to think that students choose to work in their hospital because of the excellent teaching or the supportive nature of the medical staff. In reality it may be more the distance from the student ghetto of Jesmond in central Newcastle that defines how popular a job is!

Is it better to do medicine or surgery first?

This question has taxed the minds of medical students since time immemorial. The advantage of doing medicine first is supposed to be that you will be better prepared for surgical jobs, in many of which you will be expected to look after the 'medical' needs of your patients. The supposed advantage of doing surgery first is that the workload tends to be lighter and hence more manageable and this enables you to get your feet under the table before the stress of medicine. In reality, at least one third of trainees will have to do surgery first and at least one third will have to do medicine first. It probably does not matter much which you do first – both have their strengths.

Academic posts

The new structure proposed for academic medicine in the UK (*Best Research for Best Health*, London: DoH, 2006; *Medical and dentally qualified academic staff: Recommendations for Training the Researchers and Educators of the Future*, www.ukcrc.org) is going to impact on training in many ways.

The proposal essentially seeks to select the highest performing students to pursue academic careers to support research and teaching in the universities and the NHS. There will be four research training grades to work through: Academic Foundation programme (two years), Academic Clinical Fellowship (up to three years), Training Fellowship (when you complete an MD or PhD) and Clinical Lectureship (up to four years).

Academic Foundation programmes allow graduates to begin to get experience of research and/or teaching in their first two years while fulfilling the clinical learning criteria for the Foundation programme and remaining generic in their potential. Subsequent to this there will be Academic Clinical Fellowships in specialties which will be advertised in open competition and will enable you to develop the skills needed to apply for a training fellowship with an organisation such as the MRC or Wellcome. The specialties offered will reflect the perceived gaps in academic faculty at present. For example, radiology and many surgical subspecialties have difficulty in recruiting to senior academic posts, so training posts will be offered. For post-Foundation academic posts there may well be separate education and research academic streams. The emphasis of the early Academic Foundation programmes has been on research, particularly laboratory research, but the strategy does suggest that clinical research that is directly relevant to patients is likely to be favoured in the future.

In order to get a place on these schemes you are likely to be a high-achiever and have demonstrated some propensity for research or education (e.g. through an intercalated degree). During the first year of operation of the academic programme the number of applications was disappointing, particularly post-Foundation academic posts. The academic Foundation posts are likely to be advertised earlier than the normal Foundation programme and will probably be advertised in the Academic section of the adverts in the *BMJ*, so watch this section carefully if you are thinking of applying.

'Academic medicine' will have different meanings to different people. Becoming an academic Foundation doctor will ensure that you have a lot of choice for post-Foundation posts, even if you do not pursue an academic career beyond the Foundation programme. Academic life has many advantages, not least in the variety of your working week, the chance to use your intellect to the best advantage and to work closely with students as well as to help patients through research. Because academic programmes are likely to be advertised before the normal Foundation programme, there is very little risk in applying for an academic programme – if you don't get in, you can always apply for the normal programme. If you are unsure whether academic medicine is for you, try to find out more. Attend the university's annual research day where they showcase current successes and talk to some of your senior lecturers, readers and professors. If you think that being an educator appeals, attend the annual meeting of the Association for the Study of Medical Education (www.asme.org.uk) where you can learn about what is hot in the field of teaching.

Academia provides a chance to pursue a very stimulating career in one of many directions.

Tactics

Inevitably, some Foundation schools will be oversubscribed. In particular, London medical schools generally have more students than Foundation posts and have a history of being oversubscribed. Scotland is also a net exporter of graduates. You will be asked to rank all 27 Foundation schools in your application. Clearly, there is going to be a trade-off between ranking where you wish to go and where the best applicant/post ratio is. Bear in mind that some parts of the country will be more popular with European graduates than others so the number of students in the medical school associated with a Foundation school may not accurately reflect the likely number of applicants. It will probably take a couple of years before a reliable pattern emerges.

Should I apply for a job in England, Scotland, Northern Ireland or Wales?

The health policies of the four countries that make up the UK are beginning to diverge as a result of devolution. As the gaps between systems widen, there may be reasons to apply to one country or another. These could include pay and conditions, atmosphere within the NHS in the different countries and future career prospects. Scotland has the biggest differences from the English system. Scotland is also a net exporter of graduates, so competition for places on Foundation programmes is likely to be keen. In Scotland, the NHS seems less of a political battleground than in England and has less emphasis on targets, purchaser/provider splits and alternative service providers. To those who remember what socialism means, Scotland seems closer to the original ideals of the NHS and to be adopting some progressive ideas. Scotland has, for example, decided to make social care available free for all who need nursing or residential care and has made arrangements with Voluntary Services Overseas for healthcare staff to take up placements overseas while maintaining their employment and pension rights. In England, on the other hand, the drive towards the use of private providers is bringing down waiting lists more effectively than other parts of the UK, albeit at the expense of having to live in a target culture. If the culture of the NHS is really important to you in deciding where to apply, keep up to date with the diversity within the UK's four 'national' health services.

Doing your Foundation programme in one country of the UK should not influence your chance of obtaining a specialist training post in another. Because all Foundation doctors will be working to the same curriculum and essentially the same assessments, you will be eligible for all UK posts. The system of fair and objective appointment processes should also ensure that you have equal opportunity in the future.

Salaries and work conditions should not vary much between the four countries at Foundation programme level. However, consultant salaries may vary, and more so in the future. There appears to be some evidence that pay rises in Scotland are lower than in England for senior appointments. This can be set against much lower costs of living and accommodation, however.

ELIGIBILITY – INTERNATIONAL MEDICAL GRADUATES

All medical students who graduate from UK medical schools are entitled to apply for a two-year Foundation post. Citizens of European Economic Area (EEA) countries will be eligible to work in the UK, but not all will be eligible for Foundation year 1. See the MMC website for up-to-date information, which is likely to keep changing.

If you are a doctor from outside the EEA and thinking about coming to the UK, beware. Doctors from outside the EEA have traditionally filled approximately a third of all SHO-level jobs in the UK. Unfortunately, as of April 2006 the government changed the immigration rules so that any medical job in the UK must be given to an EEA national if they are suitable for the job even if a better applicant from outside the EEA has applied. This is enormously disappointing to International Medical Graduates (IMGs), but also seems to ignore the ethical principle of justice. The UK recruited IMGs for years when they were needed and let them do the ILTS and PLAB exams right up until the announcement that slammed the door in their faces. Many doctors who had spent up to five years in the UK obtaining the necessary exams, unpaid experience and junior positions such as SHO jobs were left with no opportunity to finish the training that they had invested in so heavily. It also ignores the reality that many IMGs are educated from birth in English whereas the command of the language many EEA applicants have is poor but does not have to be formally tested.

In principle, IMGs from non-EEA countries will be eligible for standalone F2 posts. In practice, it seems likely that there will be applicants from EEA countries for all but the least attractive jobs, so opportunities for non-EEA doctors are likely to be extremely limited and will effectively be posts that no one else wants. Coming to the UK for a standalone F2 post will not guarantee the chance to pursue specialty training and opportunities for getting on to a training programme will be extremely limited.

The one exception is non-EEA citizens who come to the UK on a Highly Skilled Migrant visa. These may be available for some doctors, but the criteria for considering applicants in this category are unclear so it is uncertain what the chances are of getting a post if you are not an EEA citizen.

FILLING IN THE APPLICATION FORM

Things to remember in writing your application form

- Prepare early. Doing this the day before the entries close is likely to end in disaster as many trainees try to use an electronic system that has a history of getting over-loaded. If you prepare your application early, you will also be able to ask others to review it for you before you submit it.
- Don't lie. That goes without saying, but don't lie on your application form or embellish the facts. You'd be surprised how often this happens. Any claims that you make must be true and moreover verifiable. Do not under any circumstances make a false claim. If discovered, you will be struck off before you have even registered! And remember that the GMC is likely to be very strict in their interpretation of 'the truth'. MPs may be able to be 'conservative with the actuality' and get away with it, but the GMC will not be as sympathetic. So a claim that you 'participated in the London marathon' when your 'participation' consisted of standing in the crowd is likely to be met with the contempt it deserves, even if strictly speaking you may not have lied. It may seem to be OK to claim that you are the 'captain of the local Sunday league football team' when in fact you and your mates have a kick-around every now and then in the park and you're the one that shouts the most, but you would be guilty of trying to create a false impression. Remember, this is the earliest test of your probity. If someone you know is taking their chances and telling porkie pies, don't copy them. You never know, if you claim to be fluent in Esperanto someone on the selection panel may be as well. Then you really will be in *malfacilajo*. The MMC guidance also makes it clear that you must have documentary evidence for anything that you claim to have achieved. So, don't claim that you have achieved the Duke of Edinburgh's gold award unless you can produce the certificate.
- Your statements need to be 'individual and unique'. This is code for 'written by you' and not plagiarised from the Web or ghost-written. It's OK for footballers with half a brain to have ghost-writers for their autobiographies, but would you really wish to be seen to be as witless as them? You *must* complete the application yourself. It will sound much more personal if you do. Although there are online agencies that will help you and even write the application for you, this is forbidden by the rules of the process. Assessors may well be able to spot applications that have been ghost-written and it is likely that anti-plagiarism software will be used to detect patterns identifiable in ghost-written applications. If you are found breaking this rule, you will be withdrawn from the system and probably reported to the GMC under the 'probity' domain of *Good Medical Practice*. There is, however, nothing wrong in getting an experienced person such as your tutor to look at your application and give you some constructive feedback. They may, for example, spot spelling or grammatical errors, or suggest ways in which you can reduce

your word count so that you have space to make extra points. They may be able to advise you on which sections to use for your highest achievements. But don't let them rewrite it.

- According to the MMC team, you should complete the form in 'comprehensible' sentences, and not simply list your achievements. They will judge your grammar and spelling in this section too, so better put the computer on 'spell check'. Be assiduous when using the thesaurus to attain the zenith of your alphabetic tapestry, as a cornucopia of ecstatic prose and esoteric ramblings will appear pretentious and superfluous. OK, so we are taking it to extremes here, but do think about what you're saying, and don't go off at a tangent. Also, remember some basic style rules for English language. More than two clauses in a sentence make it hard to read and give more room for misunderstanding. You will waste words stringing clauses together when a full stop would have done the trick.

- Style issues. Do you start at the top with your name in lights or in crazy fonts like **Impact** which you've picked up off Microsoft Word? For style issues, the byword is 'keep it simple'. Just like those PowerPoint presentations with too many zany effects, you don't want your message to be lost in the presentation. So, use fonts such as Times New Roman or Arial, something the reader is familiar with. *The important thing is don't change fonts throughout the form.* Similarly, for emphasis use **bold**, not underlining or CAPITALS. Don't use colour. Justify to the left.

- Don't make jokes or put down anything that could be considered in poor taste, discriminatory or disrespectful. Medicine thrives on gallows humour in certain circumstances, but this is not the place to showcase your cynicism. Don't use the opportunity to brag or criticise others, especially the MMC!

- You must not use the same achievement to answer too many of the questions. The guidance notes say that the use of one achievement should not be 'excessive' (e.g. using the same example three or more times). It might even be risky to use the same example twice, so if you do need to, make sure you use it in a different way. For example, you could use a sporting achievement to show your leadership qualities and also how a sports injury gave you empathy with people with a chronic illness or helped you understand the role of and gave you increased respect for members of the inter-professional team (e.g. physiotherapists).

Scoring of the applications

In 2006, each of your two answers to the six questions was given a mark between 0 and 4 (0 indicates no evidence, 1 minimal, 2 some, 3 good, 4 outstanding), giving a possible maximum score of 48 marks. Each section has detailed guidance on how the marks should be allocated. General things that will encourage higher scoring are detailed in Box 2.3.

The answers you give might well be likened to the old-style Miss World competition, where candidates undertook three rounds, being judged on appearance in a swimsuit and evening wear and in an interview about themselves. Inevitably in the interview most contestants said that they cared about

> **Box 2.3   General factors that will enhance your application**
> * Good grammar and full sentences
> * Perfect spelling
> * Answering the question. Note that each question (2006 version) has two parts – the achievement itself and the significance to you. Make sure you address both aspects of the question
> * Sticking to the word limit. The assessors are under very strict instruction to ignore everything after 75 words. If your main point is not expressed until words 75–85, you will score nothing for that content
> * Make it personal. The assessors are looking for the values that you bring to medicine so it is important to give a flavour of your values
> * Give as much detail as you can on your achievements. For example, if you got a prize in pathology in year 2, tell the assessors how many other prizes were awarded that year. If you did a BSc or another intercalated degree at a university where most students don't, tell the assessors

world peace and children and had spent half their life working at the local soup kitchen. They knew what the judges were looking for. This job application is similar – a paper version of a beauty contest interview. But at least you don't have to send a photo of yourself in a swimsuit!

What are the judges/assessors looking for?

Individual guidance for each question is given below. This is not intended to be comprehensive and is not written from any particular inside knowledge of the system – I have never scored Foundation programme applications. It is intended to demonstrate that the assessors will be looking for a wide range of answers and that there is no 'right' or 'wrong' answer. The examples are also not intended as 'perfect' responses. They should be used to give you a general guide to some suitable responses and the type of information that could be used in each reply. The questions and marking system are likely to be revised in the future so you should only use these answers as models for the type of information and style to use.

Question 1: Give two examples of your academic achievements and the significance of these for you (include distinctions, prizes, etc.). At least one should be based on your undergraduate experience

The marks are given for the level of the achievement and your explanation of the significance for you. For example to achieve 4 points you need to have details of exceptional achievement with excellent insight and explanation. Major achievements with no explanation of their significance will score only 3.

High-level achievements at undergraduate level might include items generally recognised as of academic merit, such as prizes, distinctions, merits,

Box 2.4 Hierarchy of academic achievement
- PhD and/or published papers in peer-reviewed journals
- Intercalated degree or previous degree, even if arts/social science-related
- Graduating with the highest honours that your university gives
- A prize or competitive award given to few people (preferably only one person) in each year
- Getting the highest level for any stage or year of the undergraduate degree
- High marks for any one attachment, including any student-selected component (e.g. paediatrics in third year)
- High marks for a single piece of work (e.g. one essay)

etc. An example is given below. An approximate hierarchy of undergraduate achievement is given in Box 2.4. But if you have been a straight 'C', then be creative and demonstrate the talents that you do have and make the most of their relevance to your development as a health professional. Remember that the assessors come from a very wide diversity of backgrounds – they are not all university professors with incredible intellects and a stream of letters after their name. They will include people who recognise all aspects of academic achievement and in the future may include lay assessors. Therefore, unless you have outstanding grades, there might be some sense in giving one example of your highest pure academic achievement as an undergraduate and one of a more value-laden achievement.

In this section, a little planning as an undergraduate will have significant benefits for your application, particularly through the attainment of a publication or achievements in the student-selected parts of the course. For example, if you have done a mini-research project or audit, relay the findings in your application, particularly if they led to a change in clinical practice. Look for opportunities to get your views or your experience into print. There are various publications that do not require detailed studies to be accepted. For example, the *BMJ* Personal View section allows a healthcare practitioner space to express something poignant and relevant for the wider medical community based entirely on their own opinion. The weekly articles cover areas such as a doctor's experience as a patient (or those of their relatives) or their views on an ethical or controversial aspect of medicine, including educational issues. Several personal views have been published on student-related subjects. How about writing an article on plagiarism, an ethical dilemma you have faced or something that you learnt from a memorable patient? A recent one reflected on how unnecessary it should be to achieve publication and how a lack of publications was affecting their career. Very smart and ironic that one – whinge about why it is unnecessary, but use the opportunity to play the game and get something in print. The *BMJ* Careers Focus section also has many opportunities to get published. Make sure that if you do get something accepted, you highlight its importance to you.

The question specifies that at least one of your achievements should be as an undergraduate, implying that the other can be in another field. However, your A-level or Highers results are not likely to impress the assessors as most students will have had similar achievements and if they are so fantastic that they are outstanding, the assessors might wonder what you have been doing since and why you don't have anything to show for the last four years. Any academic achievement that does not relate to your undergraduate course should be something that you have achieved since leaving school.

Some examples of suitable answers to question 1:

- In my student-selected component in the fourth year I audited the use of C-reactive protein (CRP) tests in the SCBU. I found that CRP gave many false negative and false positive results for active infection. The cost was £75,000 per year. As a result of my audit, the department stopped using CRP as an indicator of neonatal infection. This project taught me that audit is a powerful tool to change clinical practice. (This example could also be used in question 3 under the heading 'Good clinical care'.)
- In first year I shadowed a pathologist and wrote an essay on 'The value of molecular markers in determining survival in colon cancer'. I was awarded the Pathology prize (only one each year). It reminded me of the scientific basis of medicine and recent developments have shown that micro-satellite instability can predict response to chemotherapy as well. My interest has encouraged me to consider a job in molecular biology.
- I am proud of the photographic skills I have developed, leading to the award of an intercalated BA (2.1) in Fine Arts and an exhibition at the Laing gallery. Photography has helped me to see things from others' perspectives and this has helped in my clinical observation skills and in the development of empathy with the patient. I also learnt to manage my time as I juggled my medical and arts studies.
- During my intercalated MRes (undertaken by 15 students) I achieved a Distinction and was published in the *BMJ*. Using thematic analysis I examined the views of medical students on the educational usefulness of their overseas elective, finding that students with clear learning objectives got the most out of their elective. I learnt how to improve my own learning and am interested in helping others develop their own learning skills by becoming an educator.

Question 2: Give two examples of your non-academic achievement and the significance of these for you

It's easy to think of non-academia. Music, sport, reading, travel, you name it, you've probably done it all. But this means that everyone else has as well. So the tricky part is extrapolating the most interesting thing that you did and turning it round so that you can get something employable out of it.

For example, you may have travelled extensively. The authors have done a fair bit of travelling but we didn't help that many people! Jonathan confused people with his north-western drawl and Mark was obsessed with seeing all the local birds. Voluntary work abroad would score more points. So, if you helped build an orphanage in Romania, that would have taught you team-work, reliability and communication skills. Extrapolate the things it taught you about life, and try to apply them to medicine.

Skills and achievements that could be relevant for this question are evidence of compassion, empathy and social conscience as well as evidence of determination, the ability to get something done, time management and organizational and entrepreneurial skills. Given that you are going to have to show evidence of your leadership and teamwork skills in questions 5 or 6, it is wise to use examples here that reflect other skills that you have or use the same examples that you will use in 5 and 6 but demonstrate a different side of you. Achievements thought to be relevant here include those in the arts and humanities, sport, innovation, design and entrepreneurial skills, experience in the community or voluntary sector or charitable work, in a spiritual context and experience in business or management.

In this category there is also a hierarchy of achievement, but it is modified by your account of its significance. For example, someone who has represented their country at their chosen sport will score higher on the achievement scale than someone who has played for the university, but the significance that you convey will also moderate the marks you achieve. As a guide, put in things that show achievements that are related to your role as a future doctor and allow you to show that to the assessors. For example, if you are particularly proud of having walked the length of the Pennine Way, emphasise your determination under difficult conditions, organizing skills or ability to keep calm in a crisis when your friend fell and broke his leg rather than saying that it was significant to you because the views were nice or it kept you fit.

This question allows you to portray yourself as a well-rounded person with lots of interests, but try to avoid putting everyday things or hobbies in this column. A lot of job applications I have reviewed recently emphasise that candidates like 'cooking a meal for friends' or 'reading'. As an assessor I would be unlikely to score those achievements very highly, no matter how special the meal. As a very keen birdwatcher, I am most proud of the fact that I have seen about half of all the world's birds, but I would strain to link this to the skills I have as a doctor. Jonathan dabbled at singing and joined an a cappella group for a while, winning a prize in a national competition with a ground-breaking medley of Queen songs. That taught him teamwork and reliability. He also managed the medics football team briefly as a student where he was ridiculed for preparing his team talks on paper but he took them to glory, winning the student equivalent of the FA Cup. That taught him teamwork (obviously), delegation and motivation skills.

Some examples:

- I have represented my university at hockey throughout the course and scored the winner in the all-UK finals in the fourth year. Keeping up my sport interest has taught me how to balance my work and personal life and plan my work effectively. I also believe in the importance of doctors leading healthy lives as an example to the general public and my hockey has helped me live up to this maxim.
- I have been involved with a project to support asylum seekers, offering a listening service and practical support. I have renewed my scanty knowledge of Arabic and feel a much greater degree of empathy to this group and a greater understanding of their health needs and poor access

to services. It has reinforced my desire to work with the most disadvantaged sectors of the community when I graduate.

- Throughout my undergraduate career I worked in McDonald's. I have been promoted through the ranks to senior manager responsible for three outlets. The training in managing people and service ethos have enabled me to see the patient as a customer and I have many ideas about how the NHS could improve its service. It has also enabled me to see some potential negative aspects of the increasing creep of transnational companies into the NHS.
- As a Queen's scout, I continued my interest in scouting and have become a scout leader. I have run two regional annual camps with 1000 scouts at each. My experience has taught me to be self-reliant and how to plan and organise large events. I have become interested in the special health needs of adolescents and am interested in pursuing a career in transitional medicine, perhaps in the area of diabetes.
- I have always had an interest in IT. As an undergraduate, I was aware that the faculty's teaching cases were widely dispersed and not easily available to students. I worked with the faculty to make these accessible to all students via the website, adding an interactive element and x-rays, etc. I used the experience to set up my own company offering revision cases to medical students and A-level candidates.

Question 3: Pick two of the GMC's principles (Good clinical care, Maintaining good medical practice, Teaching and training, appraising and assessing, Relationships with patients, Working with colleagues, Probity, Health), state the principle and illustrate your qualities

Things are starting to spice up. We've come to the freestyle event. This is an excellent opportunity to demonstrate the attitudes and skills that you have picked up in medical school and your understanding of the role of clinical governance, audit and continued education in good clinical care, maintaining good medical practice and working with patients, training others and working with colleagues. Hands up for guessing how many will choose Probity. Hmm, I think half the battle will be finding out what it means. Then again, it could play to your advantage – remember they are after your uniqueness.

'Health' is also one of the GMC principles, but we feel that you should not feel obliged to reveal any health issues that you have. For example, you might want to relate how you contracted a blood-borne virus from a needlestick injury when you were a medical student. You could probably put something in about how it's taught you the hazards of needlestick injuries, and the importance of occupational health, immunization checks, HIV counselling and the system of clinical governance. But it would be risky. Generally, best practice in recruitment and selection processes is to concentrate on picking the best candidate for the job and leaving Occupational Health to decide whether any health or disability issues will mean that the job needs to be modified or whether the candidate is suitable for the post. Certainly in the era when we interviewed candidates, we would never take health into account in a competitive interview so it seems grossly unfair to introduce it now when the MMC is trying to be less discriminatory.

Under the 'Probity' principle, it is perhaps unwise to go into any aspects of your misdemeanours. For example, if you have been subject to 'fitness to practice' procedures or have a caution or conviction, you might be tempted to put in some reflections on what you learnt. However this would be a risky strategy.

Our advice is to stick to the principles of 'Good clinical care', 'Maintaining good medical practice', 'Relationships with patients', 'Working with colleagues' or 'Teaching and training'. Your assessors will know that your actual past behaviour is a better measure of your future behaviour than a theoretical example, so it is desirable to use examples of real events you have experienced.

Some examples:

- Good clinical care: In my SSC in radiology I audited the requests for x-rays for abdominal pain for a whole year. This showed that 10% did not request an erect chest and led to two perforations being missed. The department changed its policy for the investigation of abdominal pain. I learnt always to request an erect chest, but also that better systems need to be in place to correct variations from normal practice.
- Maintaining good practice: As a student I found the best learning method to be the maintenance of a log of all the cases I saw. This helped me develop my diagnostic skills, and reading round the cases reinforced my background knowledge of pharmacology and pathophysiology and helped me demonstrate my learning. I feel that this has helped me develop my skills for portfolio learning for the rest of my career.
- Relationships with patients: In a gap year I worked with a girl with Down syndrome. I learnt to interpret behaviours and non-verbal communication in order to communicate with people who have difficulty expressing their needs. This increased my ability to communicate with people at all levels. I believe that patients, especially those with disabilities, are often underestimated, but given patience and time can gain sufficient understanding to work with professionals in determining their care.
- Working with colleagues: As a student I observed a number of disputes between nurses and doctors. Whilst the doctors understood the illness, the nurses often raised points that were important to carers and that doctors had not realised. I learnt that it is important always to listen to each others' point of view if the patient's full needs are to be addressed.
- Teaching and training: I am a qualified guitar teacher, working with people of all skill levels. I have learnt that every pupil learns differently and that to get the best of their learning the teacher needs to understand this. My pupils learn best when they can set their own goals and so are self-motivated. This has helped me to develop my own learning skills. I have used this knowledge to help friends learn.

Question 4: Identify your educational and personal reasons for applying for your first-ranked Foundation school/deanery or programme

This is one of the vaguest questions and is of dubious relevance to the selection of candidates if selection relies entirely on merit. All questions should

> **Box 2.5 Educational and personal reasons considered valid by the MMC for applying for a particular post in 2006**
>
> - Responsibilities for first-degree relatives, e.g. child, parent or children's schooling
> - A need for continuing healthcare access, e.g. regular appointments with a consultant for a chronic disease
> - Need for specific educational support, particularly if you have had progress problems during the undergraduate degree
> - Posts are relevant for your career plan, e.g. a specific F2 post you wish to experience
> - Understanding of the educational opportunities in the post
> - Specific pastoral needs, e.g. continuing counselling or chronic illness that requires ongoing care
> - Involvement in a long-term educational or research project
> - Desire to develop a specific educational interest that is available locally

aim to assess the candidate against the person specification for the Foundation programme. The interviewers aren't really interested that you want to work in Sheffield because of the massive Meadowhall shopping centre, or in Dundee because you just love Arbroath smokies. Remember they are after employable characteristics according to the person specification, so make the system work for you. We are not sure how this question achieves this, and on this basis, the question may be dropped in the future, especially as the applications are for schools not posts. The reasons that the assessors will consider relevant for you choosing a particular post or programme are specified in Box 2.5. The MMC includes among their reasons that will be accepted as valid some very nebulous factors such as 'familiarity with', 'educational continuity' and 'established support networks' or 'personal requirements that would benefit from being met from this programme'. It might be perceived that these factors will favour local candidates, could be considered discriminatory and are continuing elements of the 'old boys' network' that the system is trying to eradicate.

This question probably leads to a wide spread of marks, so, despite the difficulty in answering it, you should pay particular attention to your answers if it is retained. We suggest sticking to educational reasons for applying, unless you have dependent children or other family. Show that you have done some homework. Look up the school's compliance with the national Quality Assurance framework. If the compliance with bleep-free teaching is particularly high, mention this. If you are aware of a school-specific teaching programme (e.g. on prescribing) that is rated well and even has some evidence base to support it, then mention this. Consult with current F1/2 doctors and find out what they think of the teaching in the school. It may be that one Trust in the rotation has a reputation for excellence in a particular area that you value, such as the use of video for teaching communication skills.

Question 5: Teamwork

It is always best to give concrete examples of your experience for all of these answers. There is a mantra from psychology that 'past behaviour is the best predictor of future behaviour'. In other words, if you can demonstrate that you have been capable of good teamwork in the past and that you understand your strengths and weaknesses, this will likely predict good teamwork in the future. Keep it grounded in concrete reality and use this to illustrate general points rather than rely only on theoretical notions of what constitutes good teamwork. The 2006 question asked for your role and contribution to the team, so make sure that both are addressed. By asking about role and position, the question is seeking to assess whether you have insight into your team-work role and into your strengths and weaknesses. If you can refer to a well-known model of teamwork and relate your strengths and weaknesses to that model that will significantly strengthen your application.

By the time the panel gets to this section they'll need some caffeine to get their attention back, so make it easy for them. The first thing that springs to mind is team sports or performing arts or any job that you have had before. If you've achieved anything significant as a team, then whack that in here. For example, as mentioned above, one of the authors was part of an a cappella group. How did singing a low E make him an employable doctor? Remember that it's a paper beauty contest and you need to get into the habit of writing what the panel wants to hear. Singing could teach you about learning your role in a team and being able to strike a balance between using your initiative and following instructions for the benefit of the team. Relate an incident that occurred during the group's history that taught you something specific about your own team performance. You don't want it to sound like a hotel brochure, but you want to get your own style. Subtleties in the style of your writing make your application form memorable.

- I have been a member of an a cappella quartet. In this 'team' I learnt that my strength was in attention to detail, such as planning the year's concerts, and my preference was for a highly organised team. Other members performed different roles and some preferred a more chaotic existence. I learnt to respect the mix of types and preferences. This understanding will help me fit into teams that I work in.
- Teamwork has been essential in my previous jobs in waitressing where I have led a team of five. In both waitressing and the NHS I have observed problems due to poor communication and misunderstanding of roles. I learnt to introduce myself to team members and ensure that we had a mutual understanding of each others' roles. I recognise that there is a need for suitable structures such as interdisciplinary meetings to maintain communication.

Question 6: Leadership

Leadership is required in the NHS even of people in relatively junior positions and the panel will be looking for your leadership potential. As a Foundation doctor you will be expected to demonstrate leadership in dealing with medical students and some of the clinical staff on the ward, particularly healthcare assistants. In the early days of the Foundation programme, there was a lot of talk of 'followership' – having the skills to be good at following as well as leading. It might be appropriate to choose one example here that demonstrates that you know when to be a leader and when to be a follower, as for the most part you will be doing the latter as a Foundation doctor. It is important to understand that you have some self-knowledge of your preferred leadership style and your role in a team. This might be more important than demonstrating that you have been a leader in the past. Also, remember to use examples of things you have actually done to illustrate a general point. It is important to demonstrate that you have learnt about your own strengths and weaknesses as a leader/follower. For an interesting article on leadership and teamwork see the article on the MMC website (Nicola Cooper, Kirsty Forrest, 'Competencies for the Foundation programme – part 5: leadership and teamwork', 4 February 2006).

Example

One of my key roles as a leader was with my learning group. I used the Myers–Briggs personality inventory to discover that my preferred team role includes strengths in the sensing domain. I used my knowledge of the personality types to assign tasks to people based on my perceptions of their preferred roles. I learnt that one role of a leader is to assess the contribution that everyone can make to the team's tasks.

References

Medical students are often very concerned about their references and who will write them, assuming that the higher the status of your referee, the more likely they will be to get a post. In the past this may have been true and referees pulled strings or 'used influence' behind the scenes to ensure the appointment of 'their boy' (sorry, but it was rarely a 'girl' and therein lay part of the problem). The new system has done away with this and with the reduction in the power of patronage, the significance of the reference has almost completely died. References were never much use anyway in differentiating between candidates as almost all were glowing and 'strongly recommended' this doctor for the position. For poorly performing candidates, referees were reluctant to put pen to paper to criticise and have even been known to give excellent references to get rid of people.

In general, references are considered only after the decision to offer someone a post has been made. This is as an additional check that there is nothing unexpected that the candidate has not revealed (e.g. any disciplinary or substance abuse problems). You will note that there is no aspect of the references in the scoring system for the Foundation programme and the appointment will rely on the scoring only. So, don't worry about your references. If you do have an issue such as disciplinary record or conviction that will have to be revealed by your referees, then talk to your referees about it. For example, if you have a conviction for being drunk and disorderly, make sure that your referees know what steps you have taken to avoid a recurrence. If you have a blot on your disciplinary record, make sure that your referees know that you have responded appropriately to this with remorse and new insight into the standards expected of a doctor. I have had to write a reference for someone with these kinds of problem and it was very important to meet them beforehand and acknowledge that the issue had to be revealed in the reference, but that I could express it in a constructive manner. If you are worried about your reference, discuss it with your referee first.

Other aspects of the application form

Well, that's the main bit out of the way. There are other things that you need to make sure are done. There's the bit about the Equal Opportunities form, which is not seen by the panel but is used by the Foundation school to monitor any signs of discrimination. The information you give is voluntary and strictly confidential.

There is also the Approval form from the medical school dean. This is to say that they have approved you to be eligible for a particular school, and that any concerns about your fitness to practise are raised. This may be, for example, travel issues if you have a disability or flexible training issues if you have a dependant. If this is the case, by the time you come to apply, these issues will have been sorted out by the medical school. It is up to you to stay organised and keep everyone informed about any problems you may have that will affect your employment.

AFTER ACCEPTANCE TO A FOUNDATION SCHOOL

Once you have been accepted into a Foundation school, each will have its own method of deciding on the allocation of rotations. Some will go on the scores from your application form and some will conduct interviews within Trusts. For tips on interview skills, see Chapter 8. The reasons for choosing different rotations are discussed above.

Once you have been matched to a post by the MTAS system there is one more step. The actual job offer, in contractual terms, will have to come from the Trust, not the MTAS. They will need to complete pre-employment checks of health and Criminal Record Bureau clearance before the final job offer materialises.

SUMMARY

This chapter has reviewed the reasons why you might choose certain jobs and given some guidance on the principles behind the electronic application system and how to complete your application. Good luck in your application. Now you can start to prepare for your first day as a qualified doctor as we move on to Chapter 3.

Preparation for the Foundation programme. What do you need to know?

3

Jonathan Carter and Mark Welfare

> **❝** One important key to success is self-confidence. An important key to self-confidence is preparation.**❞**

Arthur Ashe

INTRODUCTION

So you're finally getting to that golden day, the day of graduation. By the time you read this you may have already been there, enjoyed the bubbly, donned the colourful historic robe (in my case a fluffy, pink-and-white, off-the-shoulder number) and had the photos taken with your proud parents. It really is such a relief once it's all over and you've sweated out those tense few weeks between exams and results day.

Whilst you're coming down from the graduation high you realize that you're about to start work, become a pro, mix with the big girls and boys. Just when you thought your student loan crevasse couldn't get any deeper, you are sent a letter from the GMC regarding payment to become a provisionally registered practitioner. And so begins a long relationship with all kinds of official bodies that have weird and wonderful three-letter acronyms. In fact, there is a rumour that there is an official body that spends its time making up the acronyms. It's probably called the Official Acronym Function Society (OAFS).

Transitions in life throw up exciting possibilities and potential hazards. Your transition from student to fully fledged doctor means clinical responsibilities to your patients, which most of you will be aware of. But your rights and responsibilities as an employee may well be less obvious. Working will not be new to most of you, but your experience of being an employee in the NHS is going to be very different from being a casual employee of the local bar or restaurant, not least because of the complex relationships between the different constituents in the NHS. It is definitely worth investing your time finding out who is who once you are qualified.

Your employing Trust and perhaps Foundation school will offer you an induction process when you first start work. Many of you will also have a period of shadowing before you start. Shadowing is the hands-on aspect of induction, when you get to know your base ward and are generally shown the ropes by the existing F1. You get the chance to 'try on the clothes' of being a doctor without having the final responsibility. These last few days before you hit the big time should be rewarding, with your F1 gently protecting you from the cleaner after you stepped on her newly mopped floor, and allowing you to undergo the final metamorphosis to becoming a doctor. Shadowing is described in detail below. You may need to push yourself forward in order to get the most out of it. With luck, your F1 will not have left it to the last minute to take their holiday, leaving you with a ward full of patients whilst you are supposed to be shadowing.

Induction varies from Trust to Trust, but the good news is that having a successful induction is a key quality assurance indicator for the Trusts, so there should be better standardisation in time. For some this will be a quick half-day tour through the important aspects of the Clinical Negligence Scheme for Trusts (CNST), whereas for others it will be a detailed and helpful introduction to what you need to know to do your job. In Scotland you will get an online induction which you complete at home before you arrive. This not only gives you the information you need, but also assesses whether you have completed the module and learnt it. Hopefully, the rest of the NHS will catch up with this type of system.

This chapter is designed to supplement your official induction, tell you the things that the Trust might not wish to tell you, bring you up to speed with all the official bodies and gives some top tips on the practicalities of life as a newly qualified doctor. Not only will you gain personal benefit from understanding the structures and relationships within the NHS, the curriculum for Foundation doctors includes learning objectives that are relevant to your understanding of the NHS. You could even start your portfolio now by recording the fact that you have done some background reading on this subject area by reading this chapter!

Let's take you through the alphabet soup of acronyms and common terms that make up the NHS and health environment. Once you understand the relationships within the NHS, you may be able to understand your role as an employee a bit better and also the demands and limitations on those around you.

THE A–Z OF STARTING THE FOUNDATION PROGRAMME: YOUR QUICK GUIDE

A

Accommodation

Hospital accommodation is a mixed bag and you will probably not be offered any unless your hospital is very far from the main population base or you have to move a lot in your rotation. The good thing is that the BMA will take any complaint very seriously – poor hospital accommodation is meant to be a thing of the past.

For more information, see *Living and Working Conditions for Hospital Doctors in Training*, produced by JDC (Junior Doctors' Committee) at the BMA. www. bma.org.uk

Annual leave

The first rule of annual leave is 'first come, first served', so it follows that the second is 'dog eats dog'. Don't expect others to do you massive favours so that you can take your leave if you have not planned ahead and got your request in early. You officially need to give the Trust about six weeks' notice so that there is adequate ward and clinic cover. If you don't give six weeks' notice, your employer will be within their rights to refuse your request, even if it is to be best man or for your own honeymoon. Make sure you spread your leave over the year. Even if you have nothing planned you will cherish the time off; it's what keeps you going. Don't assume that you will be able to claim financial compensation for any days off that you have not used.

B

Breaks

Research in many occupational categories such as the airline industry and mining shows that the chances of errors in the workplace are raised when employees are hungry, angry, late or tired (HALT). It's far too easy to miss breaks, but you will enjoy the job a lot more and reduce your chance of making an error if you take breaks. Remember that you are legally obliged to a break of 30 minutes for every four hours worked during a full shift thanks to the New Deal. Some Trusts are even clocking you in and out to make sure that you get your breaks, so concerned are they with your and your patients' well-being!

The British Medical Association

The British Medical Association (BMA) is basically a trade union for doctors and, like all unions, works on the premise that acting collectively is more powerful than acting alone. The benefits of membership include the weekly *BMJ* with its Careers section, access to the BMA's online teaching resources and the opportunity to take part in the democratic running of the BMA as it represents the views of the profession to the government. Perhaps more importantly, the BMA will represent you in any contractual or disciplinary dispute with your employer. The BMA is extremely helpful, replies to emails within 24 hours, takes your query seriously and will check any contract before you sign it.

The JDC represents your views within the BMA and you can get involved at local or national level.

Remember that alone you are very vulnerable to your employer's whims (e.g. on banding, hours worked, study leave allowance). If you are not a member at the time of the problem, the BMA will not defend you, so it is best to become a member from the start.

C

Canteen

Jamie Oliver hasn't got his hands on hospital food yet and so the standards are very variable, not least because the menu is mainly directed at the patients and the lower-paid staff and has a budget of less than £2.00 a day. The canteen is required to open between 11 pm and 7 am for a couple of hours, but the options and times offered may not suit you. Other options include vending machines or nearby take-aways. It is also possible to find a microwave, either in the mess or on the ward, so bringing your own food is an option if you want control over what passes your lips. For more information see *Living and Working Conditions for Hospital Doctors in Training* (produced by the JDC at the BMA).

Clean Your Hands: www.npsa.nhs.uk/cleanyourhands

A recently introduced initiative through the National Patient Safety Agency (NPSA) to highlight the massive problem of hospital-acquired spread of infection. You will see countless posters displaying the logo and further countless alcohol gel dispensers. The campaign has made a big impact on hand hygiene and will help tackle the rise of MRSA and *Clostridium difficile* infection. Did you know that you are only supposed to use alcohol gel for four patients and then you need to wash your hands? The spores of *C. diff.* are tolerant of alcohol so your hands need to be washed after attending infected patients.

The Clinical Negligence Scheme for Trusts

The Clinical Negligence Scheme for Trusts (CNST) is a group insurance scheme which NHS organisations pay into on a sliding scale. Each Trust pays many hundreds of thousands of pounds. By complying with the standards expected by the CNST, the Trust drives up standards of care, reduces risks to patients and staff, and saves money to spend on other aspects of care. One of the key standards is that the Trust must have inducted all employees into the correct policies (e.g. what to do after a needlestick injury, lifting and handling, fire safety, use of technology, etc.). The CNST has the power to change the experience of trainees in many ways. In theory, your skills should be carefully evaluated when you start in each Trust and you should not be allowed to perform any procedures until you are competent to do them. This gives the Trust an incentive to ensure that you have been taught the procedures properly.

Compassionate and special leave

This can be given for various reasons such as bereavement or your role in the armed forces. You can obtain compassionate leave with pay, for example to make funeral arrangements or to visit sick relatives. Usually you will only get a few days' paid compassionate leave (probably only three), but most organisations will give you unpaid leave if required. Human Resources (HR), Occupational Health or your operational services manager are the best people to contact to make arrangements for leave. It is polite to let your consultant know, but it is not their responsibility to sort this out.

Contract and terms and conditions of service

Unless you're a model or a professional footballer, I doubt you will have signed a contract before. When I first got my contract I skim-read it, popped my name on the dotted line and said, 'Where's the money?' As far as I was aware, that contract could have said, 'This doctor shall work for free and be required to fast for five days a week', and I would still have signed it. I had no idea about the intricacies of contracts, or terms and conditions of the job. Get the BMA to check your contract before you sign it.

Court appearances

Ideally, you will only have to make a court appearance as a witness or a juror. You can obtain leave with pay for attending court to give evidence, which may be the case if you do Accident and Emergency. An appearance in a coroner's court is also a possibility.

Giving evidence is a daunting but interesting experience. Be careful to stick to your own knowledge and don't get led up the garden path by a wily lawyer into saying something you don't mean or that is outside your expertise. The golden rule is only to comment on things you have observed. For example, if the prosecution lawyer asks you to comment on the possibility that a bruise arose from a blunt instrument wielded by the accused, you should reply that you are not qualified to comment on where a bruise came from, just whether or not it was present. In fact, if you make it clear to the police and prosecution that you are only going to read your statement and verify it in court and that you are not going to speculate on where an injury came from, they will often leave you alone and you won't be called as a witness. Remember that the GMC may well be interested in you if you give evidence beyond your expertise so do not speculate beyond what you have observed or give spurious statistical evidence.

D

Doctor

It may seem strange to have a section defining 'doctor'. But this is increasingly difficult in the modern world, with its 'medical practitioners', 'physician and surgical assistants' and the extended role of nurses. Maybe it's like an elephant, hard to describe to someone who has never seen one, but instantly recognisable when you have.

Traditional defining characteristics have been the ability to diagnose and prescribe, and the fact that you have registration with the GMC. But nurses and others can now prescribe in limited areas and nurse practitioners are able to diagnose within an area of expertise. Perhaps a defining feature is a more sustained intellectual approach to practice, supported by a deeper understanding of the scientific basis of health and a broader and deeper knowledge than our colleagues which results in a greater leadership role for doctors.

What do you think it means to be a doctor?

E

Early warning scores

There is clear evidence that trainee doctors do not always identify how sick a patient is. If you have not seen early warning scores (EWS) in action, take note now (Figure 3.1). They have been introduced to many hospitals in an attempt to prevent unnecessary deaths by capitalizing on the concept of the 'golden hour' when the patient's physiological status is deteriorating and when prompt action can prevent full-blown organ failure or death. It is characterised by some or all of the following:

- Falling BP
- Abnormality in the heart rate (too fast or slow)
- Worsening hypoxia, oxygen demand or respiratory rate
- Pyrexia or extremely low temperature
- Decreasing consciousness
- Increasing pain

If the EWS comes to more than an agreed cut-off, the nurse or healthcare assistant must call you to evaluate the patient. Do not ignore a worsening EWS. It may not be obvious what is happening, but most likely something is. If you can't work it out and come up with a management plan, call a senior. Of course, the patient may well be known to be seriously ill and even have been declared 'not for active intervention', so the EWS needs to be carefully interpreted. Remember, no one ever dies with a normal EWS so don't ignore it!

Educational supervision

Your educational supervisor is your guide through the Foundation programme and one of the fundamentals to success. A really good educational supervisor will help you plan your learning, track and feed back your assessments, give you pastoral support as needed, and give timely feedback on your performance and helpful careers guidance. See Chapter 5 for more information on how to get the best out of your educational supervisor and Chapter 7 for the trainers' guide on what they should be doing and the important differences between a clinical supervisor and educational supervisor.

European Working Time Directive

This is an agreement of the Council of the European Union and applies to all professions and jobs in the European Community. It regulates the maximum number of hours you can work each week. The aim is to bring the working week down to 56 hours by 2007 and 48 hours by 2009, with increasingly tough stipulations for the rest periods between shifts and over each month.

F

Finance and making your money work for you

Once you start earning, there will be a conflict between your desire to spend, spend, spend and the need to pay off your student loan. At some point you will also need to think about the future. It's probably too much to take in at the moment and your working hours will make it difficult to take action, but

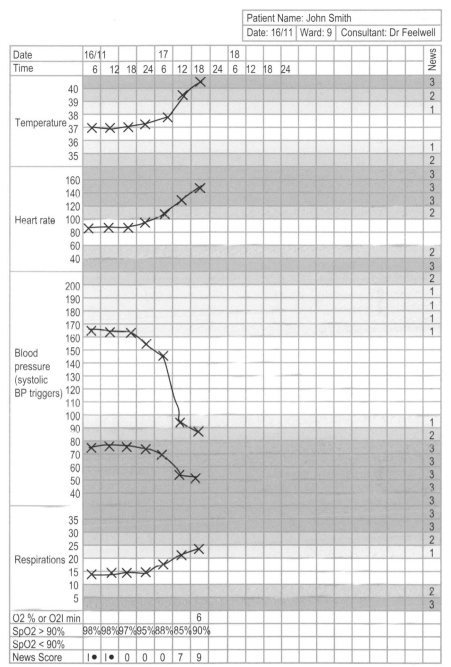

Patient Name: John Smith		
Date: 16/11	Ward: 9	Consultant: Dr Feelwell

Fig. 3.1 Observation chart for the early warning score.

If ONE or more parameters fall within the SHADED zones, perform a full set of observations and calculate a NEWS Score from values in each zone.

once you're coming down from the high of being a new doctor, make getting your finances in order a high priority.

These are the major considerations:

- Paying off loans. The rate of interest on loans from the student loan company is usually excellent. Contact www.slc.co.uk. If you have debts on credit cards or loans from commercial banks, the interest rates will be much higher so prioritise paying these off if possible. Switch debt on high interest credit cards to 0% deals.

- Income protection, critical illness cover, life insurance and drawing up a will. Taking out some form of private income protection or critical illness cover will be much cheaper for you now than later in life. For a few quid a month you could protect your income for the rest of your life if you are knocked down by the proverbial bus or, more likely, break your neck in a sporting accident. Income protection is important, especially in the early stages of working when you have not built up any sick leave rights. Critical illness cover is more expensive because it covers more. Basically, if you get one of the registered diagnoses (check exactly what is covered), then the insurance company pays out. Think about the cost of this and how likely it is that you will have a heart attack or get cancer in the next ten years. Life insurance is only needed when you have dependants, so beware of getting talked into buying it now if you don't have any. Once you own property it pays to make a will. Without a will, your estate can be very messy for your family to sort out after an unexpected death.

- Savings. It is generally advisable to pay off debt before starting to save, unless the rate on the debt is lower than the rate on the savings. You could, however, think about saving in a private pension because you will probably get a tax refund. See under Pensions. If by some amazing feat you have graduated free of debt, it is generally advised to use your tax-free savings in the form of an ISA before anything else.

- Is it better to search for financial services yourself, buy services from one of the large suppliers such as Medical Sickness or get the services of an Independent Financial Adviser (IFA), which may not be cheap? You can shop around for the best prices and the Citizens' Advice Bureau has some handy hints (see www.adviceguide.org.uk). You can buy many products by searching the Web or the finance pages of the press. If you do use an IFA, you can pay a flat fee or let them take a commission. Ask to share the commission – it may amount to thousands of pounds. Keep them on their toes by making it clear that you are seeking advice from their competitors. Shop around and don't necessarily buy health insurance from one of the medical suppliers or decide according to the amount of wine that they shower you with at promotional events.

Flexible training

There is a move towards flexible or part-time training. Your pay is banded in a similar way to full-time training, and is essentially proportional to how many hours you work and whether your hours are unsociable. Your contractual rights are the same as full-time doctors. You may well end up being paid a normal full-time salary with a small top-up for working six or seven sessions a week. Before 2005 there was top-sliced funding for flexible trainees, usually administered through deaneries. All trainees were entitled to apply for flexible training if they had one (or more) of three 'valid reasons'. These were dependent relatives (usually children), ill health and high-level sporting achievement (e.g. Olympic level). However, recently the funding has not been as forthcoming and so it has become more difficult to work flexibly in many deaneries. The arrangements for flexible training vary throughout the UK and so if you are thinking of training flexibly, seek help early on from your clinical tutor, Human Resources, Foundation school or the BMA. UK employment law requires all employers to consider seriously a request for part-time working from any worker with children, so if you cannot arrange flexible training, your employer will have to give you cogent reasons why you cannot work part-time.

Four-hour waits

If you're involved in Accident and Emergency during your Foundation programme I can guarantee you will come across this term. It is part of the NHS Plan to have patients wait no longer than four hours from when they come into hospital to when a decision is made to admit or discharge. In theory it's a splendid idea, but when it's hellishly busy and there are lots of really sick patients, this time limit can get stretched. To a bed manager the breach of a four-hour wait is like a full moon to a werewolf. I was once surrounded by bed managers during A&E when I said, 'We've got a bleeder'. They thought I had said, 'We've got a breacher' (i.e. about to breach the time limit). It is difficult to maintain ideal patient care under these circumstances and you need to be careful that government targets are not prioritised more than the patient's clinical needs.

G

The General Medical Council

I never fully appreciated the roles and responsibilities of the General Medical Council (GMC) until I qualified, when I realised that it is partly responsible for setting and monitoring the standards of my undergraduate education.

The GMC has the following three main functions:

1. It sets the standards of good medical practice
2. It assures the quality of undergraduate medical education and coordinates postgraduate training
3. It administers the registration system and examines questions of registration

This is now in a state of flux and the Postgraduate Medical Education and Training Board (PMETB) may end up with many of these responsibilities. The GMC could even disappear as self-regulation is replaced by government regulation. Currently, you need to register with the GMC if you wish to practise in the UK.

GMC guidance: The New Doctor, Good Medical Practice and Duties of a Doctor
You should be familiar with these GMC documents. *The New Doctor* sets standards for the F1 year and provides guidance on the competencies you must have to be eligible for full registration. From F2 year onwards the PMETB sets the standards as you progress towards your specialist/GP training programmes. *Good Medical Practice* is a set of standards that define a doctor's knowledge, skills and attitudes, regardless of what stage they are at in their career. It was introduced in the 1990s after consultation with members of the public to find out what they expected from the profession. *Good Medical Practice* is broken down into seven sections:

- Good clinical care
- Maintaining good medical practice
- Teaching and training, appraising and assessing
- Relationships with patients
- Working with colleagues
- Probity
- Health

These are covered in detail in Chapter 9.

Duties of a Doctor is a 14-point list and is effectively a concise version of *Good Medical Practice*. We had the 'Duties' framed on the wall of our mess, just above the pool table, in the hope that they would be absorbed as we were lining up to take a shot. So, from memory, as a doctor you must:

- Make the care of the patient your first concern
- Treat every patient politely and considerately
- Respect patients' dignity and privacy
- Listen to patients and respect their views
- Give patients information in a way they can understand
- Respect the rights of patients to be fully involved in decisions about their care
- Keep your professional knowledge and skills up to date
- Recognize the limits of your professional competence
- Be honest and trustworthy
- Respect and protect confidential information
- Make sure that your personal beliefs do not prejudice your patients' care
- Act quickly to protect patients from risk if you have good reason to believe that you or a colleague may not be fit to practise
- Avoid abusing your position as a doctor
- Work with colleagues in the ways that best serve patients' interests.

Trust plays a major part in all that the GMC advocates. We tend to see patients when they are at their most vulnerable, and unfortunately this privilege has been abused in the past. If a patient can feel comfortable with you, trust you and if you get them on your side, you'll be halfway there.

H

Health and safety at work

Your employer is responsible for ensuring your safety and that of your colleagues at work. The three main issues facing Trusts are needlestick injuries, lifting injuries and stress. These are covered in the CNST protocols.

You should be particularly aware of your responsibilities for preventing needlestick injuries to yourself and others. Follow good practice when using sharps: take the sharps box to the bedside, don't resheathe needles and take responsibility for disposal of sharps after a procedure such as a chest drain to avoid any errors by another person disposing of them for you. Don't use an overfull sharps box; change it. If you do get a needlestick injury, remember the mantra 'Bleed it. Wash it. Report it', which covers the essential first steps after a needlestick injury.

Once an injury has been reported, Occupational Health performs a risk assessment and counsels the patient about testing. It is important that you appreciate that contact with the patient should come through official channels. It is certainly not appropriate for the person who received the injury to counsel the patient; in fact, this could contravene aspects of *Good Medical Practice*. Be aware of your Trust's policy for reporting, especially out of hours.

Hospital at Night (H@N)

H@N is intended to be the answer to the problem regarding on-call rotas. Previously for night-time work there were parallel teams on call in every specialty, often with one doctor on take and one on ward cover. After fairly extensive research it was decided that you did not always need a doctor in every specialty to provide ward cover and the NHS has been trying to define the exact skill mix needed in different situations to be safe. The H@N system has not yet been fully implemented, but the reduction in hours under the EWTD from 2007 will perhaps be a further stimulus to change.

The H@N system requires close teamwork between doctors and other members of the team (e.g. specialist night nurses, medical care practitioners and others). This requires new skills in identifying the best person to do each task and in being flexible and understanding each others' roles. When it works well, the H@N system is excellent and as an F1 you have the chance to learn a lot from your colleagues.

H@N is still in its early stages and no doubt will continue to develop. If you are having a bad night and it seems that your hospital has not got the right mix of skills, remember that it is the H@N system that has allowed you to have a life and not do one in four or five of all nights for the first year or two of your working life.

I

Induction

Induction is a bit like the famous Donald Rumsfeld quote on what is known and what is not. There is stuff that you and the Trust know you need to know;

stuff that you don't know you need to know but the Trust knows you need to know; stuff that you know you need to know but the Trust doesn't bother to tell you; stuff that both you and the Trust know that you don't need to know but someone else thinks you need to know; stuff that you need to know but neither you nor the Trust know you need to know; and stuff that no one knows whether you need to know or not. Are you still with us?

The long and short of it is that induction should be a good way to get to know your hospital and their expectations of you, but at times it can seem turgid and dull because it serves so many masters, including you, the Trust or GP practice, the deanery, the GMC, various warring factions within the hospital each of whom believe that their message is the most important and, perhaps most importantly, the requirements of the CNST. (For details of CNST, look under 'C' above.)

So, induction will probably feel like an avalanche of information that you probably don't need and can't remember. The best inductions are like a map and should be accompanied by electronic or paper documentation that allows you to revisit the subjects when you need the information. The list of information that you need in starting in a new workplace is vast and induction should be spread over a period of time. The problem is that it is impossible to get all medical staff together after the first day so there is a tendency to try to force it all in one go.

There are some excellent new initiatives in NHS induction. NHS Scotland has initiated an online system for all Trusts in Scotland, which means that employees can access it at a time and place convenient to them. It also enables employers to document the fact that the trainee has received the induction, which is important for health and safety reasons and for attaining the more favourable levels of CNST status. Many English Trusts are sending induction CDs to employees before they start. If you get one, make sure you look at it before turning up on the first day.

There are essentially two levels of induction: Trust or practice induction and departmental induction. To this no doubt will be added school or deanery induction. Trust and deanery/school induction will take place once at the start of your two-year post. Departmental induction should take place every time you start a new rotation.

The following describes the essentials of each level of induction:

Trust induction
- What you need to know: which consultant you will be working with, holidays, pay, rotas, car parking, accommodation, how to get a computer login, the name of your educational supervisor.
- What the Trust needs to tell you: health and safety matters, such as what to do in the event of a needlestick injury, how to protect your back, support sources for stress, etc.; how to use the hospital notes system and any IT that is used in patient care, such as electronic prescribing or medical records and remind you to write clearly, document everything, use a black pen, etc.; IT policy, including use of the Web and pornography policy; check the level of your practical skills so that you can be signed up to practise them safely; bullying policy.

- What the deanery or education team need to tell you: the curriculum, assessment methods and usage; the name of your educational supervisor and what their role is; who administers the assessment system, the library.
- What the departments need to tell you: approach to children, radiation protection, how to fill in a pathology request form, blood transfusion policies, management guidelines for any condition likely to present to the hospital, writing death certificates, cremation forms, discharge letters, medicine kardexes and fluid, warfarin and insulin charts.

Departmental induction

This is poorly done by many departments, but probably the most important thing to ensure a happy bunch of doctors on the team and also important for patient safety. You should meet a consultant, GP or a direct representative on the first day of the job. If you don't get a departmental induction, demand one. (This is covered in Chapter 7.)

What you need to know: who you are working for, what your responsibilities are, who to call when you need help, working relationships with nurses and others, arrangements for study and holiday leave, who to tell in the event of sickness, protocols in use on the unit, learning opportunities on the unit, timetables of relevant staff, arrangements for discharge summaries.

Information

Information is the lifeblood of medicine – you need to be able to access good quality information in real time to help you in patient care. The following are some of the best and most reputable sources. You can also use the National Library for Health (see under 'N'):

- Cochrane Library – highly regarded in clinical practice. Randomised controlled trials and meta-analyses. Good, solid evidence.
- NICE – you will be able to get hold of the guidelines from here.
- Clinical Evidence – a favourite of mine. Type in 'atrial fibrillation' and it will give you the intervention (e.g. 'amiodarone'), then give you a summary and whether the evidence shows it to be beneficial. It's very helpful.
- Medline – you probably have used this database. Contains a lot of useless information, so you need to know how to use it properly.

K

Knowledge and Skills Framework and the Agenda for Change (A4C)

A4C is the new system for describing the work of everyone (other than doctors) in the health service. Thanks to the NHS Plan and the modernization of the NHS, the Agenda for Change saw the General Whitley Council terms and conditions superseded by the NHS terms and conditions of service handbook from 2004 onwards. This applies to all NHS staff except doctors and dentists, who are still governed by their own terms and conditions. Nurses and others will be developing their careers using the Knowledge and Skills Framework. Basically, the more skills and knowledge needed to do a job, the higher the pay. Your help in achieving this will be very welcome, so if they do ask for help in training or assessment, please oblige.

L

Leave

See Annual leave, Compassionate and special leave, Parental leave, Sick leave.

M

Making your life easier: getting a cleaner

A significant way to improve your quality of life now that you have qualified is to find a reliable cleaner. You are going to be working more than 40 hours a week, many of them unsociable. Your friends and support will often be working opposite shifts. You need fresh air and exercise. Your spare time therefore becomes precious. Whether you are fastidious, and clean every day or week, or whether you are more infrequent, having a cleaner frees up your time. You are moving from being someone who is (probably) cash-poor but time-rich to someone who is relatively cash-rich but definitely time-poor. A good cleaner is a godsend. I have used both private and agency cleaners. The best way is to find one through word of mouth, either work colleagues or neighbours. In reality, most good cleaners are fully booked so you need to get lucky. While you are waiting to find a good private cleaner, use an agency. This is more expensive but comes with security – any worthwhile company has excellent crime checks and systems to prevent theft, and the advantage that an agency does not go on holiday or get sick.

Modern matrons

There has been overwhelming public opinion that the NHS should 'bring back Matron', who ruled the ward with a rod of iron in days gone by. Modern matrons are meant to be an inspiration to other nurses. They ensure that the fundamentals of care are being addressed, for example making sure patients are getting their meals on time and inspecting the wards for cleanliness to prevent hospital-acquired infection. So when you see Matron, remember she was ruling the roost when you were just a twinkle in your dad's eye. Their opinion is highly respected, so if you get on with them, get a multi-source feedback form done and you will be on to a winner.

N

The National Health Service

Although I wasn't aware of it at the time, when I stepped into hospital on my first official day as a doctor, I was about to start work for the largest organisation in Europe with 1.3 million employees, spending about £2500 per household per year, or nearly 10% of Gross Domestic Product in 2006. The NHS was established in 1948 and thrives on the principle of providing healthcare on the basis of need and not on the ability to pay. The NHS needs to continue to evolve and the following is a quick guide to recent change in the NHS, particularly since New Labour came to power in 1997.

The NHS Plan

Since 1948 things have changed somewhat, and at the beginning of the 21st century the government produced the NHS Plan (www.dh.gov.uk – follow the links from Publications and Statistics), a ten-year master plan to enable reform in the NHS, by increasing the workforce, investing in more services, shifting decision-making power to the local health services and generally giving patients a louder voice. Foundation Trusts are the new style of NHS Trust set up from 2004 onwards with these principles in mind. It may come as a surprise that decentralization was an aim! Many of the following initiatives came from the NHS Plan.

NHS Direct

A dedicated 24 hours a day, easy access NHS, a bit like your GP surgery in that you spend a lot of time on the phone pushing buttons (see www. nhsdirect.nhs.uk or 0845 4647 or on digital TV). NHS Direct has largely achieved what it set out to do and relieves GPs of some of their workload. The slight disadvantage is the lack of human contact, so in effect you are losing the art of diagnosis. Diagnosis and advice are given by nurses using a rules-based system. Therefore a person who phones with a headache and a rash is going to be referred urgently to Casualty even if a doctor looking at the rash could have seen that it was not meningitis. This leads to some bizarre referrals from NHS Direct but the system may reduce workload overall.

National Institute for Health and Clinical Excellence

NICE (www.nice.org.uk) produces clinical guidance on new and existing treatments for many conditions. NICE also produces guidance regarding public health, and safety and efficacy of interventional procedures. SIGN (Scottish Intercollegiate Guidelines Network – www.sign.ac.uk) is the Scottish alternative. Both resources are useful when you are auditing your hospital policies or protocols to look for the gold standard way of doing things. They look at evidence of both effectiveness and cost-effectiveness so are at the heart of debates on rationing and resource use in the NHS.

National Electronic Library for Health

The National Library for Health is a Web-based resource that contains a wealth of information. You can browse Medline, NICE, Clinical Evidence, the Cochrane Library and much more. Definitely worth surfing next time you're online (www.library.nhs.uk). For example, say you were asked to present management of atrial fibrillation. I know, you shudder at the thought, but the National Library for Health can help you.

National Service Frameworks

These are guidelines that came into being along with the NHS Plan. Diseases and conditions (e.g. types of cancer, coronary artery disease, mental health), as well as groups of patients (e.g. the elderly) all have a National Service Framework (NSF). They are useful in that they set standards to attain within a certain time frame. They are also useful for audit purposes. Your Trust should be set up to work towards all of these goals. If you are seeking an audit subject, then choose one from an NSF – the NSF targets really matter to Trusts and they should be reasonably well aligned to patient care.

New Deal

In 1991 an agreement was reached between the government, the royal colleges and the BMA to make the crushingly intense 120-hour working weeks a thing of the past. It also looked at living standards for junior doctors (e.g. accommodation, cooking and cleaning facilities), which were thought to be far from ideal at the time but provoking outrage from the Rats in Hospital Accommodation Union. Ten years on and the New Deal was finally enshrined into contracts, and a new system of pay, known as 'banding', was introduced. The New Deal stipulates similar rules to the EWTD on hours of work and rest requirements. The differences are that doctors should not work more than 56 hours a week, and should be allowed 30 minutes' break every four hours while at work during a full shift. (The EWTD stipulates 20 minutes every six hours during a full shift day. For further details see 'Pay and your hours of work: banding and maintaining' pp. 52–53).

O

Occupational Health

Occupational Health is the division of the NHS that looks after its own staff and manages risk to patients. You will come into contact with 'Occy Health' when you start work, when you are required to demonstrate evidence of immunity to hepatitis B and rubella and be screened with respect to TB risk. Don't worry if you are unsure about any of your details – Occy Health are always happy to stick you with a needle to test you for immunity. They may offer help with stress and mood disorders, often through a psychologist. Alcohol and drug misuse are other situations where they can help, or at least point you in the right direction. (See the section on Health and stress in Chapter 9.) Occupational Health also manages illness that occurs when you are working, and if you have been off with a serious illness they will help manage your return to work and arrange any necessary modifications of your work rota or work environment.

Out-of-hours GP services

The days of calling out the family doctor when you are ill have gone in many parts of the country. With the new GP contract, GPs can opt out of out-of-hours work and primary care Trusts employ GPs to do it. They are often based in or near hospitals, making it easier to admit someone to hospital. Because the patients are seen by someone other than their GP, it is inevitable that admissions have risen by about 15% since the introduction of the new GP contract.

P

Parental leave – maternal, paternal and parental

Maternity leave

This may not be the first thing on the mind of most newly qualified doctors, but it pays to know about the provisions. As a rule, the more service you have given the NHS prior to becoming pregnant, the more generous your entitlement to paid leave. Employers are bound to keep your job for a year when you are on maternity leave as long as you have worked for them for a prescribed period of time – usually a year.

There are a number of complexities in the maternity leave schemes, but the principal system is the NHS maternity scheme: you must have continuous service with the NHS with one or more employers for at least one year, from 11 weeks before the expected week of childbirth (EWC), to be eligible. To be entitled to receive money under the NHS scheme you must return to work for at least three months after your maternity leave has ended. The 26 weeks' pay are currently broken down into 8 weeks' full pay and 18 weeks' half pay. So for potential parents out there, in theory the earliest point when you can give birth and be eligible for the full NHS scheme would be approximately 11 weeks after the start of your F2 year. Statutory Maternity Pay and Maternity Allowance apply if you have less than one year's service in the NHS.

You need to let your employers know you are planning to take maternity leave before the 15th week before the expected date of childbirth, i.e. before your 25th week of pregnancy. There is no rule stipulating when you should start your maternity leave – it depends on how you feel. One mum I knew was working nights up to the week before she gave birth. She finally gave up when her little one started joining in on chest compressions during arrests. Don't worry if you can't handle nights or can't cope with the intensity of your on calls. The Trust can continue employing you under a temporary 'pregnancy rota' with full pay, provided you get a letter from your GP which makes it clear that carrying on at the current work intensity is putting you and/or your baby at risk.

How easy will it be to get back to work?

If your job extends beyond your maternity leave, you will be able to carry on where you left off, under the same contract with the same terms and conditions. Should you want to return under a flexible working pattern (see under 'F' above), your employers are required to consider your request, and must explicitly state why if they won't agree. Be aware that you need to have a job to go to when you finish the Foundation programme if you are due to have a baby after the end of the post and you wish to claim maternity leave. I know so many women who have timed their pregnancies to points in their career when they were about to change posts and have not benefited from maternity leave. This is unfair to doctors in training who change jobs frequently. The situation will be improved by the run-through specialty training so that women are much less likely to miss out on their rightful income and job protection. The message, at least from a careers and economic perspective, is clear: if possible, delay your pregnancy until you are safely ensconced in a specialty training programme.

If you experience discrimination or unfair treatment, get the BMA on the case as they will help you deal with your employers.

Paternity leave

You are entitled to paternity leave if you have been working for at least 26 weeks in the NHS, from the 15th week before the due date of the baby. You are granted 1–2 weeks with full pay. You must inform your employers 15 weeks before the expected date of delivery. As the length of your employment in the NHS goes on, you may be entitled to unpaid leave as well. See your Trust website or ask Human Resources.

Parental leave

If you have a child under the age of 14 years and you have worked in the NHS for at least 12 months you may be allowed at least 13 weeks' unpaid leave per child per year to cope with illness, hospital appointments, etc. This is usually discretionary and you need to talk to your employer at the earliest opportunity.

Pay and your hours of work: banding and monitoring

The percentage of your basic salary that you should receive for additional hours is determined by your additional hours and how many of these are unsociable (see Table 3.1). Unsociable hours are generally regarded as hours worked before 7 am and after 7 pm, as well as any weekend work. Theoretical hours worked, and therefore pay, are worked out from the Riddell Formula, but New Deal compliance must be measured with actual hours determined by monitoring.

Remember that the punitive rates of pay of the higher banding scales are intended to induce your Trust to get your hours down to the acceptable level, not as a means of making sure that all Foundation doctors can afford an Aston Martin. These days a 'good' employer is one that has all its trainees rostered and actually working within the New Deal and EWTD limits rather than one that is paying band 3. In fact, in the Foundation programme it is extremely

Table 3.1	A guide to the banding thresholds			
Band	New Deal-compliant?	Actual hours per week	More unsociable?	Basic Salary Added %
3	No	>56	Yes	100
2A	Yes	48–56	Yes	80
2B	Yes	48–56	No	50
1A	Yes	40–48	Yes	50
1B	Yes	40–48	No	40
1C	Yes	40–48	No	20
F (Flexible)	Yes	<40	Depends	Depends

unlikely that anyone will have a band 3 payment. Deaneries have exerted a lot of pressure on Trusts to come up with compliant rotas.

You are contractually obliged to monitor the actual number of hours you work to ensure that you are New Deal-compliant and in the correct pay banding. It may seem that there is a perpetual battle raging between Human Resources trying to make sure trainees fill in and return their monitoring exercise and trainees trying to make sure Human Resources don't pull a fast one by downgrading their band scale without telling them. But this is only half the picture. Human Resources needs a certain percentage return rate from the monitoring exercise. If that doesn't occur, they can only assume that the hours you have been working are New Deal-compliant and correctly banded. So the onus is on you to fill in your monitoring to make sure you are being paid correctly. One Trust has recently introduced a clocking in and out system for Foundation doctors because it was not satisfied with their compliance with the requirements for hours and rest periods. This could become widespread in the next five years.

Payment by results

Another government initiative to allocate NHS money differently. The principles are to provide money to Trusts based on what is actually coming through the hospital doors, rather than the old style of block contracts where the Trusts were given a budget to work from – for example, the Trust will get money for every patient who has a hip replacement. Money is also given for tests performed in hospital and disease severity. This is relevant to Foundation doctors because the discharge summaries are used as a guide to how much a particular admission has cost. There is a big difference in cost between someone who has had an MI, compared to someone with acute coronary syndrome, or 'chest pain ? cause'. You will no doubt get a talk during your first few weeks from the Clinical Coding department about the correct way of writing a discharge summary. Your input into the discharge summary and logging of procedures performed (beyond routine bloods) will help to determine the hospital's finances.

Pensions scheme and getting an extra pension

The NHS pension scheme is one of the best, and you automatically qualify for it when you start work. Small chunks of your salary are deducted each month, as you will find out when you try to decipher your pay slip. Interestingly, that doesn't go into an offshore piggy bank to be stored up and given back to you when you retire, as I once thought. It contributes to paying the pensions of currently retired doctors.

The NHS scheme is rated as one of the best because it is still a 'final salary' system. At present you get 1/80th credit for each year worked and to get the full entitlement you have to work 40 years, which most of you will not. Your pension is then $x/80$th (where x is number of years worked) of your salary at retirement plus a lump sum. At present you can retire at 60 without it affecting the pension you have earned. If you retire before 60 a reduction in what you have earned as pension rights is made of approximately 4% for each year before 60 that you retire to compensate for the fact that you will be drawing the pension for longer. So, if you retire at 55 with 30/80th service and your final salary is £100,000, you will get £37,500 a year less approximately 20%. The lump sum is also reduced.

The government is planning to bring in significant changes to the scheme. This will mean a retirement age of 65 and a change from final salary to 'average earnings'. The details are not finalised and there may well be a chance to pay in a greater proportion of your salary and so buy a bigger NHS pension.

At present no competent IFA would advise you to pull out of the NHS scheme as it is very robust. Beware anyone who tries to tempt you away. But, you should consider buying extra pension provision, either in the form of a private pension, Free Standing Additional Voluntary Contributions (FSAVCs), a pension run in conjunction with the NHS scheme (AVCs) or by buying added years. Talk to your IFA about which is best for you. Remember that you get a tax refund on any money put into a pension, so putting in £100 means that you can claim back £40 if you are a higher rate taxpayer. (See the NHS pensions website: www.nhspa.gov.uk.)

Politicians: what have they done for us?

It is pertinent to reflect on the role of politicians in shaping the NHS. The NHS is one of the key battlegrounds of national politics, running close to the economy, education, law and order and defence of the realm as the most important subjects for voters. Whilst this is important in ensuring continued funding, it does put NHS employees at the centre of a maelstrom or a bit like a football to be kicked between ideologies. The only thing constant in the NHS is change. It seems that although New Labour has been in power for three terms, the NHS forms the subject of internal struggles between the modernizers and the traditionalists, so even continuity of party does not ensure that we don't live in a state of constant change. Doctors are generally a conservative bunch who don't like change and who stoutly defend their professional identity and independence. The pages of the journals and free newspapers are full of discontent with New Labour despite the fact that they have more than doubled spending on the NHS and doctors' salaries have increased considerably more than those of most other professionals. It is interesting that doctors appear to value their professional identities more than increased pay. So how have Labour managed to score an own goal in doctors' approval ratings, and who is going to come off best in the long term? There are now groups of doctors campaigning for very different models of healthcare in the UK, ranging from full privatization to a compulsory state insurance scheme. The effect of the return of a Conservative or even a coalition government on healthcare policy is difficult to predict, but it is bound to mean the beginning of another round of change. Some, including Gordon Brown, have suggested that the control of the NHS should be taken away from politicians and be run by an independent quango so that it is not subject to repeat cycles of change every time there is an election. In the end health is always going to be a big issue and subject to political influence. Doctors and other healthcare staff have to live with this inevitability no matter which side of the political fence we are on.

Postgraduate Medical Education and Training Board

The Postgraduate Medical Education and Training Board (PMETB) is a statutory body set up to regulate all postgraduate development, achievement and education. It assumed its powers in September 2005 but has had a slow start after the Chair resigned and whilst its committees were appointed. The PMETB is the gatekeeper for the Specialist and General Practice Register. It takes on many of the functions of the Specialist Training Authority (STA) of the medical royal colleges and the Joint Committee on Postgraduate Training for General Practice (JCPTGP), which previously looked after postgraduate training. The government is keen to see more power ceded to the PMETB and has proposed that it becomes responsible for the supervision of undergraduate education, a role previously performed by the GMC. Watch this space! For example, the PMETB has allegedly given specialist registration to a surgeon who had failed the final FRCS several times, much to the horror of the Royal Colleges who had previously guarded entrance to specialist status with their exams. (See Chapter 10 for contact details.)

Protection societies and medical indemnity – Medical Defence Union, Medical Protection Society, Medical Doctors and Dentists Defence Union of Scotland

Your employer indemnifies you for work in NHS hospitals, so it is optional whether you join a medical protection society or not. The arrangements for those doing primary care attachments are being revised. The question then is whether you need or wish to have indemnity insurance for any acts that you commit outside your employing hospitals. The GMC advice on helping out in any medical emergencies in the community suggests that 'whenever it arises, you must offer assistance, taking account of your own safety, your competence and the availability of other options for care'. I bet that the Good Samaritan didn't get sued by the beggar for staining his tunic, but it may be wise to be part of a medical indemnity scheme at this point, where you will be covered for any Good Samaritan acts you perform. Similarly, if you offer your services at a sporting event, make sure that you have adequate training to deal with the expected injuries and you will definitely need indemnity cover. In general, however, if you are not planning to offer your services to anyone other than your usual employer and Good Samaritan acts, you may well feel that, at this stage in your career, additional indemnity is not required. The BMA's advice is to consider Good Samaritan cover. Compare and contrast the offers from the three principal suppliers named above. The protection societies are not there to help you in disputes with your employer. You need to be in a trade union such as the BMA for this. (See Chapter 10 for contact details.)

Q

Qualifications

Now you've got the big qualification from your university, there are many more out there for you to get. As well as membership exams, why not try night classes in sign language, or a weekend course to develop communication or teaching skills? Remember to maximise your learning opportunities

– no one will be looking out for you except yourself, so be selfish! There are hundreds of things you can do in the next two years for your personal satisfaction or to enhance your application for post-Foundation training. (See Chapter 8 for further details.)

R

The Royal Colleges

The Royal Colleges are the central organisations that look after the history, current state and future of the specialties they are responsible for. There is a Royal College designated for each specialty: Physicians, Surgeons, Obstetricians and Gynaecologists, General Practitioners, etc. They are working in conjunction with the PMETB to produce the Curricula for Specialty Training Programmes and General Practice training. The Royal Colleges have many roles. As well as being historical institutions, they are responsible for publishing guidelines and statements regarding healthcare, and have an advisory role to the government and public.

The Royal Colleges are more accessible than ever nowadays. Their websites are extremely informative and keep you up to date with the latest news pertaining to your specialty. Many offer online training schemes and means of planning and tracking your learning in relation to that specialty. (See Chapter 10 for contact details.)

S

Shadowing

Shadowing can last about two weeks and is your last chance to try out the skills that you need in a safe environment. It is usually done just before the start of your post. It may seem as though you are undertaking two weeks' unpaid work, but in most medical schools it is a compulsory part of the course. The following is a list of the things you should try out in shadowing:

- Complete forms for x-ray and pathology requests
- Organize a list of contacts and phone numbers
- Become familiar with ward routines
- Practise resuscitation
- Become familiar with the way in which things are handled after death and complete a death certificate and cremation form
- Make an inter-team referral
- Complete a drug chart and any special charts such as insulin, warfarin or fluids
- Become familiar with Trust policy on things that are relevant to you (e.g. DVT prophylaxis in surgery, antibiotic policies, needlestick injury, etc.)
- Get your F1 to dish the dirt on the preferences and dislikes of other members of the team
- Get a handover list of all patients under your care and any outstanding tests, diagnostic uncertainty and communication issues
- How to use the phone system effectively

Make sure you get some feedback on how you have done these things from your F1. If you don't have the opportunity to do a period of shadowing immediately before you start, you might like to consider arriving on the ward a day or two early and using this checklist to help yourself.

Shift working

Nearly all Foundation doctors will be working full or part-shift rotas, involving nights and weekends when you will be working the whole shift. You should not expect any sleep during your rostered hours. A recent publication from the Royal College of Physicians, available as a free download (www.rcplondon.ac.uk/pubs/books/nightshift/nightshiftbooklet.pdf), details some of the measures that can be used to ensure you don't become too tired. It emphasises the risks of sleep deprivation to patients and the shift worker, whose risk of dying in a car crash when tired is doubled and whose overall performance is reduced by an amount equivalent to driving over the limit. (For simple measures that can be taken to reduce sleep deprivation, see Chapter 4.)

Sick leave

Being sick is not what you need as a doctor, especially any sickness that you acquire at work. I'm not advocating obsessions and compulsions, but rigorous handwashing will cut down on the commoner causes of taking sick leave. One such wee beastie is the rotavirus, which decimated our ward for two weeks and took out half the patients and staff, including me. (The upside was that we were closed to admissions.)

In this situation, when I was only off for a few days, I had to register my absence with my employers for their 'sickness absence' records. Once it gets to over a week you need to provide evidence that you are unwell with a doctor's certificate.

The NHS has its own policy and benefits for doctors who are on sick leave for prolonged absences, but at the beginning of employment they are rather modest – for F1 doctors this is one month's full pay and two months' half-pay; for F2 doctors it is two months' full pay and two months' half-pay.

Obviously none of us wants to contemplate going on the sick, but you never know what is round the corner. Potentially, any one of us could become sick from tomorrow. I know this all sounds pretty morbid, but you're fully fledged professionals now and you do need to protect your income. This highlights the need for income protection insurance – see the advice above under Finance.

Sister: keeping her happy

We had a talk by one of the ward sisters during induction on how to keep sister happy. This was really useful and contained practical advice on how to be a good F1 from the nurse's point of view. Things that are really important include:

- Making sure that your prescribing does not cause problems for the nurses with illegible or ambiguous instructions
- Anticipating problems so that you don't make work for others. For example, keeping fluid and insulin charts up to date and writing everyone up for prn analgesia on admission so that the nurses don't have to call you later
- Maintaining an appropriate attitude at all times to all levels of staff on the ward
- Not being dismissive, even if you think you are right
- Trying to see things from the other person's point of view
- Letting the nurses know when you are going to teaching so that they can get any urgent tasks done before you disappear. This should reduce the chance that they will bleep you when you are otherwise occupied
- Making sure that you complete important tasks (e.g. death certificates) on time

Further detail on the expectations of Foundation doctors is given in Chapter 4.

For many, the experience of working on the wards is quite difficult. It may seem that your priorities and those of others do not always coincide. You may feel that nurses act differently from doctors. Ward organisation may not focus on your needs and the lines of communication may well be poor. If you are having problems with being bleeped unnecessarily or being asked repeatedly to do the same unimportant task, ask yourself why. There may well be some simple measures that you could introduce to help with the situation. For example, would it be helpful to have a place (a book or board in the office) where unimportant and non-urgent tasks can be written down for you to do when you are free? This could save a lot of phone calls and bleeps. Try not to react to any irritations – it only makes them worse.

Remember that sisters have seen doctors come and go and know more than most about what makes a good doctor. They can sniff out a bad attitude like gastroenterologists can sniff out melaena. Keeping sister happy is definitely the 'one that got away' in the *Duties of a Doctor*.

The Surviving Sepsis campaign

It is a little known fact that approximately 20% of people die of sepsis and its complications. There has been a recent initiative to try to push sepsis up the health agenda and improve survival. The Surviving Sepsis campaign team have devised a series of measures and teaching materials (see www. survivingsepsis.org, and follow the links). The early warning scores (see pages 39–40) are often predictors of severe sepsis. This has a mortality of approximately 30–50%. The Institute for Healthcare Improvement and the SSC are aiming to reduce mortality by 25% by 2009. Remember the general measures for treatment of sepsis:

- Early recognition – measure serum lactate and BP
- Adequate resuscitation (mean arterial pressure of greater than 65 mmHg and CVP >8 mmHg) to prevent organ damage, initially with 20 ml/kg of crystalloid and vasopressors such as noradrenaline if needed

- Location of the source and drainage if it is pus
- Culture before antibiotics are given
- Early and appropriate broad spectrum antibiotic usage
- Specific measures such as use of low-dose steroids and Drotrecogin alfa (recombinant activated protein C)
- Maintain blood sugar less than 8.3 mmol and central oxygen saturation >70%

T

Targets

The NHS Plan was introduced by the government and aimed to bring the NHS into the 21st century. It set targets for NHS organisations to aim for in order to achieve this. Mainly the conversation topics of NHS managers, modern matrons, frustrated consultants or political lunchtime mess chat. Important targets include reducing waiting times for hospital appointments or operations, reducing emergency care waiting times, reducing hospital-acquired infection and those contained in the National Service Frameworks.

U

Urban medical myths

These are rumours which grow and circulate as the whole truth and nothing but the truth. Make sure that you don't believe everything you hear. A rumour circulating in one hospital was that wages were being kept low to increase hospital profits. This was in the days before Foundation hospitals, when there was no such thing as a profit for a hospital, showing a high level of ignorance on the part of juniors about how the NHS works and the managers' motives. Check the facts when you hear these kinds of stories and take a reality check from time to time. And certainly don't complain about your pay in front of other hospital workers. When you reach a senior position you will easily be in the top 5% of earnings for everyone in the country.

V

Volunteering

Consultants love keen junior doctors. There are many opportunities throughout the Foundation programme for getting your face known and helping out, e.g. teaching the new third year medical students, doing the audit that no one else wants to do, or simply doing your own ECG on take when the nurses are busy. Nothing goes unnoticed when you're at work and you will reap the benefits, whether this be a serendipitous publication, a consultant investing more time in teaching you, or just a cup of tea from the healthcare assistant.

W

Waiting times

One of the big problems in the NHS. Practically everything to do with the NHS has a waiting time attached to it. The government has produced oodles of documents and targets in order to reduce waiting times for hospital appointments, operations, getting tests done, etc. The four-hour wait in Casualty has had a big effect on medical practice. The next aspiration is that no one should wait more than 18 weeks from referral to treatment. Wow! In the out-patient setting and in primary care this is going to make a huge difference to the way we practise medicine. No more seeing someone in clinic, ordering a few tests and bringing them back three months later. It is likely that we will be working to protocols that cut across primary and secondary care. The GP who wants to refer a patient for hip replacement will no longer be able to do a cursory examination and write a leisurely and brief letter to the orthopod of their choice who will see them 13 weeks later and order an x-ray and MRI, see them again after three months, put them on a waiting list for physio, etc. No, the GP will probably have to carry out the x-ray and MRI, have already tried physiotherapy and three different NSAIDs in escalating strength and toxicity, and then make an e-referral to the orthopaedic team stating the patient's cardiorespiratory history and having already performed an online anaesthetic risk assessment. Before attending the clinic, the patient will have used an online 'you and your choice – to hip or not' decision aid tool so that they know what they are letting themselves in for. The consultant then sees the patient with a diagnosis and a decision already made and merely has to fill in the consent form and give them a date for surgery. Of course, this does not leave much chance for teaching trainees in hospital clinics because the patient will have to be seen by a consultant and the diagnostic regime will already have been carried out. Learning opportunities may well be transferred to primary care.

Such changes are going to impact on your working practices and all doctors are going to have to learn new ways of practising. (See the DoH website, www.dh.gov.uk, for details.)

X

X-ray Department

Before you start ordering tests using your newfound skills, you will get a talk from a radiologist about IR (ME)R 2000 – the Ionizing Radiation (Medical Exposure) Regulations 2000. It is there to remind you to think twice when ordering tests that expose patients to potentially harmful radiation, and you will no doubt be shown slides of patients who have developed a skin cancer secondary to being exposed to radiation. It is important that you do understand IRMER because the regulations affect how radiologists and radiographers act. Basically, IRMER dictates that all x-rays have to be justified and if they have been done unnecessarily, the practitioner can be prosecuted. So, if the patient had an x-ray yesterday but it can't be found and you want to repeat it, the radiographer will probably refuse the request.

Z

Zero tolerance policies

Violent behaviour to staff is not tolerated and the NHS zero tolerance policy is there to deal with problem patients. Violence in hospitals is not uncommon, whether this is due to medical reasons such as delirium or mental illness, or to violent or angry relatives. Staff need to feel secure in their often vulnerable working environment and each hospital should have a security team present 24 hours a day. The NHS Security Management Service (SMS) recently took over the management of this policy. (For further information see www.cfsms. nhs.uk.) If patients are violent or abusive, you have a number of options. Many hospitals have policies to deal with this – use them. Ring the general manager or your consultant for advice. If patients are rude and abusive, calmly point it out and if they continue, consider walking away. Avoid escalating the problem and make sure that you keep yourself safe (e.g. by being closest to the door, having another person present, etc.). Get your employers to issue the patient with a warning or a banning order, so that they can only attend for emergency treatment.

THE BIG DAY

No amount of induction can totally prepare you for the real thing. But the more things you have tried out before the big day, the easier it will be.

If you're lucky, the undergraduate department organises a big curry night out at the end of induction. If you're already nervous about starting work, go easy on the chilli peppers!

Surviving your first weeks and months

Jonathan Carter

4

ff Don't let the art of perfection be the enemy of the art of the possible.ff

Traditional Italian saying

INTRODUCTION

This chapter is designed to take you from induction through the first days, weeks and months of the job. It looks at 'the Fear' – the normal response of the new doctor to the first few weeks – and how to cope with it. It reminds you of your basic responsibilities and jobs on a day-by-day basis. Chapter 3 looked at the wider NHS, and this chapter puts your job into the context of your immediate working environment with a quick guide to who is who and the subculture of the hospital or GP environment.

THE FEAR

What is the Fear?

Night sweats, itchy eyeballs and running around like an idiot searching for the crash trolley when you hear the 'BEEP BEEP' at a pedestrian crossing. Ladies and gentlemen, welcome to the Fear.

You may know the Fear better than you realise. There are examples throughout life (Box 4.1). Fear doesn't arrive out of the blue. It won't come and haunt you while you're lazing on a beach during your elective or on Saturday lunchtime when you're warming up last night's pizza leftovers. The Fear arrives for a reason – to get you to respond.

Fear is adrenaline, pure and simple. This is your autonomic response (remember physiology in your first year?) in preparation for the joys of the Foundation programme. Fear is at the far end of the stress spectrum, which is around us most of the time. Without wanting to sound like a self-help book, we need some stress in our lives, but we do need to know how to manage it. This section discusses some of the sources of stress and gives a recent F1's top tips on how to manage it.

The spectrum of stress is dynamic. During a typical day you'll spend time in all zones. You might think that the zero stress zone is the happiest place (Box 4.2). But how long would that light your candle for? So how about the maxi-stress zone (Box 4.3)? Again, only so much of this is good for even the worst adrenaline junkie.

> **Box 4.1   Examples of things that provoke 'the Fear'**
> 1. Running out of small talk on the first night of Freshers' week
> 2. Taking blood from each other as medical students, knowing that your mate has the needle in your nerve, but you don't want to put them off their stride
> 3. The night before Finals, provoking a change of bowel habit most IBS sufferers wouldn't dream of

> **Box 4.2   The zero stress zone**
> * Multidisciplinary team meetings with coffee and scones
> * Surgical nights on call
> * Drug reps with free tourniquets

> **Box 4.3   The maxi-stress zone**
> * Cardiac arrests
> * Aggressive/abusive patients/relatives
> * Needlestick injuries

> **Box 4.4   Top five mini-panics**
> 1. Did you stop that patient's Sando-K?
> 2. Did you start that patient on Sando-K?
> 3. So that patient is definitely not penicillin-allergic?
> 4. Did you take that tourniquet off that patient's arm?
> 5. p-ANCA titres of 2.35 – a bad thing?

Dotted around the stress spectrum are mini-panics – harmless, nagging doubts that tend to pounce on you as you are about to leave the ward on a Friday afternoon. These are the 'What ifs . . .?' (Box 4.4).

When you become a Foundation doctor you will doubtless be exposed to countless stressful situations. Spending too much time at either end of the spectrum is unhealthy. Being aware of when this is happening and knowing how to respond when you are stressed are vitally important.

Mastering the Fear

At the risk of sounding like a kung fu Grand Master, to beat the Fear you must first understand it. Consider how you would manage the following situations:

* Mrs Jones is going for an MRI scan this afternoon and you still don't know if her metal hip is going to fly out of her body in the tunnel. It's

made of some weird new alloy put in by a professor of orthopaedics who works hundreds of miles away. You've been trying for days to contact him to clarify things, but his secretary always says he's out. The only time he was in his office he said he wasn't prepared to speak to a house officer. (We know he meant an F1.)

- You're checking the ward bloods on a Friday afternoon and dreaming of the end of the week and getting off on time. You realise that the patient with the paracetamol overdose has a nasty elevated prothrombin time. Rushing to his notes, you find out that he self-discharged this morning and his current address is NFA (no fixed abode).
- It's Monday morning and on the jobs list are two death certificates, seven discharges, three prs and a controlled drug script that keeps bouncing. Mrs Smith's family are meeting you at 10 o'clock. They're upset at the care their elderly mum has been getting. As you walk into the bay you see Mrs Smith do a pirouette and land on her hip with a shuddering crack.

In all these situations, you could lose control. The natural response is to panic, get stressed. But because you are familiar with the Fear, you can keep control. Knowing that you're not going to go insane, it's amazing how efficient you become. It's stress and you can manage it.

Keeping control is the key to 'thriving and surviving'. In 'Putting it into action' towards the end of this chapter, we will provide you with potential solutions to these conundrums.

The key areas to master to manage the Fear and stress are:

- Doing the right thing
- Doing the thing right – time management and prioritisation
- Understanding the medical subculture and the tribalism that surrounds us
- The contribution of your inter-professional colleagues.

THE JOB

Doing the right thing – ward work

Medical school, shadowing, induction and Chapter 3 should have prepared you for your first job as an F1. But there is still a lot to learn. This bit is about doing the right thing. What exactly is your responsibility as an F1? Much of the time you will feel that you are little more than an underpaid jobs monkey, but many of these seemingly mindless tasks require a high level of skill and knowledge as well as incredible attention to detail. For example, your consultant asks for an urgent endoscopy and ultrasound on an alcoholic admitted with abdominal pain who has a history of multiple admissions and self-discharge. If you are really just a mindless primate will you manage to swing the ultrasound today and ensure that this is coordinated with the endoscopy and that the patient is kept fasted for that endoscopy that you suspect will be normal?

The short definition of your first priority as an F1 is to look after the patients in your care. To do this you need to:

- Get to know about their history, current condition and their own perspective
- Monitor and document their clinical condition looking for evidence that things are not going to plan (e.g. their EWS)
- Take part in ward rounds and record what has happened in the notes – a skill in itself (see Box 4.5)
- Order, coordinate, perform, document and act on test results
- Organise treatment, including prescribing medication and fluids, and prepare the patient for surgical interventions
- Communicate with patient and carers
- Communicate with the rest of the medical team, including other specialties and GPs
- Communicate with the multidisciplinary team
- Respond to requests from nurses and others to review patients
- Plan the patient's discharge, starting from the minute they are clerked in
- Perform after-death duties, such as informing the GP or coroner, completing the death certificate and post-mortem requests

Your other responsibilities include:

- Managing your own learning (Chapter 5) and organizing your own assessments (Chapter 6)
- Participating in the quality assurance procedures of your job and learning programme (e.g. by the deanery)

Box 4.5   What should I write in the notes on a ward round?
- Patient's name, date of birth and hospital number should be on each sheet in the notes
- Date, time and name of person leading the ward round
- Content of discussion between the patient and consultant. For example, did it focus on the history, management plan, risks of treatment, prognosis, any doubts about diagnosis? Did the consultant ask about and did the patient express any preferences?
- The patient's vital signs or EWS
- Examination performed and what was found. Ask the consultant if they do not tell you – don't guess what they heard down the stethoscope!
- Test results, especially x-rays reviewed
- Any important tests outstanding that were not reviewed
- Differential diagnosis suggested by consultant, preferably in the priority order of the consultant
- Investigations ordered
- Treatment or management plan, especially any changes in medication and length of course of any treatment
- Referrals needed
- Any anticipated variations from expectations and back-up plans
- Treatment level decisions if appropriate, e.g. is this patient for resusc, are they on a palliative care trajectory, what is the ceiling of care – antibiotics, HDU, ventilation?

- Participating in assessment and appraisal of others
- Participating in the quality improvement and clinical governance processes of the NHS

So, not much to do then! How to do the thing right is the next question.

Doing the thing right: efficient working, time management and prioritisation

You will probably be regaled about the 'good old days' at some point in your Foundation years, and this will no doubt be from a retiring old boy who still performs a pleural tap through a patient's clothes. When one of the authors qualified in 1987, all junior doctors lived in hospital accommodation, were served breakfast in our own dining room by our own staff, worked for just one consultant for six months and we did a 1 in 4 rota with prospective cover, which meant at least 80 hours a week and the longest continuous shift was Friday morning to Monday 5.00 pm. There were many good things about the old system but also many that now seem bizarre and unacceptable. For many they *were* the good old days and learning from experience and your mistakes *was* the best way to learn. The radical idea now is to improve patient care by having doctors who have had enough sleep to perform well, to teach them what they really need to know to look after patients, especially the acutely ill ones, and to assess them fairly, using valid and reproducible methods. So, are the reduced hours and competency-based education and assessment politically correct nonsense or the arrival of the enlightenment to medical education? Does the new way of working live up to its billing, or is the king wearing no clothes? You decide using the comparison box (Box 4.6).

Box 4.6 Compare and contrast the old and new ways of working

Old	New
Worked for one team only	Work across teams and consultants
Knew all your patients	More cross-cover
Worked only within specialty	Cover other specialties out of hours
Teaching covered medical topics	Teaching includes generic skills
You assumed you knew what you had to know	Curriculum-led
Assessed on global impression	Assessment based on specific tools
Life revolved around the mess	There is a world outside
Slept when possible on call	Awake all night when working shifts
Worked hours needed to get job done	Work allocated hours
80+ hours a week	Maximum 48 hours a week in 2007
Expected to have full responsibility for patients	Expected to hand things over
For procedures – 'see one, do one, teach one'	Use simulation first and better supervision and feedback

Whatever you think, there is no going back, but there are a number of important skills that need to be acquired to make the new system work, particularly in the areas of time management, prioritisation, handover, personal responsibility and new methods of learning dictated by fewer work hours.

Starting the Foundation programme, the thing that strikes us most is the volume of work. It is like climbing an intellectual Mount Everest – Mount Cleverest. One response would be to implement the first golden rule: leave on time to survive. Not that I always did. It is easy to become caught on the ward like a semi-intelligent rabbit in headlights. It's not that I was kept there by a fascist dictator of a consultant – I chose to stay; I chose to 'revise' my patients, to chase bloods and to figure out if Mr Jones' Trop T-negative chest pain was purely tactical because he liked the hospital porridge so much or might be explained by deep-seated psychological processes. It was hard to draw a line in the sand and leave, even harder to hand tasks not yet done to someone who I was not sure would do them.

Time management is difficult, because it's so easy to stay late. Finishing your jobs list may seem like the bottom line, but you will never completely achieve it. How do you choose which jobs to leave? And if you do finish, would it look good to make sister a cup of tea before you leave?

From day one you need to get into the habit of efficient working, planning and prioritisation (Box 4.7). These are great skills to have and essential in your Foundation programme and your later years. Set your goals for the day and the week and try not to let others deflect you from it. Obviously, there will be some things that alter your plan – the major variceal bleed in the middle of that leisurely discharge planning meeting, for example. But if you don't have a plan or a sense of the main tasks to be accomplished, when unexpected events crop up it will be much more difficult to work out what you should be doing when the dust settles and your sick patient has been transferred to ITU. This may sound like management speak but it does work. I've had to overcome many an awkward silence on a ward round because a test result hadn't been chased up, or a hip x-ray hadn't been discussed with a radiologist.

Start to shut up shop about an hour before your finishing time. You will be able to chase up bloods during this period, and by setting an end point to the working day you will start to prioritise your jobs more efficiently. Jobs can take as much time as you allow them. Try to set reasonable limits on the time you spend on each task and if it's taking longer, ask yourself why. It may be that you are being too perfectionist in the standard you set, you may need some additional training to speed up, you may not be preparing well before starting, or you may be rushing and making mistakes. There is a fantastic Italian saying that roughly translated means 'Don't let the art of perfection be the enemy of the art of the possible', or as a psychiatrist told one of us, 'Doctors are never satisfied with good enough'. In other words, being insistent on doing everything perfectly could prevent you from even starting some of your important tasks.

Get a diary, even better an electronic PDA with numerous functions including internet access, data storage including MP3 files and photos, digital radio, phone and camera combined. Up To Date (www.uptodate.com) provides online and PDA-compatible referenced material that keeps you abreast with every field and includes medical calculators and checklists for things such as calculation of estimated glomerular filtration rates and reminders for things such as the Wells score for DVT risk. Well worth the modest cost and sure to impress your colleagues when you pull your PDA out on the ward round and help them assess the patient.

I had never bought a diary because I saw it as a sign of weakness (not quite sure why). I made the investment last year though and now I practically own memory lane. This is particularly useful for on calls. I once took part in a grand multiparous swap with about four people. Suffice to say one of us forgot we were on and the operational services manager had to get me out of bed. My name was on the rota, so it was my responsibility. If you do make any swaps on the rota, make sure you let the manager in charge of the rota and the switchboard know, using some form of traceable communication such as email. Saying that you rang and told some unnamed person is not going to get you out of the hole if things go wrong.

There are many things you can do to help the team function more effectively and time-efficiently. There is nothing worse than wasting time doing something because someone else did not do a simple task. Remember to do the following:

- Before going home, make sure that all warfarins, insulins and fluids are written up
- Make sure that any bloods requested for the weekend are absolutely essential
- Leave a list of patients for the weekend for any doctor visiting the ward. Include information on expected course, treatment levels, anyone who can go home and why

While we're on the subject of priorities, start planning your holiday and study leave now. Don't expect to get the last two weeks of July off at three days' notice because you have days owing. If you are thinking of getting married any time between now and the end of F2, book a date and request the leave now. It may even be necessary to change the order of your rotations if leave is fixed for some rotations (e.g. A&E).

In the business of the F1's life, it is all too easy to prioritise other people's needs above your learning needs. As a result of these ongoing changes, time is precious and there may not be as many opportunities for learning on the job. Previously you would have seen a number of patients with diabetic ketoacidosis (DKA) during your six months of medicine. Now you may have to look up the meaning of DKA. You may only do four months in medicine and the on call is much less intensive so you may only see one such patient. You must therefore maximize your learning from each case. Think of this as helping others because without the learning your future patients will suffer.

So, don't become a jobs monkey – put your non-opposable thumbs to good use, climb the tree of knowledge and get greedy by setting yourself learning outcomes for each day/week/attachment. Imagine you are on the Medical Assessment Unit (MAU) and there are three CT heads to book, two discharge letters to write and ten blood results that need chasing. You hear the medical registrar quietly ask, 'Does anyone want to learn how to do a lumbar puncture?' Are you the F1 who always gets the task of confronting the radiologist

Box 4.7   Eleven top tips for efficient working

1. Learn how to use the recall service on the hospital phone system. That way, when you answer a bleep and the phone is engaged, you will be able to press the recall numbers (normally R#1) and the phone will ring when the other end is free. This simple step will save you hours.

2. Multi-tasking. When on the phone, check emails, results or rewrite scripts. Females are said to find it easier to multi-task. They do it all the time – at work, at home, when driving . . .

3. Minimize the use of a 'jobs book' or lists. Every time you write something in a jobs book, you could have done half the job and it means that confirmation that a test has been requested is in the jobs book and not in the patient's notes. For example, a consultant on MAU suggests a dementia screen. Instead of writing it in the book to be ticked there and not in the notes, carry a clipboard with all the necessary forms attached. When a test is required, put a sticky on a blood form and write 'dementia screen' in the clinical information section, tick it as done in the notes and fill in the tests required at your leisure. This will also help you get radiology requests in at a time when they can be done the same day. Use a clipboard with a patient list and copies of every form you are likely to need.

4. Plan ahead and be prepared. Sounds like a top tip from someone who stayed in the boy scouts for too long, but planning is a vital time-saver. For example, keep your assessment forms handy at all times when there might be a chance to get one completed. Plan your holidays early, partly so you can arrange all the swaps before it gets tight and partly so that you are guaranteed to get them when you want. If you have to go to another part of the hospital, make sure you do all the jobs in that area to save time.

5. Don't be afraid to hand over to the on-call team at the end of your shift. This is now seen as a professional responsibility.

6. Do it now, don't delay. A good example is typed discharge summaries. If you can keep up to date and preferably dictate each one as you write the handwritten instant summary, they will never build up. When you have three 2-metre-high piles of discharges to do dating back to your first day on the ward, you won't want to start at 4.00 pm on a Friday. Keeping tasks manageable will stop you procrastinating.

7. Make an easily available list of all the phone numbers, bleeps and emails that you need. An electronic diary is great for this; file them all under 'Contacts'.

8. Adopt the habits of your seniors – and I'm not talking about Friday afternoon dental appointments. For example, if I saw someone's creatinine had shot up, it never dawned on me as an F1 to grab the drug chart and withhold any renotoxic medication, whereas it was the first thing my SHO did. The next time it happened I knew what to do.

9. Make sure you take your breaks. You are entitled to 20 minutes every four hours in a full shift. There will be more pressure on you then to complete the tasks in an allotted time.

10. Remember, blood is as blood does. If you don't find out what it's trying to tell you, you'll look like a clot. Bloods that are chased and blood forms that are ready for the phlebotomists are essential tasks for an F1, and looked on favourably if done well.
11. Be clear who is going to be responsible within the team for which tasks or which patients. If you are working with an F2, make sure that it is clear what contribution they are expected to make to routine in-patient care and keep them to it.

with a thinly disguised attempt to pull the wool over their eyes and get the CT that was requested by the consultant for no good reason? Or are you going to get to learn the LP and get another DOPS completed at the same time?

Doing the thing right: continuity of care and handover

With fewer and fewer hours for individual doctors to spend with patients there will ultimately be less continuity of care. In order to overcome this you must make handover of paramount importance.

Handing over is a skill that you become better at as you progress. In the delirium of your shift ending and the new shift starting, it is easy to forget to tell your colleague to chase up the CXR on the patient who may have a pneumonia, or to recheck the blood gases of that COPD patient.

A good idea is to keep a list of the patients you have seen on your shift and make a note of the jobs still to be done. That way you can either do them yourself during the last half hour of your shift, or hand the job over if there is no time to finish them all. It is absolutely vital and always appreciated if you let the incoming team know about the 'sickies' on the ward so they can be reviewed in a planned manner rather than when the nurses identify a problem.

Your hospital should have a policy and format for ensuring that feedback takes place and does so effectively. In advanced institutions you may have a PDA to 'beam' information from one to another and a structured document with details of each patient, particularly in high-risk areas such as SCBU. Things get a bit more complicated in large units with a lot of moderately sick patients who are unlikely to need immediate attention but any one of 300 patients could 'go off' in the middle of the night. It is always difficult to know which patients to hand over in such circumstances. If your hospital does not have a formal handover between the day and night shifts, they are running big risks. If they don't, you could always try to institute one – this would make a good subject for an audit and be a great thing to put on your CV for post-Foundation applications.

Remember that it is your duty to hand over patients to the new team. In many hospitals it is compulsory to attend handover meetings. If that's the case, you are well advised to turn up. If the format of handover sessions does not work well for you, suggest ways in which it could be improved. See guidance from the BMA (search for Handover in the www.bma.org.uk public

> **Box 4.8 Information needed in handovers**
> - Patient's name and another identifier if there are two patients with similar names
> - Where they are
> - Current clinical condition
> - Outstanding results to chase up
> - Tests that need ordering or performing
> - Anticipated problems that might develop in the next few hours
> - Treatment plan in differing circumstances
> - Who to inform in the event that the patient deteriorates
> - Any discussions that have gone on with other clinical teams, e.g. transfer to another hospital
> - What the patient and carers know about the current situation and what the patient's wishes are
> - Any problems in communication that might have occurred between the clinical team and the patient or carers, particularly if they have already complained
> - Any limitations on levels of treatment – e.g. is this patient for resusc, ventilation, dialysis, antibiotics, further intravenous cannulae?
> - Ideally all this information should be recorded in the medical notes anyway

section), the Royal College of Physicians (Continuity of care for medical inpatients: RCP London at www.rcplondon.ac.uk/pubs/wp/wp_ccmi_summary. htm) or the H@N document (*Implementing the Hospital at Night*, Section 4.1) on effective handover for more information, and Box 4.8 for the information that needs to be transmitted about an individual patient.

Doing the thing right: advice for specific situations

Being on take

Being on take puts you through your paces, and is the time when you legally work beyond 5 pm. Having just started work they can be fairly tiresome, so make sure you have a break or it will not be fun. It may feel as though no one cares if you've just done a Florence Nightingale and worked 13 hours in a row – you are a jobs monkey. Look after yourself as you would your patients. That said, I actually used to look forward to my on take days purely because one of my wards was an absolute nightmare! In my case it was out of the fire and into the frying pan.

I think the key to being on take is never to lose control. Always have an idea of who you have seen, who is on the ward generally, and the sickies of the ward (and I don't mean the porter who always stares at you after you have just done a PR).

Another skill that is handy on the Admissions Unit is learning to spot bombshells. These are bits of information such as 'His BP is 60/40' that the nurses like to drop on the doctors' office. Once that is done, the responsibility is effectively yours, as the ominous phrase 'doctor informed' will now be cemented in the nurses' notes. Remember that no one with a normal EWS ever died, so take note of the abnormal physiological parameters.

You need to remember the patients that are already there too. After the post-take ward round they tend to be forgotten, particularly as the new patients start to roll in. These can often be silent bombshells – the 80-year-old with *C. diff* who has been faecally exsanguinating for hours, but no one has stuck up any more fluids on her 'because she's going to elderly care any minute now'. Silent bombshells can blow up in your face, so be warned.

On take is where you will learn most of your acute care. I found it a busy yet rewarding time during my first year. Your history-taking and examination will become slicker than an oil spill and you will gain confidence in dealing with common patient presentations.

Handing over, delegation and prioritisation are essential skills that you will pick up. Being on take you tend to start with your head in the sand, committed to clerking but not really knowing what comes next, when the patients are seen and carted off. Every day you have to dissect a jobs list for 30 patients and rank them in order of importance. At the end of your shift you will need to toll the next doctor which patients they need to keep an eye on.

You'll probably be on take with an F2 and a registrar (or whatever they are called next year). The on-take team are the key to a successful day. Communication and teamwork are paramount. I say that because during one of my first on takes I was given a dressing down by the registrar for being 'too slow'. I'm not sure, but something about his demeanour told me he hadn't been to too many communication skills sessions. The long and short of it is I panicked, stuck my head even deeper in the sand and didn't hand over a patient with spinal cord compression who needed urgent imaging to the night team. Was that a display of good teamwork? No. Did I beat myself to a pulp about it for the next three months? Yes. I never want to put anyone in that situation. To be fair to the Foundation programme, I was able to reflect on that event and come to some kind of closure, but I'll never forget it.

Dealing with nights

Nights are weird when you first start. You spend the time wandering around the hospital being bleeped more times than a Tarantino film shown before the watershed. The wards are bathed in an eerie glow, everyone whispers and the nurses' station is turned into a newsagent's. Sadly, nights are just as busy as days, so you can't go ghost-hunting. You do get the occasional night where nothing happens, but then you can just spend your time looking at the clock.

Some of my happiest memories are from nights, because you're probably with the same colleagues for their duration. You, the F2 and the registrar are alone with the patients and if the team works, it's great. Depending on the set-up you can learn a lot from your seniors and even spend time in HDU/ITU if it's quiet. Make the most of this time to learn procedures.

Your very first night is special. For a start you have to find a way of sleeping most of the day before you start, and that can be fun for the imaginative! After the shift it feels like you've been on a long-haul flight to a different time zone. You expect to step off the plane to a welcoming embrace. All that happens is you end up trying to give your bleep away. The last 'day' of nights is also a bonus. I used to finish early on a Friday morning so it felt like a three-day weekend. So, there are many good things about nightshifts, but there are also some pretty serious drawbacks, including the risk of dying whilst driving home!

A recent publication from the Royal College of Physicians has detailed some of the measures that can be used to ensure that you don't become too tired when working shifts. This is available as a free download (www. rcplondon.ac.uk/pubs/books/nightshift/nightshiftbooklet.pdf). It emphasises the risks of sleep deprivation to both patients and the shift worker, whose risk of dying in a car crash is doubled and whose overall performance is reduced by an amount equivalent to driving over the limit. More errors occur at night, so be extra cautious when doing shifts. Check dosages and prescriptions, don't be tempted to ignore a worsening EWS and be careful with apparently simple tasks, such as fluid prescribing, on patients you don't know without fully assessing them. Sleep debt accumulates and will need to be repaid at some point. It's no good thinking that missing two hours' sleep in every 24 will not catch up as the week progresses. It is important to ensure that you do try to sleep, or at least rest lying down, for seven hours or more a day. Some simple measures that can be taken to reduce sleep deprivation are detailed in this report and are summarised in Box 4.9 (see page 76).

Dealing with a colleague who does not pull their weight

You will definitely come up against a colleague who does not pull their weight. Doctors are no different from any other group of people and there are bound to be some who are either plain work-shy or are distracted by external events. Dealing with this will probably be a new skill for you. None of us likes conflict; nor do we wish to be a nark and tell teacher. One of the key problems here is that many clinical teams do not have clear written protocols of responsibilities and your induction to your team may be superficial or even nonexistent. In a team with an F1, an F2 and an SHO/ST1 looking after 45 patients, if no one makes it clear how the work and responsibility should be divided, then your F2 and SHO may well assume that you, the F1, are responsible for all the basic patient care. Don't let them get away with it. In our experience, one doctor can look after no more than 15–20 patients effectively, especially on general medical wards with sick patients. It can be very difficult if it is left to one doctor to organise everything and the others offer magnanimously to help out with the F1's jobs when they feel like it. Much better to share out the patients equally, and each F1 and F2 doctor takes full responsibility for an agreed number of beds or patients. If this does not sort the situation out, then there are some difficult decisions to be taken. I once worked with a doctor who revised all the patients the night before and thrust herself forward at the consultant on the ward round, but was never to be seen otherwise. The consultant thought that the sun shone from her anal orifice and could not see her for the fake she was.

How to deal with it? Approaching the doctor and seeing if you can sort it out person to person seems like the best option. No matter how angry you might be with the situation, try to present it in a neutral way if possible.

Rather than approaching the doctor with a blaming attitude, put it in terms of patient safety and fairness. Try to negotiate a better division of labour that serves patients' interests. If that doesn't work, have a word with the middle grades and see if you can recruit them to your cause, offering a fair and balanced account of the situation. If that doesn't work, you may well have to approach a senior – say, the consultant on the team – but if you feel that the response will be inadequate, you could consider approaching your educational supervisor or the programme director or even Human Resources. This may well feel very difficult. None of us likes to appear weak or to snitch on colleagues, but an imbalance in the workload can compromise patient care so you always have this justification.

What to do when you are sure you are right but the SpR disagrees. Short answer: prioritise patient safety

It won't happen often, but there may come a time when you have a critically ill patient and have called a middle-grade doctor or senior and they do not respond in the way you expect. Perhaps they assess the patient as less ill or are not keen to consider the diagnosis and management plan you have proposed. You may think that if you are right, the patient is going to suffer or even die. Maybe there is conflict about the treatment level status of a patient.

You are in a difficult position – you appear to have done the right thing by calling your senior and they have made what you believe is a wrong decision. You are between a rock and a hard place. It may not feel that you have the right to question their decision, but if you don't the patient will suffer. If you go over their head and call another senior, you will have undermined the doctor's authority and potentially damaged an important working relationship. Of course, in all these considerations the first priority is patient safety. Our experience of listening to Foundation doctors' reflections is that this is a key area of concern. Their reflections show that they have always regretted not acting when they felt they were right and rarely regretted acting when they were wrong. Seniors would rather that a trainee called them and was wrong than did not and the patient died.

So, how can you go about it? The first thing is always to discuss the case again with the doctor with whom you are in dispute. Take a non-confrontational approach. Instead of questioning whether their decision is right, ask them to explain how they reached it and what factors they weighed as more or less significant. This may result in them changing their decision. Alternatively, ask them if you should, together, call the consultant to let them know what is happening. If you are still running into a brick wall and you feel that you are right, then you probably are. Recruit others to your point of view or test it on others, such as the senior nurse or another Foundation doctor. If they agree with you, you will feel supported and less out on a limb. If it is a dispute with a team member in a different discipline, call your own seniors or consultant first. In the end, if you are concerned, call the consultant. Don't feel that you have to be 100% sure to make the call – reasonable doubt will do.

Box 4.9 Top tips on dealing with nights

1. Get at least six hours' sleep during the day, including on the day you start work. Don't rely on finding a few hours during the night – chances are you won't. Make sure that your sleeping environment is appropriate – dark, quiet and the correct temperature for you. If you have kids, make suitable arrangements to get sleep – either they go out or you sleep somewhere else.

2. Make a list of who you have clerked and which jobs are outstanding. This will help tremendously when you are preparing the ward trolley round for the morning.

3. Try to fend off inappropriate ward calls during the nightshift such as re-siting unnecessary cannulae, writing up non-urgent fluids at 6.30 am, prescribing warfarin to a patient you don't know at 10.00 pm, etc. Most of these should be filtered by the nurse practitioner or another member of the Hospital at Night team. If possible, get most of the information over the phone. You will be missed on the Admissions Unit if there are a lot of patients still to clerk. Always respond positively to calls concerning a patient's clinical condition, especially if they have evidence of physiologically serious disease in the form of an abnormal EWS.

4. Drink plenty of fluids and eat appropriately (a high-protein, low-carbohydrate diet is recommended) and use caffeine prudently.

5. Take breaks while you can, you never know what's going to come up. The Royal College of Physicians advises napping for 20–45 minutes during quiet periods or rest periods at night, particularly between 3 am and 6 am, if you can. Longer sleeps are not recommended during shifts.

6. Try to get to know the patients you haven't seen. Some of them will be profoundly ill and need to be reviewed. This is a tricky but important skill, and difficult to do if there are a lot of new patients.

7. Don't hang around in the morning. People will try to get you to do jobs from the post-take round. Once your time is up, make it clear that you need to go soon, hand over anything outstanding and leave. Don't feel guilty about this and don't think that staying after shifts will impress seniors. They do/should understand the shift system.

8. Don't be afraid to ask for help. Just because your senior is asleep doesn't mean they can't be disturbed. They are getting paid, so call them if you need them, even if you are not sure they have anything to contribute. As seniors, we can happily say we would rather be called than not.

9. Own the post-take ward round. Make it yours. Know all the patients if you can. It makes it easier, even if you have but a semblance of knowing what is going on. If you are in the driving seat, you can also use it for education and for getting your assessments done. Take the consultant to the sickest patients first, even if they are at the far end of the ward, or to patients where you are not sure you have made the right decision or are unsure how to interpret an x-ray or other result. Start in HDU/ITU if you have admitted anyone there.

10. Do something with your extracurricular life before you start your shifts. It is very tempting just to work and sleep because nights are so draining, but you will benefit from seeing your friends in the late afternoon or early evening and taking your mind off work.

11. Think about how you are going to get home. If you are working far from your home, consider sleeping in an on-call room before driving or using public transport. The NHS has a mantra that doctors are like all other night workers and sometimes refuses to supply a room to sleep. However, nurses choose their place of work rather than being rotated round jobs, generally work 9 pm to 7 am rather than finishing at 9 or 10 am and they normally only work 2–3 nights maximum. Get the BMA on the case if you are required to work nights far from home or in long stretches and it is not safe to drive.

MEDICAL SUBCULTURE AND TRIBALISM IS ALIVE AND WELL IN THE NHS – A GUIDE TO NEGOTIATING THE BOUNDARIES

Understanding the differences and rivalries between departments and specialties is essential to surviving the Foundation programme. Failure here will lead to frustration and wasted time but, more importantly, harm to patients. Many hospitals sport a cast that could star in a best-selling Broadway production all year round, such is the myriad of characters. Once you get to know your friendly neighbourhood work buddies, you will feel at home as the new character in this long-running soap. Box 4.10 suggests some old fashioned and, no doubt, out-of-date aphorisms about different specialties! The following are summaries of the experience of working on the main clinical teams and how to communicate across the boundaries.

Medicine

Medicine is often 'in your face' busy: you will literally have things put 'in your face' to do NOW. You will be all systems go from start to finish. You'll be sending off batches of esoteric tests in search of equally esoteric diagnoses. There'll be times when you think you've made a real difference to someone's life, and times when you think you're nothing more than a (PR) finger, a signature (on scripts) and a pair of legs (to go to x-ray).

Box 4.10 Aphorisms about specialisms
- Physicians know everything about one thing but can do nothing
- Surgeons know nothing but do everything
- GPs know nearly nothing about everything
- Psychiatrists know nothing and do nothing
- Pathologists are always right – but by then it's too late
- What's the difference between an orthopaedic surgeon and God? God doesn't think he is an orthopaedic surgeon
- Anaesthesia is the discipline whereby the half-asleep allow the half-awake to be operated on by the half-witted
- Radiologists are like two-year-olds – they just look at the pictures

---

> **Box 4.11 Ten ways to get noticed for the right reasons in medicine**
> 1. Organize for the ward round. Make sure all tests are ordered.
> 2. Make sure all test results are back and documented where the consultant can find them.
> 3. Make sure all tests are acted on.
> 4. Think or read about interesting causes of the abnormal test results that you have found and order more tests to explain them.
> 5. Have a differential diagnosis that goes beyond 'exacerbation of COPD' or 'off legs' when necessary.
> 6. Have a problem list for each patient.
> 7. Have a clear plan of how your patient is going to be discharged, based on their activities of daily living, impressions of the physio and OT and patient and family.
> 8. Make sure you document your own impression of what you think is wrong. If you're right, you look good. If you're wrong, you'll be taught why. Everyone's a winner.
> 9. Try to pre-empt the ward round. For example, if someone has had a batch of tests at another hospital recently, get the discharge letter faxed from that hospital. It will shave days off the patient's hospital stay.
> 10. Keep relatives up to date. Sometimes I had to set aside entire afternoons to speak with relatives. But they appreciate it. A thank you card is the icing on the cake for your learning portfolio!

Twice a week you'll go on a pilgrimage with your consultant for the ward round. Along the way you will pick up many followers (medical students, the confused granny who thinks you're queuing for the bus) and be dealt a fresh list of tasks for the week ahead. Ward rounds are one of the major differences between medicine and surgery. They do actually exist in medicine. They form the backbone of ward work and get people in and out of hospital. Remember, they are a good time for your consultant to make an assessment of you as a doctor. As they say in tennis, 'The best ball boys are the ones that you don't notice'. Not completely applicable in medicine, but thought-provoking none the less. So if you are planning on getting noticed, make sure it's for the right reasons (Box 4.11).

As an F1 doing my first rotation in elderly care, I found myself doing daily bloods on a 104-year-old in her final days, asymptomatic patients were arresting for no reason and the patients we had forgotten to see were in the best health! Medicine can make your heart sink because of the workload and the outcome for so many of the patients. But that's the nature of medicine. Whereas surgery is about doing the right thing at the right time, medicine is about doing the right thing *all* the time. Sometimes you have to know everything in order to do nothing, which is often the best thing to do. Are you still with me?

When you work in medicine you will occasionally see some howlers who seem to be barn door surgical/orthopaedic/psychiatry patients but have somehow ended up in your hands (probably via a despairing A&E F2 who had been bounced from pillar to post by said specialties). I had an orthopaedic mate who had nicknamed himself 'The Wall' – nothing got past him. His GMC number is actually subliminally coded into this chapter if you would like to take the matter further. Unfortunately, this way of doing things is encoded in the DNA of the NHS and has contributed to the stereotypes of each specialty for decades. With the average surgical admissions per day running at about 25% of those to medicine, it will often feel that as a medic you are sorting out someone else's problems. If you find yourself on the wrong end of a bouncing, make sure you act in the best interests of the patient and document everything, particularly if patient safety is involved, because failure of another specialty to review a patient about whom you have concerns is frankly indefensible. Remember, when you are working in another specialty, you won't continue the situation, will you?

Surgery

When I did my surgery stint it was great. Five-minute ward rounds, sleeping like a baby when you're on nights and bouncing anything that smelt of medicine to the medics. The patients were so uncomplicated. They were in and out of hospital with us having 'fixed' them in no time at all. This was how medicine should be. There was the occasional heart-sink patient, the post-op who developed a fistula that you had been managing conservatively for the past year. But mostly it was bliss. Patients came into hospital to get better. All knife, no strife. So when you're in your darkest hour in medicine, when no *one* patient seems to be getting better on your ward, I can guarantee you will be flying the surgical flag like an extremist left-wing F1 freedom guerrilla.

Surgeons revel in having both trump cards in their hand: 'It's not surgical, it does not need an operation' or 'Operation's a success, patient's heart/lungs/kidneys are the problem now'. Under these circumstances Muggins the Med Reg will pop along to make another 'surgical save' and whisk the patient away to the medical wards. Another great thing about being a surgeon is that you can hide in theatre and leave your bleep at the desk. Sadly, there is no such solace for medics. Some hospitals now have portable phones instead of bleeps, which means when you get called, you have to pick up no matter where you are.

So, I hear you ask, why are you now doing medicine? Well, surgery has to float your boat. You have to be headstrong and basically born with a scalpel in your hand. Your first words need to be, 'Mummy, that's a poor sterile technique for cleaning my high chair'. Enjoyable as it was, my heart wasn't in it and I wasn't sure if I would fit in with the surgical team ethos.

The real skill in surgery, what makes it unique, is deciding if and when a patient needs to go to theatre. As an F1, I took it for granted when someone was whisked off to theatre, but as an F2 I realised that that judgement took guts. Can you imagine slicing open a 22-year-old's abdomen only to find a healthy appendix? Awkward silences all round. So for those skills, respect is deserved from the medics.

What you'll also find is that the surgical team is very consultant-led. Most decisions that go above the technical detail of re-siting a cannula are made by the surgeon in charge. Of course, if the patient later develops a 'medical' problem, you may be handed a lot of responsibility and feel rather isolated and unsupported. Surgeons and orthopods vary in how much they get involved in the holistic care of their patients, so you can find yourself anywhere between having no responsibility at all to being left to sort out complex post-op medical problems. Call for backup from the medical registrar if needed. You may have to work hard to feel valued as part of the team in some surgical firms – take up the challenge and make sure that you have a clear idea of what your responsibilities are and what you can get out of the job, even if you don't want to be a surgeon. Clinic and theatre will have their own learning opportunities, so if you feel undervalued and underused, go there or to ITU and get involved with the surgical patients and do some learning.

One more thing. When someone is post-op, they *will* have free air under their diaphragm. Hopefully that will ease up your sphincter tone just before you call your registrar in the middle of the night having just seen the erect CXR of the post-op patient with abdominal pain!

See Box 4.12 for the top tips in surgery.

Accident and Emergency

This has been included because many of you will have A&E experience during the Foundation programme. Even if you don't, you will doubtless come into contact with A&E doctors, or at the very least their clerkings.

A&E is like marmite – you either love it or hate it; there's no in-between. I really enjoyed it, because it was something new and you could wear cool scrubs and feel like a 'proper doctor'.

Box 4.12   Eleven ways to get noticed for the right reasons in surgery

1. Apyrexial.
2. Obs stable.
3. Plan – continue.
4. Repeat steps 1–3 *ad infinitum*.
5. You can always get the radiology requested by the consultant no matter how unlikely there is going to be any abnormality.
6. You have only one chance to suggest that the patient's abdominal pain might be due to acute intermittent porphyria. Get it wrong and never mention it again. This is surgery, not medicine, don't be flash.
7. Never forget to prescribe the TEDS and Tinz (compression stockings and prophylactic low molecular weight heparin).
8. Never forget to stop the therapeutic heparin/warfarin/aspirin pre-op.
9. If you're not sure if a new patient may go to theatre, put them nil by mouth until your senior sees them.
10. Always pr someone with abdominal pain. If you don't put your finger in it, you'll put your foot in it. Obviously does not apply if the patient has had an AP resection.
11. See the list for medicine as in reality they are pretty much the same.

The acute stuff is amazing – for example, the guy I saw who got 17 units of blood after he came in with projectile vomiting due to varices. On the other hand, there are the not so amazing bits such as minors – for example, the guy who came in with back pain for three years. He had been using cider for analgesia. That was a low point.

The tribal clash for A&E revolves around trying to meet the four-hour trolley wait and getting one of the specialties to take responsibility for someone who needs admission. Can they convince the surgeons to take a 21-year-old woman with lower abdominal pain and well-controlled diabetes, or will it have to pass via the gynae team to the medics? In fact, why not start with the medics as they are bound to put up least resistance and therefore the patient will make it into hospital before the four-hour deadline . . .

General practice

Defecting to GP land during your Foundation programme is a bit like stumbling into the wrong neighbourhood, especially as everyone gets along. I've heard GPs tell juniors arriving from hospital to forget about the traditional history-taking structure – this is the land of 10-minute consultation, when you have to make potentially life-changing decisions. Of course, it's not as dramatic as that, but there is a certain skill to knowing when to admit a patient.

You will start off observing, simply watching the GP deal with patients. Just as you're dozing off at the back of the consulting room, you'll be given your own surgery list – overseen by the GP, but a reality check, none the less. When I was a student at a GP's surgery, there was always an odd siesta time between morning and afternoon surgery when things slowed down a bit. The GP I was with either meditated or practised his rock-climbing skills on the artificial rock face on the top floor of the surgery! Awesome. In hindsight, this is the beauty of being a GP. The consultation is the tip of the iceberg, and there are numerous opportunities for your portfolio career, e.g. developing your skills as a 'Gypsy' (GP with special interest), doing hospital clinics, being doctor of the local sports club or even working in the media.

One thing is certain, you will enjoy your GP placement even if you don't want to work in primary care and cannot initially see its relevance to your future career. Make the most of the time off between surgeries (or at least try to), go out on call with your GP or work with some of the other disciplines of primary care such as the health visitor, midwife or district nurse. As with all Foundation programme placements, you get out of it what you put in and you will come back with a totally different impression of GPs' skills.

Radiology

Radiologists are the gatekeepers to all the seemingly important investigations required to establish a diagnosis. In theory, they are a fount of knowledge, happy to offer the pros and cons of each investigation applicable to solve your clinical problem. But, as gatekeepers, they can come across a bit like the teacher you never liked or seem like a group of diehard veterans who would rather irradiate their own groins than grant you a CT request. However, they are responsible for 'justifying' (a legal term) every radiation exposure in clinical medicine so their rear end is in the can if they do spray the radiation around without justification. Did you know that one CT could have a 1 : 5000 risk of giving a patient cancer?

Don't get caught in the middle of a battle between the consultant radiologist and your own consultant. You may not realise it, but Mr Jones' wish to perform every test possible on a 20-year-old with irritable bowel syndrome just in case they have an occult cancer has been the source of disharmony for 15 years in the hospital. It was made worse when Mr Jones stopped using Dr Wright as his preferred radiologist at the Nuffield, so Dr Wright has had to sell his yacht. Dr Wright is also not sure of his wife's fidelity and has caught her staring wistfully at the dashing Mr Jones on more than one occasion.

You are never going to get that CT scan. When asked to go to radiology to request it, ask Mr Jones to dictate word for word what he wants on the x-ray form in a way that will give you at least a plausible reason to ask for it. Anticipate the rejection and ask Mr Jones what he wants you to do if the request is denied. There is nothing worse than a ward round four days later when Mr Jones asks for the result and you have to tell him not only that the CT was declined, but that you have made no further progress in making a diagnosis and have been waiting for the round for his suggestions.

On a less cynical note, I did a four-month F2 stint in Diagnostic Services and irradiated myself with radiology. The radiographers were surprised at my presence and keenness to learn, but warmed to me nicely. They tend simultaneously to get on with and be scared of the radiologists. It definitely got me thinking more about why I order investigations, and I empathise more with the x-ray department now. A lot of them are understaffed and it's true, we don't know why we are asking for a test or what it might or might not show most of the time!

Speaking to a duty radiologist in the middle of the night is a bit like doing your own radio show wind-up call. I knew one consultant who used to fall asleep as you were presenting a case to him. You could tell, because he started snoring. As an F2 you may have to do this. It's certainly character-building. Like the surgical SpR, there are certain buzz-words that are likely to elicit a positive answer from your hibernating radiologist. 'We are considering a leaking abdominal aneurysm as a cause' or 'we need to exclude a space occupying lesion before going on to an LP' nearly always works, although you will need to go on and do the LP if the CT is normal so it may make a rod for your own back. Make sure that you know why you are phoning before you pick up the handset and have the notes nearby. If you are uncertain why your SpR or consultant has asked for an urgent scan, clarify it. You don't want to get stuck in between a hibernating bear with a sore head and an indignant year 1 SpR who has just got their membership and feels they know everything! Box 4.13 summarises ways of dealing with radiology and how to wangle your way into the good books of the nice radiologists and radiographers. Now you're on easy street.

Box 4.13   Top tips for dealing with radiology

1. Ask radiologists about the best way to solve a diagnostic problem rather than ask for a specific scan. They will invariably come to the same conclusion that your consultant has in what is needed but they will have felt wanted.
2. Make it a priority to get your radiology requests in early. Don't wait till the end of the ward round to write them.
3. Write 'right' and 'left', not R and L, as these can be mistaken.
4. Don't get caught in the middle between your consultant and the radiologists. See the text for full details!
5. Remember the magic words that will unlock the radiologist's frozen heart: 'Sudden onset headache' will usually get you a CT head; 'Probable obstruction' will get you an AXR; 'Tender, pulsatile abdominal mass' will get an instant CT or USS. This isn't an invitation to irradiate the whole world or lie to the radiologist!
6. Attend the cancer multidisciplinary team meetings for your patients. Now that we have such stringent targets that must be achieved for all cancer patients, the merest hint that someone has been referred as a two-week wait or is about to breach the 62-day treatment target will precipitate a flurry of activity and positive responses. You might also get to learn some radiology.
7. Don't forget to fill in the bits of the card that ask about things important for patient preparation. If contrast is needed, the scan will not go ahead if the patient's metformin has not been stopped. If a guided biopsy or abscess drainage is possible, make sure the patient is prepared for this with a normal PT and platelets and group and save in the blood bank.
8. Anticipate the implications of the result. For example, a USS of the abdomen done for fever four weeks after abdominal surgery is likely to show a subphrenic collection or liver abscess. Make sure that you request USS and drainage so that if the abscess is confirmed, you don't have to seek a further scan on another date, thereby incurring more delay and more risk for the patient as they keep waiting to go septicaemic. For a patient with a past history of breast cancer who has come in with abnormal LFTs and weight loss, will they need a biopsy as well as the scan?

How to get your patient admitted/reviewed/transferred. Or, how to polish a t**d

One good skill you will learn in any clinical situation, especially general practice or A&E, is how to get your patients admitted, reviewed and shifted out of the department. Here are some tips on how to deal with the characters involved, starting with getting the patient into hospital and ending with getting the patient transferred to another hospital.

Communicating across the GP/hospital interface

A favourite subject for any team of doctors is chiding other teams, and letters between teams are a common subject of banter. As a hospital doctor, I never cease to be amazed by the variety in quality of GP referrals to admissions or out-patients. Any budding, or indeed existing, GP reading this might be thinking, 'Yeah, our referral letters aren't great, but your discharge letters are appalling – when they actually get to us on time'. Good referral letters or discharge summaries are never talked about. You only hear about the rubbish ones. Electronic referrals and discharge summaries should help solve this problem. As a hospital doctor, I'm not sure if GPs realise just how much our opinion of them is related to the quality of their referral letter, and many hospital doctors are clearly not aware that GPs judge their performance from the quality of the discharge letters. It's virtually the only time there is any interaction between them, at trainee level anyway, unless it's an irate GP phoning you up to ask where Mrs Cannybody's discharge letter is, because the hospital started her on an ACE inhibitor and doubled her diuretics and she's as dry as a crisp.

Writing GP referrals or discharge letters as an F1 or F2 is a valuable experience and a vital issue in patient safety. A referral letter often contains important information, e.g. the 80-year-old with dementia admitted with diarrhoea who was recently on ciprofloxacin with a UTI. The fact that she was on antibiotics recently is a major clue to the possible diagnosis of C. *diff* infection.

The following are handy pointers for the two-way written communication between GP and hospitals:

- The actual presence of a letter. Make sure that you complete a referral/ discharge letter and that it's transported to where it needs to be in good time. Make sure it's either stuck to the surgery notes or in an envelope and that the patient leaves hospital with a letter.
- Handwriting. Legibility helps. You can choose how quickly you write. There's no excuse for a scrawl, unless you wrote it whilst driving or in the dark. If the feedback you get is that no one can read your writing, do something about it – handwriting is not a quirk of personality, it's a means of communication. Writing that only you can read is like talking to yourself. You wouldn't do that, would you?
- Content for referral letter. A good referral letter should have a condensed history and examination, an up-to-date list of medications and any relevant social history. Give an impression or ask a question. Not putting in your own differential diagnosis is like painting a masterpiece and not signing it. It doesn't make sense to spend half an hour with someone, crack the diagnosis, then say, 'Right, I'll see you later, someone else who doesn't know you as well as I do is going to try to figure out what is going on'. Asking a question is really useful too, even if it's the 'Off legs ? cause' sort. It makes the post-take ward round unbelievably more enjoyable when there's a clear reason for admission. A printout of drugs is helpful, but only if it indicates which the patient is actually taking rather than what has been prescribed in the last year.
- Content of the discharge letter. A good discharge letter will have details of the diagnosis, changes in treatment, outstanding investigations and follow-up arrangements, as well as any expectations of the GP. It may also contain information on what the patient knows. Many patients will seek an appointment with their GP within 48 hours of discharge and will

often need repeat scripts within a week, so the GP needs an informative letter immediately, not six weeks later. The GP does not need a summary of the clerking ('Mrs Jones is a pleasant retired post lady who was admitted with chest pain. The pain came on suddenly and radiated to the left arm. Examination showed no evidence of clubbing splinters, lymphadenopathy or lid lag. Heart sounds were normal', etc. *ad nauseam*). The GP needs: 'Mrs Jones was admitted with chest pain but had normal ECG, CXR and trop T. No specific diagnosis was made but she was started on atenolol 25 mg bd and aspirin 75 mg od and is due to have an exercise test in four weeks' time. Dr Allheart will see her in out-patients following this. Could you check a fasting glucose please as she had a random sugar of 10.'

Follow these steps and you'll be held in high regard by your colleagues on the Admissions Unit or in the community.

Getting a review by the surgical registrar

Speaking to a surgical registrar is a bit like turning water into wine; only those with divine powers can make something happen. They like to hear the words 'acute' and 'abdomen'. Constipation is a turn-off, as is '98 years old' and 'multiple medical co-morbidities'. Magic words to get them involved in the case (in addition to 'acute abdomen') include 'possible leaking aortic aneurysm', 'can't exclude bowel infarction' and 'no evidence of MI or pneumonia or any acute medical problem'. You used to be able to get a surgeon to see someone with renal colic or vascular insufficiency, but as vascular surgery and urology are now often tertiary services, surgical SpRs seem to have lost the skills of dealing with these common surgical problems.

Getting a review by the medical registrar

Speaking to a medical SpR is a bit like ending a relationship, and you're the one doing the dumping. They are generally nice but harassed individuals who like to blindside you with questions such as 'Why has the patient got a raised anion gap?' Much as you would love to, you cannot avoid admitting tricky patients to medicine. It may only add to its reputation of being a dumping ground, but in the end patient safety demands that the patient has to go somewhere and medicine is often the path of least resistance. Think about what you want from the medical team. It can be better to ask for a consultant specialty opinion rather than the SpR, particularly if it is a problem that will not clear up in 24 hours. The SpR may not be able to come back and review them the next day and it does not serve the patient well to have a series of medical SpRs seeing them on subsequent days. Also, the GI consultant will, for example, have much better access to tests such as endoscopy than a non-specialty SpR.

Successful tertiary referrals

What is it that turns even the most benign of SpRs into strutting cockerels when they go to work in a tertiary centre? When you take off the window dressing they are just like any other doctors. But getting someone past them can be well nigh impossible. I once had the experience of phoning a nearby neurosurgical centre about someone who has disseminated cancer and who could not stand up or pee. I was 'bumped' on the grounds that I was not able to describe an exact sensory level and therefore the SpR felt that cord compression was unlikely. When the consultant phoned back a short while later, they accepted the patient immediately. You only speak to these individuals if your patient is really sick and they need treatment that your hospital can't offer, for example angioplasty, haemodialysis, neurosurgery or liver transplant.

Here are some hints on making a tertiary referral:

- Plan for the phone call. Have the notes to hand, summarize the main points, be near a computer screen so you can quickly look up any results asked for
- Decide what you want to get out of the referral – is it advice or a transfer?
- Make the reason for the referral clear in the first sentence
- Make sure they know that your consultant has asked you to phone
- Use the language that they use and can understand and can't ignore. Which of the following would you respond positively to?

'Hi, I am Dr Jones from Fulbeck General. The gastroenterology consultant has asked me to phone because we have a patient with fulminant liver failure due to a paracetamol overdose. It is 40 hours since OD and the PT is 65 seconds and the pH 7.2. We believe he fulfils the Regional shared care protocol for urgent transfer and he is a potentially suitable case for transplant with no significant past medical history and no persisting mental health problems.'

Or:

F2: 'Hi, I've got a patient with liver failure that might need transfer.
SpR: Why?
F2: Well, he took a paracetamol overdose and he is not doing very well.
SpR: Does he fulfil any of the criteria for transplant or transfer?
F2: Er, what are they?'

If despite your clear communication the person still gives you grief and you feel that the patient really does need urgent transfer, the only card you have to play is your consultant:

F2: 'Well I can see that you don't think the patient needs to come over but my consultant was sure that he did. Which consultant are you on with? I think it's best if my consultant rings yours directly so they can decide at the highest level.'

YOUR QUICK GUIDE TO DEALING WITH THE DEPARTMENTS IN THE HOSPITAL

Increasingly, many jobs previously done by doctors are performed by others and the role of the multidisciplinary team is now paramount in patient care.

No doubt your undergraduate career will have furnished you with some understanding of the role that each member performs, but new health professionals are springing up all the time so here is a short reminder if you are not up to speed.

Pharmacy and pharmacists

These are your guardian angels because they are responsible for checking drug charts and discharge scripts. They've saved my bacon once or twice and will continue to do so. They seem to be the only people in existence who can consistently write a controlled drug script correctly. I think they should have special licence to call you a plonker every now and then, because of the number of prescribing errors doctors make. For our top tips for prescribing, see Box 4.14.

I'd better mention the controlled drug script. This is like the Mount Everest of the prescribing world – only mastered by a few, with the danger of getting someone higher than they need to be if done incorrectly. I still get it wrong. If it wasn't for the Zen-like patience of the pharmacists, we would not be allowed to do controlled scripts (see Box 4.14).

Also worth a mention is the *British National Formulary* (*BNF*). This was like a holy text when I first started. OK, it is a bind at first because you're constantly checking things like how much codeine you can have in 24 hours, and why there are so many similar names for long acting diltiazem. Once you're

---

Box 4.14   Top tips on prescribing and using pharmacy

1. Controlled scripts: The patient's name and address must be in your own writing, the form must be given and the TOTAL dose must be in words and figures. Easy really. For example, MST tablets, 10 mg bd for 10 days = total dose; 200 mg = two hundred milligrams.
2. Do your warfarins every day: saves the hospital at night team time.
3. Check medication on admission with the GP if the pharmacist does not do this. GPs really don't like it if patients are sent home without the levothyroxine that they have spent two years adjusting.
4. Clarify the reasons for any changes in medication on discharge summary.
5. Include an anonymized sample drug chart in your evidence in your portfolio.
6. Remember it's gram and not g, microgram and not µg or mcg.
7. Always prescribe oxygen. It's a drug after all and given wrongly can be harmful!
8. Use the notes section on the script to clarify whether people are on the medication long term or not, or to indicate that it has been stopped or the dose changed temporarily, e.g. stopping metformin when a patient comes in with renal failure, an increased dose of steroids during an exacerbation of COPD, etc. This saves time and errors when doing a discharge letter/script.
9. Write 'one' or 'two', instead of the numerals.
10. For inhalers, write the actuation dose, e.g. with salbutamol, always write 100 microg/puff. Inhalers come in different strengths.

used to it though, it's a revelation. Keep one handy. And no, pharmacists are not walking *BNF*s – look it up yourself.

Do know what you are prescribing. If someone comes in on a drug that you have never heard of, look it up. Chances are no one else will have heard of it.

Medication histories from GPs are invaluable and pharmacists often do this, but if they don't, chase it up yourself. Once you get past the multifaceted automated telephone voice, you can get some worthwhile information.

Ward clerks

Ward clerks range from surly old dragons to Valkyrie temptresses. Very useful people for doing the secretarial things that you didn't have time for because of all your other meaningless tasks. They will pester you for the right things at the right time (e.g. death certificates in the morning). I was repeatedly asked to do these first thing and never knew why, until I realised the family come into the ward to collect it for funeral arrangements and have to sit in a dour relatives room until you've got it sorted. Not a nice thought and definitely a task to prioritise.

Ward clerks can be very helpful in locating patient notes, getting requests to and from radiology or x-ray, sending specimens, etc. If patient notes are overloaded or falling apart, they should be able to arrange for a new set to be created and the old notes re-housed. It is your responsibility to file your own medical notes, although the ward clerk should/might file results if asked nicely.

Switchboard

Helpful voices on the end of the zero. Quite a good game is to wander to their headquarters to get a new battery for your bleep and try to match the face to the voice. Remarkably useful if you're having a blank and can't remember the extension for biochemistry. Also handy for knowing bleep numbers, home numbers of doctors who have forgotten to turn up for work and GP surgeries. Get them to give you a short tutorial on how to use the phone system effectively.

Porters

Doctors and porters are at opposite ends of the job spectrum and many times they seem above you in the hospital hierarchy. They often double as bouncers/security guards. This is good for helping you with a psychotic or delirious patient, but bad if you've upset them. If you befriend them, you're in the money. Good for betting tips, getting gossip from other wards and finding a decent garage/plumber/hit-man/second-hand car, etc.

Nurses

Nurses are badly paid for working themselves into the ground and doing the jobs that high-quality bleach would turn its nose up at. They are true lifesavers for newly qualified doctors – probably the most important people in the neighbourhood. They will save you on numerous occasions. Ignore their advice or concerns about patient status at your peril. Their training may be different from yours, but they often have vast experience and a common-sense approach to clinical management. They will also know a lot about the personalities and rivalries between people and departments that will impact on your working life.

Nurses are definitely under-appreciated and disrespected by many newly qualified doctors interested in the three 'S's: status, style and s*** (you know the third one). For an example of status, there was one female doctor who, when asked by the nurses why she wanted a particular sliding scale of insulin put up on a patient, said, 'Because I'm a doctor'. Now that isn't right, is it! And with regard to the third 's', always remember the old Chinese saying: 'Don't crap on your own doorstep'. There is nothing more certain to turn the nurses against you than you behaving badly towards one of their own, whether you or they are male or female. You have been warned.

If you actually listen to a nurse you're on the right tracks. The good ones are usually on the money when they say a patient 'just doesn't look right'. It may be a grey term, but by the time you've seen them, you may well come to the same conclusion.

Specialist nurses, nurse consultants or nurse practitioners play many different roles in modern healthcare. They are a vast repository of knowledge and skill and will almost certainly know more about their specialist area than you do, and often more than the SpR. If a patient turns up on your ward with a problem cared for by a specialist nurse, it is often valuable to let them know. The patient will often expect to see their specialist nurse and because of their knowledge of the patient, they will often have a unique insight into their care. You will also learn about the optimum management of the patient's condition. Have you noticed how much easier it is to ask a nurse about something that you don't understand than to ask a senior doctor?

District nurses

These are experienced nurses in primary care who are the equivalent of hospital sisters. Handy for facilitating patient discharge, e.g. giving daily tinzaparin to the patient with a DVT whose INR is sub-therapeutic, but well enough to be discharged. They have a range of roles not seen by the hospital and also work closely with GP surgeries. Learn more about their role when doing a GP attachment.

Midwives

Highly skilled nurses, with calm heads under pressure. They've carved out their own niche in the Delivery Suite. You will meet them if you do Obs and Gynae on the Foundation programme. Can be intimidating, but they're genuine and warm-hearted under the surface.

AHPs (allied health professionals) or PAMs (professionals allied to medicine)

PAMs is a rather derisory acronym for the therapists discussed below. Not only does it give you a clear expectation that they are professions suitable for women only, but they also seem to subjugate their role under that of medicine. We prefer allied health professionals as a more accurate and less value-laden term. They have a key role in deciding when patients are fit to go home or on the type of placement needed.

Physiotherapists

Multidisciplinary magicians who get to work on the lame to get them back on their feet. A friendly bunch who can probably outdo you in a neuro exam and are pretty handy with a Bipap machine and lung suction. Have an insider's knowledge on the terms for the different appliances older people use – zimmer, wheeled zimmer, delta frame, rota stand – and other phrases to keep you bemused during multidisciplinary team meetings on elderly care. Chief roles are in assessing, maintaining and improving mobility and in working on patients' respiratory status, ranging from post-op chest care to delivering non-invasive ventilation. Also have key roles in rehabilitation, sports injury clinics and pain teams. Not to be confused with . . .

Occupational therapists

OTs can get someone out of hospital when it matters most, and so are highly valued. They have a key role in the multidisciplinary team, especially in elderly care, and an estate agent's knowledge of what's hot and what's not in the residential home market. OTs are more concerned with activities of daily living and adaptations to a patient's living environment than physios and are not concerned with mobility as such.

Speech and language therapists

Do what it says on the tin, but also play a key role in assessing and treating swallowing difficulties due to pharyngeal problems. They can teach you to do a basic swallow assessment for patients who have had a stroke, for example. Can help people with speech or language problems to communicate when in hospital, which will help to reduce their fears and worries. Spend a bit of time with them to learn some basics.

Social workers

Often talked about, but seldom seen. Key members of the multidisciplinary team who can get a bit of stick from all concerned when it comes to discharging a patient, mainly because the work they do is behind the scenes and never witnessed on the ward. Usually employed by the local authority rather than the health service so there can be a culture clash between their values and those in the healthcare system, particularly around the time it takes to arrange a discharge and the seemingly arcane procedures that have to be gone through to resolve what seems an easy problem. They don't really have much contact with doctors except to get your opinion on a patient before a case conference. A lot could be done to improve communication between doctors and social workers, so talk to yours regularly, not just at a weekly meeting. We have all seen the case where a social worker is trying to arrange for a patient to go home despite the fact that the patient's clinical condition has deteriorated to the point where they are on a syringe driver. Keep them informed. Social workers have a role in helping patients plan for discharge in terms of sorting out care packages, funding for residential or nursing care and making sure that patients are receiving the appropriate benefits, especially the special care allowances that patients are entitled to if their expected prognosis is less than six months. Social workers can also be very helpful in developing discharge plans for patients with complex psychosocial problems such as eating disorders and alcohol problems.

Junior doctors

Yes, you have your own subculture too and it pays to be aware of some aspects of it to help you understand those around you. Medicine can be like the military – Foundation doctors can be compared to new recruits on their first mission. Like the military, there is also a very strong hierarchy in the NHS. There is a robust culture of survival and a degree of togetherness which is helpful to cope with the transitions you are facing. In general, this cocoons you at a time of difficulty. But, like the military, doctors do not always react positively to someone who steps outside their norms. These include being competitive, succeeding, coping, keeping things within the team and not complaining. Doctors therefore tend to react poorly to colleagues who show behaviour interpreted as weakness. Be careful about your responses to anyone who is struggling – we have all seen less than supportive behaviour to people who needed time off or emotional support. Like new recruits, there can also be a danger of overdoing things when off duty – be prudent in your drinking and other behaviours. Part of the togetherness can also be a 'they are all against us' attitude, which can be quite destructive and sometimes makes people see things from a rather jaundiced perspective. The loudest voices amongst any group of workers will be those who are least content. You will have observed the attitude: all managers/consultants/politicians are bastards; we never get any training in this job; in the other Trust they get paid much more for the same shifts, etc. Take a reality check from time to time and examine the facts. (See Urban medical myths in the A–Z section of Chapter 3.)

Healthcare assistants

HCAs, or auxiliaries, are extremely handy and fun people to work with. They are often local and have lived near the hospital for years, and at any one time have a member of their extended family in hospital as a patient, so tread carefully. Seem to know just about everyone in the hospital, including who is courting whom, so to speak. HCAs probably see you more as the average patient does, so respect their feedback. HCAs do most of the patient observations these days and are likely to be the people who spot the worsening blood pressure or high temperature. Many HCAs are working towards entering nurse training and doing vocational exams and so need small projects. If you want to complete a small teaching project the HCAs are a great place to start and will almost certainly value genuine interest in their development. Talk to the nurse in charge about how you can assist them develop their role. Help them by washing your own cups and keeping the doctors' office tidy.

Phlebotomists and ward assistants

Working for a service driven by demand, the 'phlebs' are genuinely helpful people who often get a poor deal. They get you thinking about why you're ordering a test and tend to kick up a fuss when you over-request bloods, and rightly so. Do you ever find yourself throwing away the forms if the phlebotomist cannot obtain a sample and you will have to do it? Shame on you. They were obviously not *that* necessary. In some Trusts the role of phlebotomists has become extended as 'doctors' assistants' or similar. Their general role is to help in all the admin, act as a runner, fill in forms, perform simple tasks such as phlebotomy and inserting cannulae or doing ECGs. More Trusts should be and are developing these roles.

Medical and surgical practitioners

Many new roles are being created to get the skills mix in the NHS right and fill gaps or create efficiencies. They are generally recruited from the life sciences and many have had three years' full-time training on top of their first degree, so have actually spent longer getting trained than doctors! At present the Midlands seems to be the core territory of medical practitioners, but a new government policy seeks to create courses throughout the land. It may seem a daft question, but if there is a need for their skills, why not train them for five years instead of six and call them doctors? At present the proper name for this new cadre of workers has not been finalised and they may end up being called physicians' assistants. They will, however, be trained to a nationally agreed curriculum and standards (unlike medical students for whom medical schools set their own curriculum and standards) and will be coming to a hospital near you within five years. They will have a role in evaluating patients, diagnosing and initiating treatment. They are likely to be broadly trained and have excellent skills in acute care and will be able to work under the supervision of a senior doctor. Does that sound familiar? If not, you obviously have not looked at the Foundation curriculum.

Psychologists

Psychologists have a key role in helping people with many types of problem, ranging from the more obvious mental health issues that you would expect to adjustment issues, living with a chronic disease or grieving. Psychologists are subdivided into myriad sub-specialists. Health psychologists usually work with people who have a physical health problem and so are most likely to be the type of psychologist you come across in hospital. Health psychologists might be helpful in dealing with a man with difficulty in adjusting to a heart attack, an adolescent girl who has weekly admissions with uncontrolled diabetes or a woman with breast cancer who is preparing her children for life without her. There is often a specific service in primary care and mental health teams have specially trained psychologists, including those who specialise in the assessment of people with cognitive problems. When referring a patient, make the reason clear to the psychologist and let the patient know that you don't think they are 'going mad' and describe what help a psychologist might be able to give.

Summary of the multi-professional team

Understanding the training, roles and professional attributes of your inter-professional colleagues is essential if you are to play your part in the team. Understanding their training and the limits of what can be delegated to them is vital. To check that you have been paying attention, answer the MCQs in Box 4.15. Now reflect on it in your portfolio and put it in the evidence section of your end-of-year assessment.

PUTTING IT INTO ACTION

This chapter has given you some advice on how to cope with the demands of your new job and explored the issue of tribalism and subculture in the NHS. Obviously, the rivalries and tensions generated in the system impact not just on your working life but also on patient care. We would all like to see these conflicts reduced and the patients' needs put first. Become part of the solution to this, not part of the problem. So how do we put all this information into practice? To answer the difficulties raised by our three original cases:

Mrs Jones and her new alloy hip going for an MRI

The key here is the most appropriate means of communication. Some professors may lack verbal communication skills but they love email. Ask the secretary for the professor's email address, email them, not revealing that you are an F1, and you will be guaranteed a reply. Also, the professor will not be able to deny electronic advice as easily as verbal when the hip does fly out.

The paracetamol overdose who self-discharged

Difficult one. The fact that the patient self-discharged makes it their responsibility. But was their capacity properly assessed? Overdose patients commonly self-discharge, and many do not have their capacity fully assessed. To be honest, most of the time we are glad to get rid of them because they can cause chaos on the ward. But I have heard of a patient who came in having taken an overdose, then absconded and was found decomposing in a field two weeks later. In terms of this case, involve your seniors early on. If they

Box 4.15 Self-assessment of new health service roles

1. The following have a medical training and are registered with the GMC:

   a) Medical practitioner
   b) Clinical assistant
   c) BST
   d) Podiatric consultant

2. The following are allowed to prescribe:

   a) Healthcare assistant
   b) Charge nurse
   c) Medical practitioner
   d) Specialist nurse
   e) Pharmacist

3. A 75-year-old with diabetes has recently had a myocardial infarction and has reduced mobility and difficulty in vision. Match the profession to the role.

   a) Specialist nurse in diabetes
   b) District nurse
   c) Occupational therapist
   d) Social worker
   e) GP

• Assesses the home to make sure the patient will be safe and arranges necessary modifications
• Monitors the patient's home progress and the interactions of all the new drugs on their function
• Attends daily for first week of discharge to ensure that patient can prepare and give insulin and anticipates problems that may occur
• Advises on suitable Digami regime for patient to be discharged on
• Liaises with family to check that the patient's shopping and cleaning really will be done by family for first six weeks

Give three ways in which you can contribute to the smooth function of this 'team'?

1
2
3

like to leave early on Friday afternoons, it's your responsibility to ensure that they fulfil their contracted hours. Can the patient be contacted? True, he has no fixed abode, but scour the notes for a mobile phone number or a next of kin phone number. In some situations you will need to inform the police so they can help you locate the patient. Once you have found a way of contacting the patient, you have to convince them to come back to hospital for further tests. This is easier said than done. But the main points are that you found an abnormality on the bloods, acted swiftly, have informed your seniors and have located the patient. This may seem like it's straight out of a detective novel, but it does happen!

How do you balance the Monday morning jobs list of two death certificates, seven discharges, three prs and a controlled drug script that keeps bouncing and a 'serious clinical incident'?

Clinical needs come first, so give Mrs Smith some analgesia and arrange an x-ray and orthopaedic review and personally ring the family to let them know what has happened, whilst simultaneously filling in the death certificates, having politely asked the ward clerk to get all the notes and the death certificate book together for you. If you had been planning better, you would have filled in the discharge summaries last Friday so that would not be an issue. But if you have not done them, recruit the pharmacist and/or medical students to fill them in for you or ask the F2 if they will help. You can now do a controlled drug script first time correctly. Nothing stresses more than to have to repeat a routine task when you are very busy, so get it right first time. Finally, are those prs really a high priority? Could they be done by the nurses or a medical student? If you go off duty without doing them, will it alter the patients' clinical outcome? If asked repeatedly to do things of little value, ask why. If they really are needed, best to get on with it as soon as possible as there is nothing like the thought of three prs to induce procrastination.

MEDICINE IS ALSO ABOUT VALUES

So, you have the skills of survival. But for the most part, survival is not just about the first month or about knowing the magic words to ask a radiologist who is 30 years your senior. That will come with time. It's more about getting the basics right. The fundamentals are to be thorough, assume nothing and be genuine. This makes everything else easier. Assumption and arrogance are unhealthy attitudes that you will experience, albeit fleetingly, as you progress. But they're often harbingers of a fall. The minute you start assuming things in medicine, a big dog will be guaranteed to bite your behind.

After your first month you'll be thinking, 'What the hell was all the fuss and worry about?' Actually, you will probably be thinking, 'Why the hell have Finance put me on emergency tax banding?'

BEYOND THE FIRST MONTH – KEEPING TRUE TO YOURSELF AND REMEMBERING WHY YOU STARTED

Now that you've got through the first month and acquired the basic skills, how does it look? Are you enjoying yourself, or do you wish you had pursued that childhood dream of becoming an astronaut? It may feel that the student in you has been kicked out in a bumpy ride and you will not be alone in wondering whether you made a good decision to invest 4–5 years in studying medicine. Working as a new doctor is a big wake-up call and most doctors have dark moments when they wonder if they should be doing something else, so don't think that you are alone. Those 'financial planning' lunchtime meetings do our philosophical ruminations no good either. 'Planning your time in the NHS for the next 40 years' was the title of one seminar. But by that time we will be 65, with a catalogue of good and bad memories! You may

> **Box 4.16   Ten top homilies on how to thrive**
> 1. Treat yourself as you would your patients
> 2. Don't be a hero
> 3. Assume nothing
> 4. Be a genuine customer
> 5. Leave at 5 pm (or thereabouts) to survive
> 6. It's OK to hand over
> 7. Never be afraid to call for help – it is big and it is clever
> 8. Listen to sister
> 9. Be consistent in filling out your portfolio. And I don't mean by consistently not doing any of it
> 10. Remember the patients that made a difference – to your life or to your practice

be beginning to realise the scale of your commitment to being a doctor and the NHS.

Perspectives change as an F2 and you begin to piece it all together. You're no longer the rabbit in the headlights, but the driver, looking out for the rabbits. Today, I am a medical SHO on a rotation who like you, is involved in run-through specialist training. The career doors are opening and I'm glad I stuck at it. Becoming a doctor does not happen overnight. OK, so your job title does. But your development and the art of diagnosis take a long time.

Beyond the issues of the rapid changes that you have faced and the stress of coping with your new role, it is easy to lose sight of why you are there. Can you remember why you started in medicine all those years ago? Concentrating on your core values is a good way to counter stress, fear and disillusionment during F1. It may feel that the system is set up to erode your core values and to frustrate your attempts to live up to them. Go back to the 'Targets' section in Chapter 3 if you need reminding of the factors that might erode your values. As the old saying goes, don't let the bastards grind you down. Try to avoid cynicism.

What are your core values? Try writing them down.

What do you do, though, if you're only just surviving, let alone thriving? Chapter 9 looks at what to do if things are not what you want or if they are going wrong. This chapter concludes with top ten homilies to help you thrive (Box 4.16).

Taking control of your learning: getting the most out of your learning opportunities

5

Mark Welfare

" Engineering is not a science. Science studies particular events to find general laws. Engineering design makes use of these laws to solve particular problems. In this it is more closely related to art or a craft. As an art its problems are under-defined. There are many solutions, good bad or indifferent.

The art is by a synthesis of ends and means to arrive at a good solution. This is a creative activity involving interpretation, imagination and deliberate choice. "

Ove Arup, Newcastle born engineer-philosopher

INTRODUCTION

I came across the above quotation in the engineering department at Aberdeen University when attending the annual scientific meeting of the Association for the Study of Medical Education and it set me thinking about the aims of medical education. The quotation could easily be paraphrased as:

'Medicine is not science. It is the art of using your imagination and applying scientific principles to find the best solution to clinical problems.'

Medical education can therefore be viewed as a two-fold task: learning the scientific principles and learning the principles of applying them. Hopefully, your undergraduate career has taught you the former. Now you have to consolidate your learning in the latter.

The Academy of Medical Royal Colleges has emphasised that your Foundation training is designed to develop 'medical practitioners who are judgement-safe, patient-focused and accountable to the public for delivering evidence-based effective medical care' (draft revision of the Curriculum for the Foundation Years; www.aomrc.org.uk, accessed 25 September 2006).

The incline of the learning curve for F1 doctors is probably the steepest that you will ever experience. You are moving rapidly from a state of 'knowing' to 'doing', translating the scientific principles that you have acquired as an undergraduate to actions, with the added complexity that those actions have direct consequences for the health or even life of your patients. It will seem that you do learn just by being there, on the ward, in admissions, in practice, seeing patients. And of course you will learn by this passive osmotic process. But the challenge is to maximise the learning that you get out of each and every day and every clinical encounter. This takes a more proactive approach.

There are many challenges to learning in the healthcare environment. You and those around you will be busy and sometimes tired. Your seniors will have different levels of interest and skills in teaching. Your role models may model behaviours that run counter to the ideal that you are trying to learn. There may be times when you want to ask for help and no one is available. The working practices of the NHS may frustrate the feedback loop that is so essential to learning. So you need to learn ways in which you can overcome these hurdles.

The aim of this chapter is to alert you to the best ways of learning and help you to take control of your learning and get the maximum advantage out of the opportunities that you do get.

KEEPING THE PATIENT SAFE WHILST YOU LEARN

The chapter begins with a brief reminder of the importance of patient safety in your learning. In times gone by it was reputedly common for trainees with little experience of a procedure or technique to develop their skills on a patient without supervision. This is clearly unacceptable. In developing your diagnostic, prescribing, management, procedural, communication or other skills, always make the patient's safety, dignity, comfort and well-being your main priorities. Harm can come to a patient by a poorly delivered piece of bad news as well as by a mishap during the introduction of a central line. If you are in doubt that you are well prepared for a clinical encounter or do not have adequate supervision, do not proceed. With the Clinical Negligence Scheme for Trusts, trainees are increasingly being assessed as competent to proceed autonomously with each procedure. If you have not been signed off as competent to perform a procedure, you should not attempt to do it alone. Also, remember that basic competence does not translate into expertise in all circumstances. It is one thing to be able to insert a central line in a pre-op patient under controlled conditions, quite another to do it in a restless delirious patient with low intravascular pressures and a PT of 25 seconds.

The new curriculum from the Academy of Medical Royal Colleges (AoMRC) outlines the need for the practice of skills using simulation or role play initially and then practising with less and less supervision until you have achieved full competence and expertise. Simulation is likely to become a growth area.

Learn to recognize when you are working within your limits and when you are in danger of going beyond your level of expertise. This is the judgement-safe domain that the AoMRC defines as one of the key skills of being a doctor and it applies at all levels, from F1 to professor.

HOW DO YOU LEARN?

There are many theories about learning in medicine and all probably have some truth to them. This section relies on three main theories which seem to have a lot of common sense and resonance to the way in which I have observed my trainees learn and to my own learning and development. They are Kolb's learning cycle, the visual–aural–kinaesthetic learning styles model and models which rely on the development of differing layers of skill. Understanding of these three bits of educational theory and jargon may help you see why learning is not always maximised and what you can do to improve your learning opportunities. The new curriculum also suggests that we should change our vocabulary from 'learning' (which perhaps implies mainly a cognitive change) to 'developing' (which implies a more global change in behaviour).

Kolb's learning cycle

Learning in medicine is often summarized by the aphorism 'see one, do one, teach one', which reflects an approach to practical learning that seems to disregard patient safety! However, with slight revision it may not be too inaccurate or unsafe. Adults are thought to learn by reflecting on experiences, coming up with possible alternatives, making a plan, trying it out and then starting again with reflection. So, the old aphorism could be rephrased from a three-step model to a seven-step model:

Step 1: See one (or more)
Step 2: Reflect on what went well and what could have been done differently, informed by feedback from a more experienced person so that any errors are corrected
Step 3: Seek additional information (e.g. by background reading) to make sure that you know what you are doing
Step 4: Think about when you might get a chance to do it yourself in a safe environment and how you will approach it
Step 5: Do one under supervision
Step 6: Repeat from step 2 until competent under a variety of conditions
Step 7: Teach one

This is the essence of Kolb's learning cycle. The problem in clinical learning is that the links between observing something or doing something (step 1) and then getting the chance to practise it again (step 5) are often missing:

- Trainees do not always get feedback on their performance in a clinical case
- Trainees do not actively reflect on what went well or not so well
- Gaps in theoretical knowledge remain unplugged
- The next time they face a similar situation they have not planned for it and so are unprepared
- They still do not get adequate supervision

The implications of Kolb's learning cycle to your learning are therefore pretty clear. It is vital that you get accurate, timely and relevant feedback on your performance in each case and that you have the insight to identify your weaknesses and accept feedback so that you can develop. It is important that you process this feedback and your own reflections and use these to plan further learning opportunities and get more background information so that when an opportunity comes along you are well prepared. For further detail see Chapter 7, pages 154–155.

Types of learners

Learning styles models suggest that people have a preferred way of learning. One of the best known is Honey and Mumford's four classic learning styles: Activist, Theorist, Reflector and Pragmatist (see www.campaign-for-learning. org.uk, or assess your own learning style at www.peterhoney.com). Whenever I have done this with doctors they have been overwhelmingly activists – they just want to get on with it. This is a potential problem when we are mainly asking you to be reflective learners!

The visual–aural–kinaesthetic model seems to have the most validity and is easy to understand. It is based on the way people prefer to process information. It has helped me understand my strengths and weaknesses in learning and may be useful to you too. Three things have taught me that I have a mixed style, but that primarily I am a visual rather than aural learner, although I also like the practical side in some circumstances. First, I have a problem remembering people's names when I'm told them. But if they are wearing a printed name badge I will probably remember it for ever. Second, I have always been poor at spoken languages and music. Now I know that this is because of my lack of aural learning skills. Third, as a keen birdwatcher I have always been able to identify a bird on its 'jizz'. This is an indefinable visual quality that sets one species apart from another. Even a brief glimpse of, say, a sparrowhawk is instantly identifiable. But, when I am confronted by the wall of sound of the dawn chorus in the Amazon where a hundred or more species may be calling at once, I cannot pick out the song of even one species and I will instantly forget a song if I have heard it only once. When I have seen the bird I can usually match up its song with my visual memory, showing that I need the visual connection to learn aural information.

So what are the implications of this model for learning in medicine? Visual learners may, for example, benefit from being able to see notes or pictures when being taught and so learning on a ward round with no visual aids may not suit them. Aural learners are presumably good at taking in information mentioned on ward rounds or clinics, but will not be so good at 'spot diagnoses' or in specialties such as dermatology or endoscopy, which rely on good visual memory. Kinaesthetic learners are likely to be good at learning in practical situations such as ALS courses and in learning practical skills on the job, but will not get much out of a prolonged ward round where many esoteric diagnoses are discussed and obscure tests ordered.

You can see that your preferred mode of information processing may affect your learning and your future career choice. Perhaps it is not by chance that I am an endoscopist and don't have to rely on listening to heart sounds to earn my living.

Are you aware of how you process new information? Are you better at learning from visually received data, heard information or action? And if you can work this out, what is the impact on your learning needs?

In reality, things are not that simple and many learners adopt mixed learning styles or adapt their learning style to the task at hand. It also seems that learning that occurs through a variety of methods will be deeper. So seek out multiple methods of learning key skills.

Building layers of skill

Another key concept in learning that may be helpful is the progression in your depth of learning and practice.

The development of layers of skills is traditionally expressed in Miller's pyramid, which traces practice from the level of 'knowing', through 'knows how' and 'shows how' to 'does'. This parallels to some extent the general progression from undergraduate pre-clinical (who perhaps 'knows'), to clinical student ('knows how') to trainee ('shows' that they can do – competence) to expert ('does' – performance). Although the assessments in the Foundation programme focus mainly on 'competence' (the ability to do something when supervised in a controlled environment), the new curriculum recognises that trainees need to move towards a position of expertise (demonstrate that they can do something in difficult circumstances and that it has become intuitive and is a part of everyday practice). The new curriculum also recognises that no matter how competent someone might be, they must be able to maintain that competence when extraneous factors, such as stress, fatigue or adverse personal circumstances, interfere.

Finally, remember the Chinese proverb about teaching and learning that can be paraphrased as: 'Give a man a fish and he has one meal, teach him to fish and he will never be hungry'. There are clear parallels in the way in which you interact with your teachers. It is all too easy for your trainer to teach you the right answer to the clinical problem.

Imagine a presentation of rectal bleeding in a 25-year-old. Your trainer's response to your presentation of the case could be: 'In this position I would do a sigmoidoscopy and leave it at that. It's almost certainly piles but we need to rule out proctitis.' This style of teaching is the equivalent of giving you a fish. You will be able to solve the same problem next time providing it appears in the same form, but you are no further forward in learning the general principles surrounding the problem.

A better approach would be for your trainer to ask you how you might solve the problem and tease out your diagnostic reasoning. If you can't get to the answer, they could teach you the general principles while giving the answer. 'Well, with this clinical presentation the chance of piles is highest because the patient does not have any diarrhoea and it has been going on for two years and blood drips in the pan. If they had a family history of inflammatory bowel disease it would make colitis much more likely. Cancer is very unlikely because of the patient's age. Even in the older age group a sigmoidoscopy is normally enough to rule out cancer for rectal bleeding alone. If the patient had recent change in bowel habit I would think about a colonoscopy instead, and definitely so if they were over 40.' This style of teaching will have taught you how to fish – you should have grasped the key evidence-based principles behind the investigation of bowel symptoms and you will be able to deal with most subsequent referrals.

So in your dealings with trainers react positively if they seem to be asking probing questions. If they always give you the answer without asking questions, make sure you learn by turning the tables and asking the probing questions yourself. So, extending the example above, when told to do a sigmoidoscopy, ask why. Would it be the same for all age groups? Was there any evidence base for doing sigmoidoscopy rather than colonoscopy, etc.?

The implications of this layered understanding of development for your learning are many. It is clear that repetition of clinical experience is not only desirable but necessary to develop full expertise. As teachers we are often confronted by trainees who report they have 'done that'. This particularly applies to generic skills such as communication skills and consultation techniques. But the model suggests that no matter how many times you have 'done' something, there is still more to be learnt. Learning and development continue for all skills throughout your career.

PLANNING YOUR LEARNING

It is a mark of an effective learner that they show evidence of planning their learning. This should enable you to spot learning opportunities, target your learning to particular goals and have written evidence of your planning. This could well prove very beneficial when you go for a post-Foundation interview. The job specifications for all specialties are bound to include the need to be a good learner, so if you have evidence for this, you should be able to present it at the interview.

The structures for planning your learning are the use of your portfolio and sharing it with your educational supervisor to make a learning plan.

Use of educational supervision

You may well find it helpful to read the chapter for trainers (Chapter 7) for further information on the educational supervisor's role, how they should conduct a meeting and the difference between educational and clinical supervisors.

As I see it, the educational supervisor has five main functions. They:

1. Help you plan your learning
2. Check that your assessments are progressing and feed back the results of some
3. Help you with career management
4. Provide pastoral support
5. Send completed documentation to the deanery

The way in which an educational supervision session is conducted should give you a chance to focus on your key concerns, review your portfolio (including your development since the last meeting), discuss your career aspirations and help you set learning objectives for the next post.

In helping you develop a learning plan, the educational supervisor needs to evaluate how you are doing for each of the main competencies, work with you to identify any obvious learning needs and help you develop a plan with SMART objectives: Specific, Measurable, Achievable, Realistic and Timely.

The responsibility for the success of the educational supervision relationship is mainly yours, not the educational supervisor's. It is your responsibility to organise meetings, prepare properly, bring the appropriate documentation and follow the plan through. The educational supervisor has the responsibility to provide you sufficient time for your meetings and offer alternatives if they have to cancel.

Trainees need varying amounts of support from their supervisor. You are supposed to have three meetings for each four-month post, although realistically this may well be less for most trainees. If, however, you are having problems, you may need to meet more frequently. Negotiate the frequency and length of meeting that you need. Paradoxically, it is my experience that the more competent trainees, who perhaps need less guidance, are better at organizing and attending their educational supervision meetings. If you are not progressing well, make sure that you see your educational supervisor regularly – they are there to help you!

Matching your learning to your career aspirations

In the early stages of your F1 job your learning needs will reflect your inexperience and will be broad. However, as you progress into F2, you will need to develop your learning plan to match both the learning outcomes of the Foundation programme and your career aspirations. As discussed in Chapter 8, you need to develop evidence of the competencies required for entry to the future post. The competencies required will be published in the national job specifications and should be referred to via the MTAS or MMC websites.

Making a learning plan and SMART objectives

Making a learning plan is probably the most important aspect of the management of your learning. It involves five basic steps:

1. Understanding what you need to learn
2. Assessing where you are now
3. Identifying the key priorities for development
4. Identifying how you will get there
5. Determining how you will know you have got there

1. Understanding what you need to learn – the syllabus for the Foundation programme

The Foundation curriculum contains the detailed list of competencies that Foundation doctors are expected to acquire (the syllabus). This is the official account of the knowledge, skills and behaviours/attitudes that you need to aspire to during Foundation programme. You should be familiar with the syllabus as it should form the basis of your learning. The current syllabus is arranged under the seven headings of *Good Medical Practice* with the addition of an eighth – acute care – and can be found in detail on the MMC website under the section of documents available for download.

This book will not go through the syllabus line by line. You should become familiar with it and plan your learning as much as possible against these competencies. The key thing that you need to be aware of is that you will be assessed against the broad range of the competencies but will not be expected to demonstrate competence in all the skills.

At present the syllabus is not given to trainees as a hard copy and is not presented with the rest of the portfolio on the portfolio website. Instead, it is accessed through the MMC website. It would be highly desirable for the revised syllabus to be given in hard copy to each F1 so that you are guaranteed to have an easy-to-use format of the essential guide to what you are supposed to learn in the next two years. If you are not given a hard copy, I urge you to download and print one for easy reference and cross-checking.

The first iteration of the curriculum for the Foundation programme is currently being revised and there is a draft version 2 available on the Academy of Royal Medical Colleges website (www.aomrc.org.uk), which acknowledges that the Foundation programme is a work in progress and will continue to develop. For example, the new version appears to take account of key issues such as chronic disease management omitted in the first version.

You may be surprised to learn that the new syllabus has over 300 separate competencies listed for you to develop (and be assessed against) in the next two years.

In general terms the key 'headline' objectives for F1 will be:

- Clinical accountability and risk management
- Safe prescribing
- Evidence and frameworks for patient safety
- Clinical governance and accountability
- Legal responsibilities in ensuring safe patient care
- Effective time management, prioritisation and organisational skills
- Recognizing diversity and gaining cultural competence

And for F2:

- Decision-making with patients
- Team working and communicating with patients
- Understanding consent and explaining risk
- Managing risk and complaints and learning from them
- Ethics and law as part of clinical practice
- Using evidence in the best interest of patients
- Understanding how appraisal works to promote life-long learning
- Taking responsibility for the future of the NHS
- Teaching others effectively

These objectives are highly idealised and it would be reasonable to ask how many consultants or GPs could fulfil them. For example, how can an F1 or F2 doctor be expected to have responsibility for the future of the NHS? Surely, this is a political aim rather than an educational one. It also raises the questions, who will be able to teach these diverse and aspirational goals and is there any realistic chance that they will be achieved in a meaningful way or will they lead to the 'blind leading the partially sighted' model of medical education where teachers know less in realistic terms than trainees? Without denying the importance of teaching skills and acting without prejudice, how many seniors have actually had significant training in patient safety or understand the concept and practice of cultural competence? (For interesting articles on patient safety and cultural competence, see R. Glavin, 'What every clinical teacher should know about patient safety', *The Clinical Teacher* 2006: 103–107; and J. H. Roberts, 'Cultural competence in the clinical setting', *The Clinical Teacher* 2006: 97–102). The Royal College of Physicians has also developed a teaching programme ('Safe foundations: junior doctors and patient safety') which focuses on this important issue. There are some excellent articles on other aspects of professionalism on the MMC website. Search for the series 'Competencies for the foundation programme' under the New Articles section. The *BMJ* Careers Focus section also carries regular articles on the subject.

My experience is that Foundation doctors will generally excel in many of the important areas of clinical practice, even if these are not key aims of the syllabus. Most are indeed polite, considerate and generally reasonably competent at history-taking, at least within moderately straightforward consultations. The vast majority learn the basic procedures and are able to manage stable patients reasonably well. Their written records and legibility could improve, but they certainly do no worse than their seniors in this regard. The vast majority of trainees start out with a lot of respect for patients, are appropriately cautious in their approach to new skills, have a very sound approach to patient safety and governance, and take appropriate action when they make a mistake. However, they may develop less good attitudes over time due to the modelling around them.

Reflecting on the significant weaknesses (or development needs!) that I regularly see in Foundation doctors, I suggest that you concentrate on the following areas of the syllabus:

- Diagnostic reasoning: Incorrect or missed diagnosis is clearly a problem for the patient. At best they may have been prescribed an unnecessary tablet. At worst they will die. Diagnosis is more than just recognising a symptom pattern and ordering the confirmatory test. It involves high-level analytic skills which can be taught and learnt. It is only covered superficially in many undergraduate courses and is probably done 'intuitively' by seniors so that it is hard for them to teach. Knowing how we make a diagnosis is an essential cognitive skill. There is a chapter in Nicola Cooper, Kirsty Forrest and Paul Cramp's *The Essential Guide to Acute Care* (Oxford: Blackwell, 2006) that covers this subject. I urge you to develop your understanding in this area.
- Selection and interpretation of appropriate tests: The approach of trainees and seniors to diagnostic testing is similar to their approach to diagnostic reasoning – haphazard at times, poor at others. The teaching of the principles of selection of appropriate tests is taught largely theoretically in many medical schools at undergraduate level, although those that use a problem-based learning approach may deal with it more effectively. So, all the theory behind sensitivity, specificity, positive predictive value and Bayesian statistics that should help you decide on the use of appropriate tests has probably been forgotten, even if it was ever understood. This is the time to dust off your old textbooks and revise the theory as well as learn from practice or online learning. Past papers from college exams include many questions based on the

rational use of tests. Guidelines such as those issued by NICE or SIGN also contain sensible analysis of the rational use of tests. Probably the best way of grasping the principles of the appropriate use of tests is to undertake a project that assesses the use of one test in routine practice in your locality. Suitable tests that have interesting patterns of use where pre-test probability strongly influences the performance of the test include D-dimer, troponin T and ferritin. One of the worst problems in clinical practice is to have a 'positive' test result from a test that should never have been done because the probability of the disease was very low. You know the result is almost certainly a false positive but you feel compelled to take it seriously because of the consequences of the diagnosis.

- Prescribing: Poor prescribing is common at all levels of the NHS despite its huge implications for patient safety. It is such a key area of 'doctoring' that we simply have to improve. There will be formal teaching on prescribing within your Trust and you should also refer to Chapter 4.

- Handover skills: Another key area in good practice in this era of shift working. Participate fully in your Trust or practice handover procedures and seek to improve them. Identify your strengths and weaknesses and seek feedback on your performance. This is an interesting area for applying clinical governance and audit procedures. It is now seen as professional to finish your work hours on time and hand over any important, unresolved clinical issues to the next shift. But this does take some skill and requires certain attitudes and behaviours. For instance, you do have to be able to communicate the urgency and importance of the problems to the next team in a way that will enable you to trust that they will act appropriately on unexpected results, for example. And if you are the doctor being expected to carry things on, you need to be able to record information accurately so that you don't forget. You also need to be able to prioritise your work so that you have time to follow up information you have been given and not be distracted by other 'emergencies'.

- Acute care: Recognizing symptoms and signs of severe acute illness. This is a key area and hugely important to patient safety. There are well-established courses in acute care (e.g. ALERT and ILS) and you will no doubt be offered something equivalent. However, this does not guarantee that you will put the skills into practice. Make awareness of abnormal bedside physiology one of your key clinical skills. Respond to the physiology and make broad diagnostic sweeps for the cause. Make sure that you give enough fluid for adequate resuscitation and give it rapidly initially. Be particularly careful of patients with septic shock and resulting organ failure and be aware of the principles of managing shock (see www.survivingsepsis.org). Be especially aware of your limits in managing the seriously ill and when to contact the senior. No harm can come from seeking help when you could have managed alone, but if you do get things wrong, the patient could suffer.

- Nutrition: Anyone who wants to specialise in an underdeveloped area would be well advised to think about nutrition. Obesity has become a huge public issue, but under-nutrition is a serious problem for people with many chronic diseases. There are many excellent short courses in nutrition each year. The use of screening tools to identify patients at risk of under-nutrition would make a very good area for audit, particularly if you examine whether there is appropriate follow-up action.

- Advice on drinking cessation and supportive measures: Facilitating behaviour change is a key skill for doctors and one that is not prioritised by the curriculum. Problem drinking is becoming the national disease. Understanding the so-called 'cycle of change' (see Figure 5.1) will help you understand what approach to take to people at different stages of change and help you move away from the 'advice' model that appears to be endorsed by the curriculum towards a patient-centred approach. In whatever specialty you work, you will see the effects of alcohol on health and you should have basic skills in managing alcohol and drug dependence.

- Legal framework: Many trainees are anxious about the legal situation in which they work and in particular the issues related to consent, particularly in delirious or intoxicated patients, and the risks that they might be prosecuted. The legal framework is also rapidly changing and you need to keep up to date. Ethics and legal issues frequently interact, so understanding the legal framework will enhance ethical understanding. Consider online learning (e.g. on the Royal College of Physicians website) in this area as it is mostly fact-based.

2. Assessing where you are now

The current (2006) national portfolio gives you just 2–3 lines to identify your learning needs for each of the eight domains of the curriculum. This is woefully inadequate. To identify your learning needs you need to match your current level (self-assessed or externally assessed) with the more than 300 competencies required in the syllabus/curriculum. Obviously 300 competencies is too many to focus on. The Northern deanery developed a self-assessment tool that is mapped to the key areas of the curriculum and should help you to identify where you feel you are with approximately 80 key competencies. It can be used by anyone. Go to www.mypimd.ncl.ac.uk and search for 'self-assessment', then click on the document marked 'self-evaluation (salaries)'.

In my practice of educational supervision, I normally suggest that trainees complete this self-evaluation several times during the year. This can be done on the same hard copy using different coloured pens. This may seem childish, but it means that you can easily track your learning through the year which should enable you to identify your progress and the areas where you still have learning or developmental needs.

3. Identifying the key priorities for development

Having performed your self-assessment you can translate the areas of need into a learning plan. Concentrate on areas where you self-assess as poor or

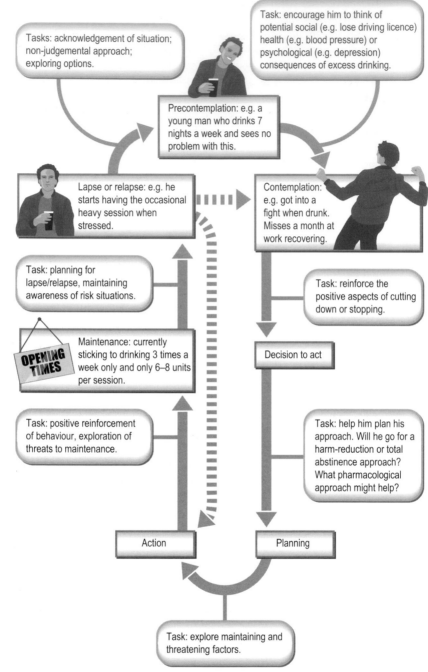

Fig. 5.1 Working example of the cycle of change.

medium and which you also think are important in clinical practice. Identify between three and ten key learning needs and make some SMART objectives. For example, an F1 at the beginning of a medicine attachment is likely to self-score as low at advanced life support (ALS). A **S**pecific objective would be to become competent in ALS and in defibrillation. It could be **M**easured by passing an ALS course and by seeking feedback through a DOPS assessment after an arrest. It is probably **A**chievable and **R**ealistic within four months in a medicine attachment (but unlikely to be achieved in a surgery or GP attachment, for example) and it is **T**imely because when you enter F2 you may be in charge of an arrest team.

It is important to keep your learning plan focused and not be too ambitious. Ten key learning needs in a four-month attachment are going to stretch the **A**chievable bit.

4. Identifying how you will get there

You should review your key learning objectives with your educational supervisor and plan how you will achieve the development needed. Take into account all the learning situations available to you, as described below. Your educational supervisor should be able to give you feedback on whether you will be able to access the learning needed in a particular attachment or whether it would be better to wait for another attachment. For example, if learning to suture is a key aim, it is unrealistic to expect to achieve it in medicine; it should be deferred until a surgery attachment.

5. How will you know you have got there?

There are a number of ways in which you could monitor your progress and work out if you have arrived, including your confidence level, self-assessment of competence, others' assessment of your competence or day-to-day performance and by achieving a pass mark for a course (e.g. ALS or online learning).

Many trainees use confidence as a measure of progress. As a measure it has a lot of validity and is clearly an important motivator. Generally, most trainees are good at assessing their own confidence, but the problem with using confidence is that it can be misplaced – you may be confidently doing the wrong thing or you may remain under-confident but actually be quite competent! The same applies to self-assessment of competence. It is therefore important to check your assessment against others. Do you generally under- or over-assess your confidence/competence?

Assessment by others includes the formal assessment tools of the Foundation programme – DOPs, mini-CEX, CbD and the multi-source feedback tools. But you can also get informal and verbal feedback. It is advisable to get formal assessment of the competencies you have achieved, particularly those you have identified as important. This will provide useful evidence for your Foundation assessments and for job applications. (See Chapter 6 for more details of the assessment process.)

The influence of assessment on learning

Another useful aphorism is that 'assessment drives learning'. Given that your assessment is work-based and involves mainly the use of the four assessment tools, this is important to understand. At present there are no formal assessments of your background knowledge in the Foundation programme. Your application of knowledge is tested to some degree in the Case-based Discussion (CbD), but that is all. There could therefore be a temptation not to seek further formal knowledge-based learning during your two years on the Foundation programme unless it is essential for your job. Knowledge, including background science, is tested in Royal College exams, which you will probably be facing in the near future after F2, so if you do no work on your knowledge for two years, you may struggle to re-engage. In planning your learning, take future learning needs and 'gates to specialization' into account.

The other key point to consider is how you can use the assessments to enhance your learning. They are designed to perform this function (see Chapter 6 for details). In particular, the CbD can be a very powerful learning tool as it gives you the chance to discuss in detail difficult cases with a consultant or GP. If you choose the cases wisely and the review is done in a meaningful way, that will maximise the learning opportunities, so this could be the most significant learning method in the programme. I would encourage you to obtain as many CbDs as possible. For the multi-source feedback, mini-CEX and DOPs (directly observed procedures), it is important that people give you constructive feedback if you are to maximise the learning opportunities from them. Choose people you know will do it most effectively.

SPECIFIC LEARNING OPPORTUNITIES

The health service exists primarily to serve patients, so it should be no surprise that service comes before education most of the time, even if this is a rather short-sighted approach. In the service environment you need to plan to get the most out of your time. When you have completed two or three ward rounds, clinics or theatre sessions, think about the way the session is structured and whether you have maximised your learning. Approach the consultant or GP to change small things and improve opportunities.

Ward work and ward rounds

For your day-to-day ward work, the consultant is not the only person who can give you feedback. The nurses will often accompany you on critical events such as breaking bad news, dealing with an angry relative or explaining treatment to a patient. The pharmacist will be able to feed back on your prescribing. Seek their views on how you did each time. Your feedback will be much more accurate and meaningful if you receive it immediately. Use the assessment forms to stimulate discussion.

If your ward is not busy, seek out learning opportunities elsewhere rather than allowing work to expand to fill the time available or sitting with your feet up reading a newspaper. Plan with your colleagues so that you all have time to seek opportunities away from the ward (e.g. in clinic or coronary care) and accompany the doctors there. Use the library or go online to check the evidence base for the treatment of the conditions you are seeing. Use the patients' drug charts as a stimulus to learning. I have never met a Foundation doctor who could go through the chart and describe the main indications, side-effects, contraindications and interactions of the drugs on a single chart!

Ward rounds have great potential for learning, but this often goes unrecognised. The seniors make decisions and order tests, but you are often none the wiser why they thought diagnosis A was more likely than diagnosis B. The main element of teaching may be delivered after three hours of rounds, when your concentration and ability to absorb new information are lost. The learning from each case, particularly those you have been most closely involved in, needs to be made more explicit and clearer.

For a very interesting model for ward rounds, see Gordon Caldwell's article ('Real time assessment and feedback of junior doctors improves clinical performance', *The Clinical Teacher* 2006: 3: 185–188). He presents a technique and documentation that can facilitate learning and lean on the ideas behind the formal assessment process.

The post-take round is also a very potent source of untapped learning. If you only have an hour to do the round before the end of your shift, plan to review the patients you and the rest of your team have admitted. The consultant can then see the patients you have not seen with the next shift.

Box 5.1 has some top tips on making ward rounds more productive for your learning.

Box 5.1   Top tips on improving learning on ward rounds

- Plan ahead. Identify cases where you are uncertain and ask the consultant to spend time on them.
- Use the first minute or two to agree with the consultant and others how learning will be fitted into the round.
- Ask questions that help you understand the consultant's thinking – for example, their diagnostic reasoning or therapeutic decisions or ethical reasoning.
- Don't concentrate exclusively on knowledge – ask for feedback on prioritisation, time management, recognition of the acutely ill patient, documentation, prescribing, etc.
- Make time to be watched doing a physical examination on a difficult case (e.g. neurology or mental state).
- Make sure that when you have completed relevant tasks you get someone to complete one of the formal assessment forms for your portfolio.
- Seek feedback from nurses and patients as well as from seniors – they often have a different perspective.
- Keep a written note of important learning outcomes using a reflective diary or just keep a notebook. For most people writing things down fixes them in their mind and this might be particularly important for learners who prefer a visual source of information.
- Try to spend three minutes at the end of the round on learning – clarifying anything you don't understand, checking the evidence base, getting further feedback.

Acute care, including admissions and A&E

Acute care is such an important part of the syllabus that you will have much to learn whilst working in A&E or on any other type of admission, but time pressures will be intense. Make sure that you attend the induction sessions designed to teach you about cardinal symptoms that should never be ignored and the common causes of medical error in the acute area. Examples of things that are easy to miss include scaphoid fractures, subdurals, pulmonary emboli, complications of pregnancy including ectopic, non-accidental injuries and atypical presentations of myocardial infarction.

Acute care is an excellent opportunity to learn and practise procedures such as blood gases and lumbar punctures and get them signed using your DOPs forms. In acute care you have to be self-directed and a little selfish if you are to get the most out of it. It's very easy to get stuck doing routine post-take tasks rather than things that help your development.

See Box 5.2 for top tips on learning in acute care.

Out-patient clinic and GP surgery

Seeing people in a clinic setting, either in hospital or in the community, brings a different set of skills into play. New patients test your history-taking, examination and diagnostic skills. Much of out-patients and, in particular, general practice is chronic disease management and so requires a very different approach from what you will have become used to when dealing with in-patients or emergencies.

Box 5.2 Top tips on learning in acute care

- Select the acute cases to match your learning needs, not your comfort zone.
- Let people know which practical procedures you wish to learn and need supervising for (e.g. suturing, aspirating joints or the chest or abdomen, chest drain or central line insertion, delivering a baby, etc.).
- Concentrate on getting your DOPs and mini-CEX assessments done.
- Make a commitment in your clerkings – it is much better to list a series of probable diagnoses and reasons for and against than to finish with a vague problem. For example, don't finish with 'emergency admission – fall ? cause', make a proper differential diagnosis that might include 'postural hypotension – likely drug-related, need to exclude cardiac arrhythmia'. This will help your diagnostic reasoning and enable the consultant to feed back to you in more detail.
- Make sure you get feedback on your clerkings. If your shift has finished before results are back or the patient is transferred elsewhere, keep a note of the name and find out the next day. This is vital because without it you will not learn from all your hard work.
- Share the learning from interesting cases with the rest of the team – if you see someone admitted with acute porphyria, make sure your colleagues learn about it too. Hopefully, they will let you know about interesting cases too.
- Use on-call and acute care experiences to learn about generic skills such as prioritisation, delegation and working in teams.

Box 5.3   Learning in clinic

- Plan your learning and service. When joining the team find out from the consultant or GP what the opportunities are; check them against your own learning needs.
- Try to get a good mix between new cases and follow-ups or chronic disease management problems. If a particular clinic has just one type of problem, go to another session (e.g. join the practice nurse for the diabetic follow-up clinic or the midwife for antenatal).
- Consider sitting in with a senior as well as seeing patients on your own. You can learn about consultation skills and management from the senior.
- Seek deep learning – it is better that your trainer teaches you general principles about diagnosing chest pain rather than telling you what the most likely diagnosis is and what tests he wants done.
- Make sure that you get the opportunity to present all new patients to the consultant for patient safety and learning reasons.
- Seek a three-minute round-up at the end.

In primary care things are usually very well organised. You will have one primary trainer who will supervise most of your work and you will build up your skills and confidence from an initial period of observation followed by long appointments and eventually to fairly independent practice. In hospital clinics such structure and support are the exception and you are expected to see people from day one. This reflects in part a difference in financial arrangements (GPs are paid to have trainees, hospitals are not), in history (the GP training scheme grew from nothing in the last 30 years, so could be organised afresh with specified trainers) and culture (hospital doctors expect you to be able to cope and get on with it).

Make sure that you always present new cases to the consultant to avoid making an error. Follow-up cases may need to be discussed with the consultant initially, but after a while you may have confidence and competence to see many yourself and make decisions. See Box 5.3 for further tips on learning in the clinic setting.

Theatre

Theatre and other procedure-based environments such as endoscopy and radiology are a setting rich in learning opportunities, but need to be used wisely. It is likely that in the Foundation programme you will not be at a level where you need to learn actual surgery or endoscopy, and you certainly will not be inserting angiographic catheters. So, you need to be able to define the learning opportunities and match them to your needs. See Box 5.4 for top tips on learning in these environments.

Ambulatory care settings

Increasingly, care is being given in day centres, such as medical investigation units and day case surgery units. Patients are pre-assessed by a nurse specialist

Box 5.4 Top tips on Foundation doctor learning in theatre (or investigative situations, such as endoscopy or interventional radiology)

- Plan by talking to your clinical supervisor. What type of lists do they have? What are the opportunities for you – is there any spare time for you to develop your skills or are the lists very time pressured?
- Identify appropriate generic learning goals (e.g. sterile procedure, theatre safety patterns, planning an emergency case).
- Identify specific learning goals appropriate to your stage and your career intentions, e.g. practical skills relevant to surgery (start basic from incision and suturing at closure to the use of a laparoscope before working up to intra-abdominal action such as appendicectomy); more factual learning (such as revising your anatomy); or learning about appropriate behaviours in theatre.
- For trainees who know they will not do surgery, surgical learning goals might include learning about indications and contraindications for specific operations and pre-hospital work-up and late complications to watch out for in primary care, rather than actual 'cutting'.
- Use active observation techniques when watching. How are the team communicating? What is good and what doesn't work? What is the nature of the relationship between all the staff present?
- Ask questions, but be careful to respect the surgeon's and anaesthetist's need to concentrate more at some times.
- Don't forget the anaesthetist. Perhaps the most critical area of theatre work is the anaesthetic. You can achieve factual learning (e.g. revise the drugs used in anaesthesia), some skills (ventilation, intubation, cannulation, arterial and central venous lines) and some behaviours (anaesthetists have a very strong safety ethos with strict protocols to follow. Do other specialties have anything to learn from them?).
- Avoid going to theatre for theatre's sake if the learning opportunities do not match your needs. Don't go just to impress the surgeon with your keenness or simply because it is on the timetable. There is a danger that you will waste a lot of time sitting around seeing and learning nothing. Never get trapped into being a retractor holder for hours on end.

and the anaesthetist and the learning opportunities available from these cases are often lost because trainees don't work in these environments. There is much to learn in these areas, such as practical procedures, post-op analgesia, inter-professional care, the selection of patients for surgery and type of anaesthetic, the explanation to patients and the process of informed consent. If your timetable allows it, try to attend these settings and see patients alongside the other clinicians working in the area.

ITU, HDU and CCU

The opportunity to work in these settings in F1/2 has to be one of the big advances that the Foundation programme has brought about. The opportunities for learning in the critical care area are fantastic, particularly in the acute care domain of the syllabus and in developing your procedural skills. They are also excellent places to learn about patient safety, communicating with patients and their families, teamwork and inter-professional working. As an F1 or F2 you will not usually be expected to have much expertise and will often be supernumerary so you can focus on your learning.

Make sure you plan to get the most out of even a short attachment in ITU. You may well have a role communicating between different clinical teams – for example, a single patient will have input from surgery, medicine, radiology, microbiology and the anaesthetic or intensivist team. Getting them to work together and coordinating actions is a challenge. How did you manage to prioritise which of three urgent procedures should be done first and make sure that the patient was safe during a CT scan? How do you find working with nurses who are far more expert than you are in managing many aspects of care? How do you learn from them and their approach? You should also take the opportunity to observe seniors speaking with families about levels of care, prognosis and appropriateness of treatments. Reflect on what you learn from these experiences. Were there any general lessons from these experiences?

Finally, critical care is an excellent place to get your assessments up to date.

Laboratory and radiology settings

Increasing the numbers of F2 doctors means they will have the chance to experience working in diagnostic specialties (e.g. radiology) or laboratory specialties (e.g. microbiology, biochemistry, histopathology and immunology) and again these are full of learning opportunities. Some of the key learning outcomes that can be addressed include the rational use of laboratory tests, interpretation of test results, use of audit and clinical governance procedures. By the end of these posts you should understand the terms 'sensitivity', 'specificity' and 'positive predictive value' and even have a working knowledge of Bayesian statistics so that you can put it into practice.

Working in these specialties provides an excellent opportunity to improve your CV and obtain evidence of competencies for your post-Foundation application. You should aim to complete an audit or research project during this post – a detailed piece of work that will allow you to use the literature and develop your skills in evidence-based practice. There is a great opportunity to get your project published.

The place of diagnostic specialties at the interaction between different specialties will also give you a different view of medical practice. You will be able to see the complex interactions between teams and how the way they work affects patient care. You will witness communication styles, including written requests, across teams that help or hinder care – all of this without even mentioning any learning goals related directly to the actual laboratory work.

With good planning, all doctors should be able to learn much that is relevant to their future in medicine in any of these specialties.

Study leave, tasters, college exams and private study

Effective use of study leave is vital to your development. Your study leave in F2 is for approximately 30 days (equivalent to the old SHO grade), subject to approval, and you should have an allowance of approximately £650. There will be a number of courses that you have to attend and most of your budget will be used for these. In F1 you do not have formal study leave, but the programme will organise teaching in generic skills that will correspond to approximately three hours a week. Part of your F2 study leave allowance and budget may be used in F1 towards courses such as ALS.

So, how can you use the rest of your F2 study leave effectively with little available funding?

Tasters are a relatively new format. The idea is that you can have some time (usually up to a week) to try out a specialty that you would otherwise not experience. This will help inform your career choice. To be used effectively, tasters need to be taken before your application to post-Foundation posts in February. So, you need to plan tasters carefully, in discussion with your educational supervisor or careers adviser, and with the trainees that you are working with to ensure that you can get the leave.

The issue of college exams is going to be a key battleground in the future. The MMC has made it clear that passing college exams will not be an essential or desirable criterion for entry into specialist training. But they certainly cannot stop you taking the exams if you are eligible and there may well be sound educational reasons for doing so at this stage. For example, the basic science questions and learning may be easier now rather than later. I would encourage you to look for formal courses with recognised qualifications that will enable you to demonstrate your development in the future. These might be college exams, but they could equally be university courses or a higher degree such as Masters, which can be completed in two years' part-time study. Any qualification that you obtain during the Foundation programme will give you an edge in future applications. On the FAQ part of the MMC website there is a response to the question 'What if I satisfy the Foundation competencies before the end of the two years?', which basically says that you will not be able to leave the post before the end of the two years but 'you will have opportunities to. . . . acquire new [competencies]'. This seems to me to sanction the pursuit of the competencies associated with college exams! Inter-mediate-level exams (e.g. Diploma in Child Health) are worthwhile pursuing as evidence of your commitment to and aptitude for a specialty.

Private study has always been a legitimate reason for study leave for SHOs, particularly when studying for college exams. It is uncertain if this will be allowed in the future for F2 doctors, but it is certainly worth a try. You will need to make a case to your educational supervisor to be granted private leave and it will have to have clear goals.

Investing in your future is something that you will be used to as an under-graduate, but has not been required at postgraduate level. There has been a great reluctance by some trainees to spend money on their own development in the past. This may well have to change, but you can be sure that if you do invest £1000–£2000 on developing yourself in your Foundation programme, it will be well spent.

Formal classroom teaching

The deaneries and Trusts are working to develop the education programmes offered to you. The teaching programme at present is not well developed but in the future it is likely to become more streamlined and to use standardised and evidence-based teaching sessions common to all units across the country. In Scotland there is already a more common approach, organised by NHS Education for Scotland under the banner 'Foundation Education Programme' through the Doctors Online Training System. This seems a coherent and useful approach, which could be developed in the rest of the UK.

You will probably be offered two types of formal learning opportunities: short lunchtime sessions and longer sessions (a half- or full day or even several days) that focus on professionalism topics.

In most hospitals there will be a weekly series of lunchtime teaching sessions delivered by a consultant or expert in their field, such as a pharmacist or specialist nurse. In general these will cover the diagnosis and management of fairly common presentation and conditions. The information presented will often be visual, so easy for visual learners to access. To make it most effective it should be a mix of case-based discussion with a mention of the evidence base on which the management is based. It should involve learners rather than being delivered as a lecture. There should be a chance for you and the other Foundation doctors to influence the content of the sessions so that you can cover subjects that reflect your learning needs. The sessions should be evaluated, either individually or collectively, so that the speakers can get feedback on their teaching.

These sessions are often difficult to organise because the teachers are generally busy and it is not uncommon for them to be cancelled or for sessions to be missed. Make sure that you and the other trainees are alert to any gaps in the programme, especially no-shows, and that you keep in touch with the teaching programme organiser, particularly the clinical tutor, to make sure that the outcome from the sessions is maximised.

Initially, there will be a variety of approaches to the professionalism sessions, which will be compulsory. These should cover ethics, communication, time management, teamwork and leadership, communication, clinical skills, prescribing, risk management, etc. There is already a reasonably well-developed module on prescribing. This is being rolled out nationally and the RCP teaching on patient safety is also likely to be run nationwide. Other standardised sessions will follow.

Trainees and others often emphasise formal teaching but this over-values the learning that takes place for an hour a week in the lecture room in comparison to the learning that takes place in the other 47 work hours. It is certainly a style of teaching that allows an expert to convey a lot of facts in a short time to a moderately sized group. It is useful to supplement your factual knowledge and to revise the management plans that you should have learnt as a student but which inevitably need reinforcing once you are in practice. It allows you to build on the knowledge that you already have and make your learning deeper, even on common conditions that you will have learnt many times before. But you still need to put it into practice and that can only be done in the workplace.

Online learning

Online learning is expanding and becoming much more sophisticated. It is likely that in five years' time much more learning will be available online. The *BMJ* is developing considerable resources and the NHS has developed a series of sites devoted to diverse subjects, including cultural awareness and communication skills. (See Chapter 10 for contact details.) There are many other providers. Online learning is likely to be effective for factual-based learning such as drug side-effects, legal issues and causes of, for example, splenomegaly. Clearly, there are limits to how well you can develop skills using online resources and there will always be a gap between learning facts and protocols in the abstract and putting them into everyday practice. One of the advantages of online learning is that it can be accessed whenever you want and can be taken at your own pace. It can be covered repeatedly and in a variety of depths. It can also be assessed easily and evidence of your learning provided for your portfolio.

Simulation

The field of simulation in learning clinical skills is another area that is likely to grow considerably in the near future. Simulation ranges from the use of sophisticated multi-tasking models that can simulate every known heart sound and medical emergency to the use of trained role players and actors in the teaching of consultation skills. The use of simulation is still in its infancy. There are numerous advanced simulators around the country that languish in cupboards and are brought out for just a few days each year. In postgraduate education the role of professional role players has yet to be fully developed and is confined to a few pilot sites and interested centres. Few seniors have the skill or time to devote to these time-intensive methods.

Simulation using models is ideal for learning about acute care and the scenarios and procedures associated with it. But it has many other possibilities. Use of video during simulated emergencies is ideal for getting feedback on how you behave in an emergency or how you work within a team. Professional role models can be used for teaching communications skills and patient-centred consultation as well as how to deal with a difficult or angry patient. If you are offered the chance to take part in teaching sessions involving simulation in any form, you should jump at it.

SUMMARY

Your two years in the Foundation programme will see you progress from novice to limited expert. It is an amazing change and you will hardly recognize where you were two years before. These years are the chance to develop the life-long skills of continuous professional development. Planning your learning, using your educational supervisor appropriately, being tactical in what and how you learn, maximizing your learning opportunities, being able to use reflection as a key learning skill and providing evidence of your learning and your learning skills are the key indicators of the fully fledged professional.

Good luck in achieving those 300+ competencies.

Assessment in the Foundation programme

Mark Welfare

66 Competence, like truth, beauty and contact lenses, is in the eye of the beholder. 99

Laurence J. Peter

INTRODUCTION

Having survived the first month and contemplated the numerous outcome measures in the curriculum that you must achieve by the end of the two years, you will now be thinking about how you are going to pass the exams at the end of the course. After all, as an undergraduate you probably carefully planned your learning to do the minimum to achieve the pass mark! Prepare yourself for a shock: there are no exams! This may seem like wonderful news, but there is a catch. You have to organise your own assessments and record them in your portfolio. The purpose of the assessments is to help you pass, not to trip you up. Good planning will reduce any anxieties you have about the system. The assessment process will also help you focus on planning your learning. This chapter will take you through the principles of competency-based assessment and the use of the portfolio and help you to plan your evidence gathering so that your end-of-year assessment is a doddle.

WORK-BASED COMPETENCY ASSESSMENT

In Chapter 5, we reviewed the competencies you are required to develop in the Foundation programme. We will now review these to look at:

- Why we have this system of assessment
- How you can demonstrate your competence

Chapter 1 gave some background on why the assessment system has been changed. Prior to 2005, house officers were required to get a certificate signed by their supervising consultant, the clinical tutor in the hospital and the post-graduate dean to say that they had completed their unmapped journey from Land's End to John o'Groats (or satisfactorily completed their posts – see Chapter 1). For the most part this was not a problem. At least 96% of trainees performed satisfactorily and were signed off appropriately, although they were often disappointed about the lack of positive feedback that they received. For the small minority of trainees with problems, there was no clear guidance as to whether they had reached the standard required or not. There was no curriculum, no competencies to aim for and no written outcomes; it all depended on the word of three people, two of whom may rarely have met you. The general criterion applied was that 'if it wagged its tail and barked, it must be a dog'. In other words, if you looked and behaved like a successful house officer, you probably were. This left problems for trainees who might be unfairly failed (particularly if this was based on prejudice) and for the NHS and patients when poorly performing doctors were let through because of lack of clear pass/fail criteria against which they could be assessed. Those doctors with problems might also have missed out on the chance for rehabilitation or extra training if their poor performance had not been recognised early. Prominent cases of failed systems for ensuring competence in consultants such as the Bristol paediatric cardiac surgery case and the gynaecologist Rodney Ledward meant that doing nothing was not an option.

So, there has been a radical shake-up in standard-setting throughout the profession, affecting everyone from medical students to professors. The Postgraduate Medical Education and Training Board (PMETB) is now in charge of all medical assessments and they have defined the principles which any assessment should meet (See Box 6.1 or go to www.pmetb.org.uk and follow the links). All assessments take place against the GMC's *Good Medical Practice* framework with its familiar seven headings (outlined in Chapter 3 and discussed in more detail in Chapter 9).

We are now all obliged to demonstrate our fitness to practise in these seven areas and there are increasingly well-defined criteria for career progression we all need to meet.

Box 6.1   Paraphrasing of the PMETB principles for an assessment system

1. The assessment system must be fit for a range of purposes, which must be openly documented, match career progression and should add unique information and build on previous assessments
2. The content must be based on curricula referenced to *Good Medical Practice*
3. The methods used will be chosen on the basis of validity, reliability, feasibility, cost-effectiveness, opportunities for feedback and impact on learning
4. The methods used to set the standards for classification of trainees' performance (i.e. whether they pass or fail) must be explicit, transparent and in the public domain
5. Assessments must provide relevant feedback to trainees on their performance and the performance of their education and training
6. Assessors must be properly trained, especially in equality and diversity, and demonstrate their competence in their role
7. There will be lay input in the development, implementation and use of assessments and lay people may act as assessors in some areas
8. Documentation will track progress and enable trainers and trainees to access it as appropriate, be transferable and also provide evidence for revalidation
9. There will be resources sufficient to support assessment e.g. for training assessors, developing and implementing assessment methods and providing infrastructure

WHY WORK-BASED ASSESSMENT?

Increasing academic study over the last 20 years has added evidence to the best method of assessing doctors (much of which is summarized in B. Jolly and J. Grant, *The Good Assessment Guide*, Buckingham: Open University Centre for Education in Medicine, 1997; and Van der Vleuten *et al.*, 'Assessing professional competence: from methods to programmes', *Medical Education* 2005, 39: 309–317). The result has been a move away from exams, initially to objective structured clinical examinations (OSCEs) but increasingly to work-based assessments.

In summary current thinking suggests that:

- Exams assess what you KNOW
- OSCEs assess what you CAN DO
- Work-based assessments are meant to show WHAT YOU DO in everyday practice

The emphasis now is on developing a programme of assessment of professional competence and behaviours that taps many different areas of a doctor's work and that answers two questions:

1. Are you fit to progress to the next stage, or do we need to look more closely at your skills?
2. What are your strengths and weaknesses?

After all, it is your everyday practice that counts.

As a consultant I maintain my own portfolio using tools similar to those that you will be using in the Foundation programme. As a consultant, my performance is reviewed each year in an appraisal meeting and the results will be used by the GMC to assess my suitability to stay on the Medical Register. Therefore, the Foundation programme assessment provides you with a good opportunity to get up to speed with the use of a portfolio and work-based assessment because it is going to stay with you for the rest of your career.

A PMETB review of work-based assessment delineates some of the advantages of work-based assessment in comparison to exams:

'the emphasis is moving rapidly away from gaining a certain number of marks in high-stakes examinations and more towards gathering evidence of clinical competence and appropriate professional behaviour and attitudes. Much of this evidence cannot be captured in the kind of formal examinations that have traditionally been the primary focus in postgraduate training. It is demonstrated, day in, day out, in the workplace and seen by educational supervisors, other team members, fellow healthcare workers, patients and their relatives and carers. Since it is both demonstrated and observed in the workplace, then it stands to reason that the workplace is where the evidence can be gathered. This is why workplace based assessment will become increasingly important over the next few years.' (*Workplace-Based Assessment*, PMETB, 2005, p. 4: www.pmetb.org.uk)

Assessment in the Foundation programme

THE PURPOSE AND USE OF YOUR PORTFOLIO IN DEVELOPMENT AND ASSESSMENT

So, your future is now in your own hands. Yes, it really is up to you to demonstrate that you have reached the appropriate level to move on to the next stage. You have to gather evidence over the course of each year to demonstrate your development. That will determine whether you pass or fail and whether you can progress to the next stage of training. The evidence will include the four or five 'approved' tools in your portfolio, but you are free to add more evidence. But the portfolio is not there simply to provide summary evidence. It is also supposed to aid your development by helping you plan your learning and reflect on events so that you can learn from both positive and negative experiences.

THE NATIONAL PORTFOLIO

Portfolios have been used widely in academia and industry for some time. They are designed to help people develop (formative) and to assess performance (summative). The two roles are quite confusing and some people believe that the formative and summative functions should be completely separated. For example, you may well feel inhibited in writing an honest account of a medical cock-up in your formative reflective practice document if you think that your final assessor is going to read it. Others believe that the two are so intertwined that any distinction is meaningless and that all assessments should have a formative element. The Department of Health has decided to have a national portfolio that combines the two functions and this fits very neatly with the two questions outlined above – 'Are you fit to progress?' and 'What are your strengths and weaknesses?' In reality the reflective bits may also produce evidence of competence (e.g. evidence of being able to plan your learning) and the summative elements will give you feedback that you can use to develop.

In the pilot years of the Foundation programme, several deaneries developed their own portfolios with differing emphases and documentation. At the launch of the full programme in 2005 a national portfolio was designed which attempted to use the best from each local portfolio. Inevitably, some of the best bits were casualties of the consensus needed to develop a single national document and, as a result, some deaneries, including the NHS in Scotland, are continuing to use variations of the UK national document. In principle they all have similar functions and structure, even if the detail differs. The 2005 national portfolio is acknowledged as being a transitional document and further developments will take place in the coming years. Because of its importance the Foundation portfolio is being subjected to a high level of evaluation so any developments will be evidence based.

Many of you will be familiar with the use of portfolios to help development and some of you will have used portfolios for assessment in your undergraduate course. In more traditional medical courses students will not have used portfolios, so this may represent a greater challenge to them.

Initially, we will review the formal assessment tools provided by the DoH and then discuss other types of evidence you can present.

The assessment tools

The Foundation programme's *Rough Guide* and the portfolio give reasonably comprehensive details of the use of the assessment tools, including trainees' experience of using them. Further information can be found on the MMC's website (www.mmc.nhs.uk/assessment and www.mmc.nhs.uk/pages/foundation/rough-guide). Box 6.2 summarises the characteristics and use of the portfolio and the numbers of each assessment required for 2005/6, but things are changing rapidly so check the website for future years. The figures given are minimum numbers – there is no upper limit on the assessments that you can collect.

In most deaneries, the use of the four assessment tools is being coordinated nationally and you will need to register with the coordinating centre to give permission to hold your data electronically. None of your assessments can be entered until you have done this. The portfolio has mainly gone electronic and this will undoubtedly be rolled out nationally in the near future. If your deanery or school has not gone electronic, you may be given a book of triplicate copies of the assessment forms or you may have to print them from the website. Every month you should receive a summary of your current completed assessments and how you are doing compared to the national mean of all Foundation doctors.

For the DOPs, mini-CEX and CbD, you will collect completed forms in your own time as the year goes by. You need to plan your collection of these assessments to cover all clinical areas and body systems and make sure that

---

Box 6.2 Key facts about your portfolio
- Your portfolio is designed to help you learn (formative) and for you to provide evidence for your later assessment (summative)
- The self-appraisal, learning plan and reflective practice documents are mainly formative
- The CbD, MSF, mini-CEX and DOPs are mainly summative
- There has been confusion about the number of each assessment tool required
- Remember the sign of the devil (6-6-6) for mini-CEX, CbD and DOPs. Six of each, each year
- 8-8 for mini-Pat: 8 in October/November and 8 in April in each year; 10 for TAB
- Don't forget that evidence will probably have to be collected before the end of May, so in effect you only have 10 months each year to gather your evidence
- Remember: no evidence = no pass. Start now
- If not using the e-portfolio, carry forms with you or put in an easily accessible place in your work area
- Photocopy everything and keep it in a separate place in case of loss
- Evidence other than the standard assessment tools can be added to your portfolio

you gather evidence in as many of the competency domains as possible from as many people as possible.

Case-based discussion

Case-based discussion (CbD) is designed to test in depth what you do in routine, everyday practice and so is based on cases you have been involved with. It is mainly used to assess clinical reasoning, but aspects of legal and ethical practice will also be covered. CbD is a chance to demonstrate your skills in making a differential diagnosis or management plan from the information you had at the time. It is not designed to test your knowledge about obscure conditions or be the format for an examiner to demonstrate all that they know on the subject. You should expect to be tested on why you have chosen your options, given the information available at the time, and whether there were any other diagnoses or interventions you could have considered. For common conditions, you should be able to discuss the evidence base behind the standard treatments.

You will need to arrange a minimum of six CbD discussions in each year (two per four-month attachment), each with a different assessor, one of whom should be the supervising consultant or clinical supervisor. Other assessors should be middle-grade doctors or above (SpR, clinical assistant, staff grade, GP or consultant), not SHOs, ST1/2 doctors or your Foundation peers. As for the mini-CEX and DOPs, you need to choose cases that cover the range of systems. CbD should assess a case where you have had significant input and where you have been involved in decision-making. Your feedback will not be worthwhile if your role has been only to document the ward round decisions and results of investigations. Some suitable cases for CbD are shown in Box 6.3.

As discussed in Chapter 5, in our experience CbD is used by trainees not just to gather evidence on their performance but to learn and to talk through unresolved learning issues with a senior colleague. You will get more out of the process of CbD if you take challenging cases to your assessor rather than straightforward ones, especially as your confidence grows. Don't be concerned that challenging cases will make you look less competent. Most assessors will prefer to see someone who is closely examining their own practice, challenging their thoughts and being a reflective learner. You are being

---

Box 6.3   Suitable cases for CbD assessment
- An emergency admission that you clerked
- Your assessment of a patient that you reviewed who has deteriorated on the ward
- An episode of care in general practice that could include several short consultations in a defined time period
- A new out-patient you have seen
- A pre-admission clerking

assessed on your thought processes mainly, so using a challenging case will enable you to demonstrate a deeper level of decision-making.

The process for CbD is that you select two cases that you have been involved with and take the notes to your assessor, who will select one of the cases for discussion. In addition to reviewing your record-keeping, you will be questioned about your involvement with the case under the following headings:

- Clinical assessment
- Treatment and follow-up
- Investigation
- Future planning
- Referrals

Aspects of professionalism and overall clinical judgement will also be recorded. The assessor will record your strengths and weaknesses demonstrated by the case and you will then agree an action plan with your assessor which will help you plan your future learning.

Directly observed procedures and mini-clinical evaluation exercises

These two assessment tools tap similar areas of doctor–patient interactions, directly observed procedures (DOPs) concentrating on procedural skills and mini-clinical evaluation exercises (mini-CEX – with a 'hard C' pronounced mini-KEX not SEX) on a procedure or a consultation. Both rely on direct observation and on your choice of time, place and assessor. The obvious difficulty here is finding someone with the time to observe you and getting them to write the form immediately. DOPs can be done by anyone above you in the medical or non-medical hierarchy, including an F2, but mini-CEX should be done by a consultant, GP or SpR equivalent. You should plan to sample all clinical areas and different types of problem using both tools. In particular, you must get examples from each of the main areas of the acute curriculum for the mini-CEX:

- Airway
- Behaviour/psychological
- Breathing
- Pain
- Circulation
- Gastroenterology
- Neurological

The main challenge for the DOPs is to make them interesting and meaningful. The list of procedures given by the original MMC document includes everyday things (e.g. venepuncture, blood culture and IV cannulation) and others that are not done regularly by doctors (e.g. subcutaneous and intramuscular injections).

One of the problems is that there is no gold standard to be marked on for these simple procedures. These are simple tasks that the average medical student should be able to do. They don't really test you after the first month or two unless there is a very stringent marking schedule. For example, do you always take the sharps box to the bedside? Do you record when a cannula has been put in and when it should be removed? Do you know whether a cannula should be flushed with saline or heparin, and how often? As other people's practice is likely to be substandard, or not following evidence-based practice, you are likely to receive glowing marks and little constructive feedback. Having some standards for the ideal technique would be helpful for these seemingly simple procedures.

Because of these limitations, you should aim for a range of DOPs assessments, starting at the lower end of the skills ladder and moving rapidly towards those at the higher end. Learning procedural skills is at the top of the learning agenda of F1 and F2 doctors and you will probably not be satisfied by being able to show that you can put in a cannula, take blood and give injections at the end of F1. In our experience, most trainees have had the opportunity to do two or more of the more advanced procedures during F1.

Always remember that when you go for a post-Foundation job, the evidence in your portfolio is one of the best things you have to convince your future employer of your suitability. Increasingly, the requirements of CNST (the NHS insurance scheme – see Chapter 3) mean that you will not be allowed to do procedures unsupervised until you have been signed off as competent. If you finish F2 with evidence that you are competent in lumbar puncture and inserting a chest and abdominal drain, you will be well placed at the beginning of your specialty training. The revised curriculum suggests that higher-level skills relevant to the specialties you have worked in, including lumbar puncture, central line insertion and pleural or joint aspiration, will be relevant.

Suggested encounters where you could have your performance assessed using the mini-CEX or DOPs are shown below.

Airway mini-CEX or DOPs
- Managing a choking incident
- Cardiorespiratory arrest
- Intubation in theatre in anaesthetic rotation
- Routine tracheostomy care

Breathing mini-CEX
- Ask consultant to watch you take a history from a patient with breathlessness in clinic
- Get your SpR to watch you doing a respiratory examination, even on a healthy volunteer
- Assessment of radiology such as CXR

Breathing DOPs
- Obtaining a sample for and interpreting a blood gas
- Teaching a patient to use an inhaler
- Performing and interpreting spirometry or peak flow

Circulation mini-CEX
- History or examination in a suitable patient
- Immediate treatment for abdominal aneurysm
- Assessment of a patient with acute limb ischaemia
- Acute LVF or chest pain: explanation to patient about current problem (e.g. myocardial infarct (MI), atrial fibrillation (AF), shock)

Circulation DOPs
- Perform and interpret ECG
- Assessment for and prescribing of thrombolysis
- Performing an exercise ECG (F2)
- Cardiorespiratory arrest, including defibrillation
- Insertion and use of a central line to monitor circulatory status

Neurological mini-CEX
- History from an appropriate patient, including confused elderly or patients with falls
- Full neurological examination. Our experience is that medical students and trainees find the neuro exam the most difficult of the systems examinations (one of the authors admits that he did not learn to do a competent neuro examination until his second SHO year) – so, go on, give it a go!
- Explanation to a patient (e.g. stroke, MS)

Neurological DOPs
- Performing and interpreting Glasgow coma scale or similar
- Assessing cognitive function using an appropriate assessment tool, such as the MMSE
- Explaining to patient, getting consent for and performing a lumbar puncture
- Requesting and interpreting radiology such as a skull x-ray or CT head

Pain mini-CEX or DOPs
- Immediate management of a patient with trauma or MI
- Use of patient controlled analgesia
- Assessment of a patient's palliative care needs

The original syllabus missed out some areas of acute care that are of vital importance, particularly the care of septic patients. Gastroenterology as a discrete entity also appears to have been neglected. The first version of the curriculum had little emphasis on chronic disease management. The medical schools are making a major shift to educating undergraduate students in the area of chronic disease management, so undervaluing it in the Foundation curriculum seems a wasted opportunity. The draft revision of the curriculum does address chronic disease management in more detail. Antibiotic prescribing, poor treatment of sepsis and hospital-acquired infections are a major concern of the public and the government and so were a surprising omission. We recommend that these areas could be included in your mini-CEX or DOPs as well as those in the 'official' acute care curriculum.

Care of septic patients mini-CEX
- Assessment of a patient with post-operative fever
- Clerking a patient with suspected exacerbation of COPD or community-acquired pneumonia
- Examining someone with fever of unknown origin

- Assessment of the febrile child or febrile convulsions
- The use of the Surviving Sepsis protocol in management of an acutely ill patient

Care of septic patients DOPs
- Antibiotic choice
- IV access and antibiotic administration for pneumonia
- Gloving and gowning procedure for barrier nursing
- Blood culture from peripheral or central access

Chronic disease management mini-CEX
- Explaining a new diagnosis to a patient, or breaking bad news
- Discussing patients' ideas, concerns and expectations about a particular clinical problem
- Health promotion in the form of discussing smoking cessation or harm reduction for a heavy drinker or drug user
- Discussing the risks of obesity and strategies for weight loss with a patient
- Discussing risks and benefits of warfarin for a patient with AF

Multi-source feedback (MSF), mini-PAT (peer assessment tool) and self-PAT, Scottish Workplace Assessment tool and TAB (Team Assessment of Behaviour)

The purpose of this aspect of assessment is to see what your colleagues think of you in global terms, not just in relation to the one encounter assessed by CbD, DOPs and mini-CEX. The self-PAT also allows you to assess yourself using the same format as the mini-PAT and find out how accurate you are in assessing your own performance. You need to get a range of people to do these assessments, one of whom must be the consultant you are working most closely with. There are some differences in the way the three tools are used, so refer to the specific sections on each depending on which option you have. Some deaneries or schools have chosen one tool to use, some another and some have given trainees the choice.

One characteristic these tools share is that you receive anonymized and accrued data, not the individual forms. There are some potential advantages in using anonymised feedback for assessment. For example, it is thought that people are more likely to raise concerns if they know that you will not see the feedback. Critical comments, even if fair, could lead to difficult relationships at work if not anonymised. The disadvantage is that people may write things under the cloak of anonymity that are hurtful or vengeful and that you cannot learn from. In particular, if the free text comments are not constructive or do not have sufficient context, it may not be possible to know which behaviour has prompted the comments and therefore needs changing. For the moment this is what we have. Box 6.4 is a summary of the similarities and differences between the mini-PAT and TAB. Usually your multi-source feedback will be sent to your educational supervisor and it will be your responsibility to arrange a meeting to review the results.

Box 6.4 Summary of mini-PAT and TAB

Mini-PAT summary:

- Assesses five areas of 'Fitness to practice', including clinical skills
- Twice a year
- 8–12 assessors nominated on each occasion
- Clinical colleagues only (i.e. doctors, nurses and allied health professionals)
- Not suited for clerical, secretarial or managerial feedback
- Results come from range and averages for each question, overall average score and free text comments
- Results compare to your self-evaluation and national mean
- Feedback from your educational supervisor

TAB summary:

- Assesses two areas of 'Fitness to practise'
- Minimum of ten assessors required during the year. They need to be found as you go along
- Consultant plus any other colleague including non-clinical such as ward clerk, lab staff and secretary
- Feedback from your educational supervisor
- Style of form encourages behavioural feedback
- Results in the form of 'concern' levels and free text comments
- Feedback from your educational supervisor

SUGGESTED SCHEDULE FOR GATHERING YOUR FORMAL ASSESSMENTS

Realistically, few people will gather much evidence in the August of their first year. Most of you are coming to terms with 'the Fear' (see Chapter 4) in August. Besides, as the standard assessed against is 'at the end of the Foundation year', you may be uncertain about obtaining assessments when you have only just started. In addition, your evidence summary will have to be submitted in June so you really only have nine months between September and May to gather your six CbDs, six mini-CEXs, six DOPs and ten TABs if that is the MSF tool that you are using. Mini-PAT is easier to complete because it takes place at two defined time periods and reminders will be sent to you.

Some rotations will offer you more opportunities for assessment than others and there may be other things that will affect your schedule. For example, if you are working in A&E you are likely to have a lot of opportunities to obtain DOPs assessments, but the ratio of seniors to trainees means that you are less likely to be able to get many CbD assessments. Similarly, if you are working in general practice, you may have the chance to do many mini-CEXs but you may have to be creative to find some DOPs and you will need to approach more than one GP to do your two CbDs.

So, planning and keeping a check on where you are at is going to make your life much easier. Decide a schedule near the beginning of the year based on your placements, your knowledge of yourself and the advice of your educational supervisor or a colleague with experience of these assessments, such as an F2.

The bottom line is that you will need at least two assessments each month (from the CbDs, DOPs or mini-CEXs) and you need to keep up with the MSFs at the appropriate time of your placements.

SCOTLAND

In Scotland the assessment system is developing some different streams. In particular, they are using their own MSF system and are also using an interesting method of formative learning using critical incident analysis.

EXAMPLES OF OTHER TYPES OF EVIDENCE THAT YOU CAN GATHER IN SPECIFIC COMPETENCY DOMAINS

Experience suggests that a minority of Foundation doctors will find it hard to synthesise their thoughts and reflections using the written tools available. One comment made in our evaluation of the local pilot of the Foundation programme was: 'I think there's too much emphasis on writing it down because it happens anyway and we do it almost without thinking about it through talking things over with our colleagues. . . . Doing it informally is almost better for you.' In a sense we can see the trainee's point of view but, just as in record-keeping, 'if it is not documented then it did not happen'.

So, find innovative ways of documenting your informal reflections. You could tape or video your reflections or you could do a group reflection and complete the documentation together. Alternatively, you could ask your peers to document your attitudes to and practice in patient safety by recording discussions you have had with them. Many other methods of gathering evidence exist and they do not need to be paper-based. Treat your assessors to a multi-media synopsis of your competencies. The PMETB mentions many other types of evidence that can be included in a doctor's evidence of fitness to practice. These include examinations, trainers' reports, audit, research, critical incident review and video.

Here are just a few examples of other types of evidence for specific competency domains.

Good clinical care

History-taking, examination and record-keeping

- Anonymised clinical notes
- Video of a history or an examination, with patient's written permission

Safe prescribing

- Some completed anonymised drug charts you have filled
- Completed 'Yellow Card' (every doctor should do at least five a year)
- Audit of prescribing in your clinical area
- Reflections on prescribing errors you have made or 'near misses'
- DOPs completed by a pharmacist

Makes patient safety a priority in own clinical practice

- Completed audit presentation in PowerPoint
- Reflective learning tool on a critical incident
- Completed anonymised hospital incident form (preferably not one for someone who fell out of bed with 'no bony injury')
- Record of attending meeting on patient safety and clinical governance and reflections on what you learnt

Understands and applies the principles of medical ethics

- Certificate from completed online medical ethics course
- Reflections on reading book of ethics case studies
- Reflections on ethical dilemmas you have faced and how you dealt with them

Maintaining good medical practice

- Results of examinations
- Your learning plan and progress against it
- Trainer's report
- Evidence of online factual learning, e.g. www.BMJlearning.com

Teaching and training

- Evaluate your teaching using any standardised evaluation tool designed for the appropriate purpose. A simple tool could just ask for the best and worst aspects of a teaching session and 'how it could be improved'
- Personal reflections on a teaching episode using a formula such as 'What went well, what did not go so well, what would I do differently next time?'

Relationships with patients

- Communication skills: make a video of consultations (using your Trust's consent form for recording)
- Thank you cards from patients

GIVING AND RECEIVING FEEDBACK

Giving and receiving feedback is one of the hardest aspects of medicine, especially if the feedback is not good. Medicine has an inglorious history of giving mainly negative feedback and using sarcasm and humiliation as learning tools. Not surprisingly, people do not respond well to feedback delivered in this way, even if the content is correct. Increasingly, you will be asked to provide feedback on the performance of colleagues, including consultants and your fellow Foundation doctors. Multi-source feedback to doctors as part of their assessment is high stakes because it can determine progress and continued registration with the GMC. As you would hope to receive constructive feedback, it is your responsibility to give constructive feedback.

Box 6.5 Things to remember in giving feedback

Do:

- Make the feedback balanced: the recipient needs to know which behaviours to keep as well as those to change
- Give positive feedback, frequently and unreservedly and be fair and supportive rather than critical
- Base your feedback on specific examples if at all possible
- Make your feedback behavioural not subjective. This means giving feedback about something that is directly observable (e.g. 'badgering the nurses') rather than any assumptions you have made about why they did what they did ('she thinks she is above the nurses') or meaningless generalizations ('rude', 'irritating')
- Offer positive suggestions of alternative courses of action
- Beware the use of humour – this may well come out as sarcasm
- Own the comments
- Make it timely. Feedback about an event that occurred six months ago is not helpful!

Don't:

- Be afraid to make it unreservedly positive if there are no significant negatives. We tend to qualify even excellent performance with a big 'but'
- Be censorious
- Humiliate
- Use sarcasm

How can we ensure that feedback is fair but objective and that it is useful to the recipient?

The simple rules to remember are described in Box 6.5.

This section advises on how you should give feedback in your assessments of other Foundation colleagues (through mini-PAT or TAB) and suggests some ways of dealing with negative feedback that you may receive.

In this exercise, we will attempt to give feedback to one of our colleagues via the mini-PAT assessment and then put ourselves in their shoes.

Exercise

Your view as an assessor:

Jill is an F1 whom you have known as an undergraduate. She has been a high achiever and got a distinction. She has a lot of knowledge and can always answer questions on the ward round, but when it comes to an emergency she does not always choose the right option or always recognise that she is out of her depth. She is well known as being conscientious, spending a lot of time with patients and families, and frequently leaves work at 8.00 pm. In your dealings with her you have on occasion felt demeaned by her response when you have asked her for help and you have seen some irritation between Jill and the nurses at times, specifically around the issue of care of IV access lines. You have been asked to do a mini-PAT assessment four months into F1.

The completed mini-PAT form (Figure 6.1) shows that you have scored her well for her ability to diagnose patient problems and communication with patients and note-keeping. However, she is placed as borderline or 'below expectations' for time management, knowing her limitations and some aspects of working with colleagues. Your assessment is in keeping with others obtained on this occasion, particularly the nurses on the ward. Her educational supervisor receives the summary data and the free-text comments (Figure 6.2). How will she respond and will this feedback help her?

Jill's view:

You have always wanted to be a doctor and started off with much excitement and a passion to help your patients. Your hard work has paid off because you mostly understand what is happening with the patients and you have been able to find a couple of rare diseases that had not been thought of by the admitting medical team. The NHS is proving to be a tough place to work in and you frequently go home late. Standards are not what you had expected, but you are trying to improve things on your own ward. You are aware that this is creating some discord with the nurses but feel it is important for patient care.

You get the feedback from your mini-PAT and are really upset by it. Despite your conscientiousness you are rated as 'below expectations' in some areas and you are not sure what the free text comments mean. You see your educational supervisor who is supportive but cannot clarify what has led to your low ratings and the hurtful comments in the free text section.

Alternative scenario:

Jill's mini-PAT is completed with exactly the same scores but with new free text comments (Figure 6.3).

Jill is still concerned that despite her hard work she is 'below expectation' in some areas. However, she now has a better idea of what could be improved. Specific examples put things in context and help Jill see what is going wrong. Helpful suggestions are given of alternative ways of looking at the issues. The balance between 'doing well' and 'could improve' is much better. The writer has owned the comments and by putting things in the first person ('I would have . . .') will help Jill have permission to do things differently on future occasions.

Follow-up exercises

Try filling out some sample mini-PAT or TAB forms (download from www.mmc.nhs.uk/assessment) for people that you work with, or try the following case and stick to constructive, behavioural feedback.

6

Mini-PAT (Peer Assessment Tool)

How do you rate Jill in:	Below expectations for F1 completion		Borderline for F1 completion	Meets expectations for F1 completion	Above expectations for F1 completion		U/C*
	1	2	3	4	5	6	
Good clinical care							
1 Ability to diagnose patient problems	○	○	○	○	✓	○	○
2 Ability to formulate appropriate management plans	○	○	○	✓	○	○	○
3 Awareness of their own limitations	○	✓	○	○	○	○	○
4 Ability to respond to psychosocial aspects of illness	○	○	○	✓	○	○	○
5 Appropriate utilisation of resources e.g. ordering investigations	○	○	○	✓	○	○	○
Maintaining good medical practice							
6 Ability to manage time effectively/prioritise	○	✓	○	○	○	○	○
7 Technical skills (appropriate to current practise)	○	○	○	○	○	○	✓
Teaching and training, appraising and assessing							
8 Willingness and effectiveness when teaching/training colleagues	○	○	○	○	○	○	✓
Relationship with patients							
9 Communication with patients	○	○	○	✓	○	○	○
10 Communication with carers and/or family	○	○	○	✓	○	○	○
11 Respect for patients and their right to confidentiality	○	○	○	✓	○	○	○
Working with colleagues							
12 Verbal communication with colleagues	✓	○	○	○	○	○	○
13 Written communication with colleagues	○	○	○	✓	○	○	○
14 Ability to recognise and value the contribution of others	○	✓	○	○	○	○	○
15 Accessibility/Reliability	○	○	○	○	○	✓	○

* U/C Please mark this if you feel unable to comment.

Fig. 6.1 Mini-PAT scores for Jill.

134

Anything going especially well?

Jill is very conscientious – perhaps too so at times. Sometimes I think that Jill needs to 'get a life'.

Jill's knowledge is good but ...

Please describe any areas that you think she should particularly focus on for development:

Jill is irritating in the extreme. She makes me feel like a complete idiot and she thinks she is above the nurses.

She goes to pieces under pressure and has only been saved by the registrar turning up just in time.

She is not practical at all.

Your Signature: .... Date: ☐☐ / ☐☐ / ☐☐

8727612698

Fig. 6.2 Mini-PAT for Jill. Original free-text comments.

Anything going especially well?

Jill is very conscientious – in particular she is well known for spending a lot of time explaining things to patients.

Jill sets herself high standards. Her knowledge is fantastic – I would never have thought about Addison's for that patient last week. I am learning from her.

Her note keeping is meticulous – it's always easy to work out what's going on with her patients if you are called to see them out of hours.

Jill is the only F1 doctor I know who knows the positive predictive value for a D-dimer test.

Please describe any areas that you think Jill needs to particularly focus on for development.

I am a bit concerned that Jill tries to do too much alone. One example was the GI bleed last week. Jill was trying to sort everything out herself but the patient was getting worse. I would have called the registrar or F2 for help.

Jill's approach to others can get their backs up. Sometimes you have to tread gently. I agree that we should take people's iv access out when it is not needed but she upset the nurses in the way she suggested this. It might be better to take out the drip herself as an example or talk privately to the sister about it rather than badgering the nurses every day. I have noticed that the nurses are starting to make her life tough.

Jill – you are in danger of burn-out soon. It's OK to hand over the tasks at the end of your shift and go home on time!

Your Signature: .... Date: ☐☐ / ☐☐ / ☐☐

8727612698

Fig. 6.3 Mini-PAT for Jill. Revised free-text comments.

Joe is an F1 whom you have known as an undergraduate. He has always been a bit of a lad and wants to be a surgeon. He is popular with the nurses and other trainees. You are working together in a stroke unit. He is very helpful with procedures, and when patients are sick he is very proactive and knows exactly what to do. He is also very proactive in seeking agreement on treatment levels and 'do not resuscitate' orders from his seniors but does not always agree with the consensus. He attends the multidisciplinary discharge planning meeting every week, but often leaves to attend to acute problems on the ward such as patients going into AF. There have been several instances where you have not been able to contact him to hand over patients when you go off shift and when you share out tasks after the ward round he does not always do his fair share. On occasion he is late to work and complains of having a hangover on occasion.

Responding to feedback, or 'The most dangerous doctor is one who is not aware of their own weaknesses and limitations'

We have all received negative feedback at some point. It may have been from teachers, friends or parents, or indirectly when we did not succeed at something we thought we should have. Generally, as high achievers in academic life, doctors have received few knocks, but no matter how many times we have experienced it, it is still hard to take negative feedback. At some stage in your Foundation programme it is likely that you will get some.

Twenty years' experience working in the NHS shows that the most dangerous doctor is not the one who makes a mistake or does not know things, but the one who does not understand their weaknesses and does not learn from their mistakes, errors or mishaps. There is no shame in getting feedback that identifies areas where you need to develop or mistakes that you have made. Your assessors are not looking for a perfect portfolio. What they are looking for is someone who has achieved the basic competencies and shown they have the necessary learning skills and professional attributes to respond appropriately to feedback. Here is an exercise and some tips to help you deal with this and turn a negative experience into a positive experience.

Exercise

Jill has received the second set of feedback from the previous exercise on the use of mini-PAT. Put yourself in her shoes. Take a few minutes and think what you would be feeling and thinking when you receive this feedback.

- What are your possible emotional responses?
- What are your possible practical responses?
- In the long run, how could you use it to your advantage?

Emotional responses
Your initial response to negative feedback could include virtually any of the human emotions and in fact may go through several in a few minutes. You might recall Elizabeth Kübler-Ross's five stages of grief defined in her book

On Death and Dying (London: Macmillan, 1969) – denial, anger, bargaining, depression and acceptance – to help you understand what is happening. To these we might add a sixth emotion: blame.

Here we look at these responses and ways of dealing with feedback and some of the potential consequences if they go unchecked.

Denial or 'only seeing the positive': In general, Jill has done well and she should be pleased with her feedback. She already meets or exceeds performance in some areas and the feedback has identified some areas where a relatively small amount of development work could resolve the problem areas raised. It is great to get positive feedback and this will help Jill's confidence enormously. However, if she concentrates only on the positives she will fail to learn from the negatives. Jill may not see or may not accept the negative feedback she has received. She may explain it away by feeling the assessor has not been fair, or deciding they do not know all the facts, etc. There might be a temptation to try to bury the bad news by not entering the assessment in her portfolio. Be aware that 'burying bad news' is dishonest and would give rise to questions about your probity. If Jill does not listen to this feedback and work out a way forward, the areas of her practice that give rise to concern will not go away and could threaten her career or her happiness at work in due course.

Anger and blame: Negative feedback, even when balanced with positive, might well make Jill feel angry with her assessors. A degree of anger may be normal but there is a need to move on and try to assess the meaning of the feedback. Don't shoot the messenger. It is not going to serve Jill well if she blames others or seeks revenge, even if subconsciously. It is also dangerous to assume that certain free text comments came from one individual. Don't harbour a grudge and certainly don't let your feedback influence what you write for someone else's feedback.

Bargaining or 'explaining away': In this context, we can view bargaining as explaining away or being due only to a particular circumstance or from a particular individual and therefore of little significance. This may allow Jill to justify her actions and ignore the feedback. We must accept that feedback is, in the majority of cases, given honestly and fairly, even if we disagree with it. This is part of 'being able to see ourselves as others see us'. Again, there is significant risk in assuming that negative free text comments must have been written by a particular individual and therefore have little meaning. In my experience, people's assumptions about who has given feedback are often wrong and can lead to resentment towards an individual whom we wrongly blame for another's comments.

Depression or 'only seeing the negative': Doctors tend to be quite critical of themselves and others and frequently over-weigh negative comments rather than accept positive comments. Jill sets high standards for herself and there is a danger of generalizing from comments that say she is not perfect and therefore feeling that everything must be bad. Jill may well see the scores of 'below expectations' in four areas and not acknowledge the seven 'meets expectations' and two 'exceeds expectations', even though she is only four months into post. She may ignore the very positive free-text comments.

Jill must keep things in perspective and see that there is a way out of any situation and concentrate on turning this into a positive learning experience.

Acceptance: We may not like the feedback and our initial responses may well be denial, anger, depression or bargaining or a mixture of all of these. In time, Jill will benefit from accepting the constructive feedback and learning from it. It may well be that she will need to take additional actions before she can do this. It can take quite a long time to understand the feedback we receive and its meaning, and to work out a way to respond to it.

Seeking further feedback

If Jill does not believe this feedback or if negative feedback has not been specific enough to know its meaning she should seek more feedback, either through the use of more assessments or by talking to a trusted colleague, to add greater meaning or verify it. Her educational supervisor or clinical tutor should be able to help her. Alternatives include peers or a trained mentor. Nurse educators have often got a lot of training in giving feedback and helping learners reflect on it, so choosing a nurse you work with may also be helpful.

HOW WILL ALL THIS EVIDENCE BE ASSESSED AND WHAT IS THE PASS MARK?

At the end of each Foundation year you will need to demonstrate your competencies and have them assessed. This is one area where the Foundation assessment finds it difficult to live up to the fourth PMETB criterion for assessment, that the standard for passing an assessment must be clear and transparent. The criteria for passing the Foundation programme assessment remain a 'global assessment' of the evidence offered in your portfolio by someone with expertise.

The process for final assessment may vary and has not yet been clarified at a national level, but in general will rely on four stages:

1. Completion of a summary of the evidence of your performance by you or your educational supervisor, using the evidence from your portfolio
2. Your educational supervisor signing off that it is an accurate summary
3. An assessment of that summary by a panel of assessors in a process called a Record of In Training Assessment (RITA)
4. The issuing (or not) of a certificate of satisfactory completion of Foundation training or one of several other possibilities, described below

The second version of the Foundation curriculum makes the assessment process a little clearer. It states that 'there is no expectation that a formal assessment of every detailed competence will be undertaken, rather the assessment will involve sampling from among the detailed competencies' but that 'a doctor who is experiencing difficulty . . . will require more of their practice to be sampled than one who is performing consistently'.

COMPLETING YOUR EVIDENCE SUMMARY

You are required to offer evidence that you have attained each of the competencies. Much guidance has been issued in the Foundation *Rough Guide* and in the guidance for the portfolio. You need to describe what the evidence is for each domain and what it shows. For example, for evidence of your skills in the acute management of chest pain you could specify that you have DOPs, mini-CEX, a representative anonymised clerking and drug chart that show that you make a full assessment, do a comprehensive examination, fully inform the patient of treatment options and prescribe appropriately.

Once you have completed the evidence summary your educational supervisor will need to sign off that it is an accurate record of your achievements, but in most deaneries the final assessment is made by a RITA panel. In specialist training the RITA is usually completed face to face, so that you have a chance to explain your evidence and so that the panel can help you plan your learning for the following year. It is unclear whether Foundation RITAs will be face-to-face or paper exercises. Certainly in some deaneries the line being taken is that verbal evidence is not rigorous enough to be taken into account in decision-making so only the paper-based summary and the portfolio are being used with no personal meeting. Only trainees who are borderline or are going to get a RITA C or D are invited for interview.

OUTCOMES FROM THE ASSESSMENTS

In F1 the outcome is merely 'pass or fail' in terms of being signed off for full registration.

The outcomes from RITA are expressed in legal terms for SpRs and subject to legal statute (Box 6.6). There is not, as far as we are aware, any legal statute for the RITA process in the Foundation programme, but the possible outcomes are the same. Basically, a RITA C means 'carry on full steam', a RITA D that there is some aspect of your practice that requires closer attention and there should be clear and specific targets for you to achieve in a specified timeframe. You will probably be allowed to continue to the next step of training. A RITA E means that you have not finished the period of training satisfactorily and that you need to repeat some of the training or practice with closer supervision for a period until reassessment indicates that the competencies have been reached. In effect, a RITA E is likely to mean that you will not be able to progress to specialist training immediately until competency has been demonstrated.

Box 6.6   The three possible outcomes from the RITA panel

RITA C Record of satisfactory progress

RITA D Recommendation for targeted training

RITA E Recommendation for repeat of experience or intensified supervision

Reasons why you may get a RITA D or E:

- Generally poor scores on assessments
- Very poor scores on one of the assessments
- Anything that indicates that your practice is not safe
- Insufficient evidence presented to the panel in the evidence summary
- Lack of engagement with the teaching process, particularly attendance at organised teaching
- Concerns raised by your educational or clinical supervisors even if assessments appear satisfactory
- Outstanding grievance procedures

You should arrive at your RITA panel knowing roughly what the assessment is likely to conclude. The dual formative/summative nature of the Foundation programme assessments means that you will have had many results fed back to you and you will have been able to see how your performance relates to that of your peers around the country. If you are having problems, your educational supervisor and probably programme director will have been speaking to you on a regular basis.

Provided that you have engaged with the teaching and assessment process, gathered the minimum dataset, presented it satisfactorily and been reasonably competent, you are highly likely to get a RITA C. Less than 5% of Foundation doctors are predicted to be given D, and E should be very rare indeed.

If you do get a RITA D or E it is not the end of your career. Treat it as a wake-up call and learn from it. The most important thing is that you know exactly why you have been given the D or E and that the panel helps you to sort out some SMART objectives to rectify the problem and carry on with training. At the panel you may be too upset to take this in and to discuss the future coolly. If you do not get clear reasons why you have not been given a C, make sure that you follow this up. This is the time that you really do need SMART objectives to know where you are going and how you will get there.

There will be an appeals process for people who get a RITA D or E and some trainees have taken legal action to review their assessments. Appealing or challenging the assessment carries risk. It seems likely that the appeals process will only overturn decisions that are based on factually incorrect data (e.g. if you were downgraded because of poor attendance at teaching but can demonstrate that your attendance was satisfactory). If you are considering appealing, seek advice or mentoring from a senior colleague you respect.

NOTE ABOUT THE FUTURE

The draft revision of the Foundation curriculum published for discussion in September 2006 outlines a few problem areas with the assessment system. In particular, it appears to question the grading system for the formal assessments that appear to give the same meanings for grades 1 and 2 ('below expectations') and that the use of 'borderline' as a descriptor for grade 3 means that the assessor is relieved of having to decide whether the trainee is satisfactory or not. In particular, the AoRMC is concerned that these grades will not prove defensible in a court if challenged by a trainee who has been failed. They also suggest that the current assessments do not assess probity and that several of the domains of *Good Medical Practice* are not well covered. They also assert that most of the assessment methods tap competence (what you are observed doing under controlled conditions) rather than performance (what you do in everyday practice) because they take place in specially organised formats (especially DOPs and mini-CEX) outside of normal working practice.

SUMMARY

This chapter has taken you through the background to the new assessment system, why it was introduced and how you should approach the task of gathering evidence for the assessments. Good luck in your assessments. Remember to hold on to your portfolio for ever. If you ever want to seek registration in another country it will demonstrate the competencies you have achieved, and if your registration here is ever challenged you will have a ready-made bank of evidence to defend yourself.

A brief account of the Foundation programme for people involved in the training of Foundation doctors

Mark Welfare

> **❝** Give a man a fish and he is fed for one meal, teach him to fish and he will never go hungry.**❞**
>
> Chinese proverb

INTRODUCTION

The only constant in the NHS is change, and the shake-up of doctors' training reflects that culture. Many of you will not like some or all of the changes that have come about through the Foundation programme and the rest of the Modernizing Medical Careers initiative. We can argue that they have led to problems in workforce planning, that they were rushed and lacking in evidence, that they have thrown the baby of experience out with the bathwater of competency, that shorter training will damage the consultant system and many more issues besides. This book does not argue for or against the changes, but acknowledges that, like it or not, they are here to stay and we have a responsibility to engage with the process to the benefit of our trainees. We cannot turn the clock back, and our trainees need our support to negotiate the system and get the best out of their learning opportunities.

This chapter gives some background to the changes of the Foundation programme and covers the practicalities of how to help your trainee through educational and clinical supervision, developing an educational plan, reviewing their assessments and giving effective feedback, and outlines your responsibilities in signing training off.

You may find other chapters relevant to your needs as a trainer. Chapter 1 reviews the changes that the Foundation programme has brought about and why they were made to give you the historical context. Chapter 5 reviews the curriculum for the Foundation programme and what trainees are expected to learn and advises them on planning their learning and maximising educational opportunities. Chapter 6 describes the assessment process in detail and in particular looks at better ways of giving feedback. Chapter 8 looks ahead to the rest of Foundation doctors' career and how they can use the Foundation programme to progress. It may be helpful to you in offering careers guidance. Chapter 9 looks at performance, being a doctor in difficulty and when others make trainees' lives difficult. The last chapter is a resource of contacts and potted summaries of each specialty.

Trainees may choose to read this chapter if only to get a feel for what the main issues are for trainers and an idea of what they can expect from an ideal or idealised supervisor.

SO, WHY GET INVOLVED IN EDUCATING FOUNDATION DOCTORS?

There are many motivations for getting involved in the education, support and assessment of Foundation doctors. Being active in teaching also ensures that we keep up to date and often results in our learning more about our own practice and learning needs. We can all remember one or more clinicians who supported us in our younger days, who nurtured us and gave us timely and appropriate feedback. Without their support, we may not have made it to where we are today. Many of us will wish to repay that debt by helping those who follow us. Bringing on a trainee can give us intense personal satisfaction and more positive strokes than our clinical work. We may also be concerned to maintain the standards of our profession, to smooth out the changes in the education system and make sure that we improve the delivery of education to these doctors. Finally, we may be motivated by a degree of self-interest – education is fun and provides us with variety in our working week, or we may be seeking recognition, such as for discretionary points or academic promotion.

DEFINITION OF THE TERMS INVOLVED IN SUPPORTING A TRAINEE

Traditionally, trainees had a different supervisor for each post that they worked in and house officers in particular had individual supervisors for each of their six-month posts. The title of this role could have been educational supervisor, clinical supervisor, plain old supervisor or even appraiser. These terms were used interchangeably and without a clear understanding of the responsibilities. For example, in psychiatry an educational supervisor was supposed to deliver two hours' teaching a week to an individual trainee. When trainees were attached to one consultant firm and worked day and night with them, the old models may have been adequate. However, revised work practices, shift systems and changing expectations have meant that the old system needed to change. Trainees need direct clinical supervision whilst in a post, but they also need continuity as they go through the two-year period. It would, for example, be difficult to plan your career if you had to start discussions on career options with a new supervisor every four months. This continuity is given by the educational supervisor. Box 7.1 reviews the main functions needed in supporting a trainee. The Operational Framework for the Foundation programme gives helpful definitions of the different supervisory and support roles based on *The New Doctor*.

Educational supervisor

This is the doctor responsible for making sure that the Foundation trainee receives appropriate training and experience. They are responsible for simple

> **Box 7.1 Summary of the main functions required to support and supervise an individual trainee**
>
> | | |
> |---|---|
> | Help them plan their overall learning | ES |
> | Monitor their overall development | ES |
> | Help them plan and manage their career. Careers advice | ES |
> | Sounding board to deal with pastoral issues and allow reflection on own overall performance | ES |
> | Help them plan assessments and keep them on track | ES |
> | Feedback assessments such as mini-PAT or TAB | ES |
> | Help them reflect on overall assessments | ES |
> | Let them know what is expected. Induction at departmental level | CS |
> | Help them plan learning in a particular clinical environment | CS |
> | Teach them clinical medicine based in service | CS |
> | Monitor their performance on a day-to-day basis in terms of patient safety | CS |
> | Feedback on their day-to-day clinical performance | CS |
> | Complete assessments | CS and others |
> | Sign off that they have completed an attachment satisfactorily | CS or ES |

ES = educational supervisor; CS = clinical supervisor

careers advice and guidance in most circumstances. Education supervision meeting is probably the best descriptor for the unit of time devoted to educational supervision. In some areas this is also referred to as an education review. In most parts of the country the Foundation trainee has the same educational supervisor throughout the two years. Together with the clinical supervisor, the educational supervisor decides whether individual placements have been completed successfully.

Clinical supervisor

The professional (not necessarily a consultant or even a doctor) responsible for teaching and supervising the Foundation trainee in the everyday working environment. They can sign off the form at end of post to confirm its satisfactory completion. The clinical supervisor should meet the trainee when they start a new post and induct them into the department and ward. One person may well be clinical supervisor for several trainees, so making the induction process more efficient. The information required for departmental induction is listed in Box 7.2.

Mentoring

Mentoring is a specific type of confidential support characterised by a non-judgemental and supportive relationship with someone who has no responsibility for progress or assessment and who has usually been chosen by the mentee. Mentoring usually helps trainees deal with more complex issues that

---

Box 7.2 What is needed for departmental or practice induction

- The type of clinical problems they are likely to encounter
- The protocols in use on the unit/practice and any variation between seniors
- Day-to-day responsibilities
- The division of labour between F1, F2 and specialty trainees
- Relationships with other staff members, including the manager who is responsible for them during the attachment
- The level of clinical responsibility they are expected to reach during the post
- Who to contact for clinical advice when needed
- Arrangements for ward cover during holidays and study leave, including clear guidance on how many staff members can be away at any one time
- The learning opportunities in the post
- The weekly timetable for the rest of the team, including GPs, consultants and career grade doctors if they are responsible for providing clinical advice
- Relationships with other professions that are key to their work and learning, including district and specialist nurses, health visitors and midwives and the learning opportunities provided by allied health professionals
- On-call arrangements
- Procedures for reporting sickness absence

---

cannot be dealt with by their educational supervisor or that they do not wish to be dealt with by their educational supervisor.

Coaching

One of the seven pillars of the Foundation programme is that it should be 'coached'. There does not appear to be a universally accepted definition of coaching as applied to the Foundation programme. It seems to imply an active role in encouraging and building skills with the trainee. Essentially, coaching seems similar to educational supervision.

Appraisal

This term has been used in the past to refer to the process of feeding back to a trainee on their performance and helping them to plan their learning. As appraisal now has a more specific meaning in the context of consultant performance review and does not incorporate all elements required for the support of a Foundation trainee this term has been superseded.

Assessment

Assessment refers to the process of judging the trainee's performance against set criteria or competencies. The trainee is responsible for organizing their own work-based assessments which contribute to the final assessment of attainment (or not) of successful completion. There are two stages of attainment – at the end of the first year the trainee has to have evidence that they have met the criteria for full registration with the GMC, and at the end of the second year they have to have evidence of reaching the Foundation competencies. The evidence is presented in their portfolio. They are required to detail the evidence that they have gathered towards each competency in the summary of evidence, and the educational supervisor is required to sign off that this is an honest and correct record. A third party, usually in the form of a Record of In Training Assessment (RITA) panel, is then required to assess the summary of evidence against the competencies and judge whether the standard has been reached.

TRUST RESPONSIBILITIES

The Trust has a number of roles in ensuring that the trainee's experience is maximised. These are described formally by the MMC under the Quality Assurance procedures for the Foundation programme and are monitored annually. They include the provision of Trust induction, the appointment of the educational supervisor, the provision of an adequate teaching programme and the implementation of policies relating to hours, pay and the prevention of bullying.

Trust induction

MMC requires that Trust induction covers three main points: training in the use of the portfolio and assessment tools; infection control standards; and the use of the hospital handbook. However, induction to the Trust serves many masters other than the requirements of the Foundation programme, including those of the CNST, which requires at a minimum that healthcare workers' skills are checked and signed off before they perform a procedure and that they are trained in any technology that they use. The Trust will want to ensure that trainees have been given information related to health and safety, such as what to do in the event of a needlestick injury, and lifting and handling. Clinical governance will want to inform trainees about the reporting systems and audit protocols. Radiology will want to mention the regulations on requesting and authorizing x-rays. Human Resources and Occupational Health will have their own agenda. Education, research and many other departments will find there is something that they need to tell all new doctors. Finally, trainees will want to know about their pay and conditions, contract, IT access, use of IT systems, geography of the workplace, etc.

It is easy for Trust induction to grow and grow and for a full day of induction to be stuffed full of facts that cannot all be taken in. Increasingly, induction is being delivered as an ongoing process involving a number of innovative methods. Some Trusts send new employees a CD or DVD with much of the information on it. In Scotland a Web-based system is used. One of its strengths is that it also records the fact that trainees have received the information, which is essential for legal and governance reasons, and can even test them. Another innovation is to get rid of lecture-style presentations and provide a multi-station roadshow-type presentation which utilises small-group teaching methods (*BMJ* Careers Focus, 16 September 2006, pp. 106–107).

TEACHING AND LEARNING IN THE FOUNDATION PROGRAMME

The curriculum for the Foundation programme was put together by the Academy of Medical Royal Colleges and is based on the GMC's seven components of *Good Medical Practice* with the addition of a supplementary component: Acute Care. The curriculum is described in detail in Chapter 5. It has a strong focus on 'professionalism' and could be viewed as rather light on knowledge-based outcomes, particularly if they do not relate to acute care. Hospital teaching systems for house officers used to rely on a weekly tutorial designed chiefly to impart factual knowledge to new doctors, mainly to help them shift their skills from history-taking, examination and diagnosis, which they should have learnt at medical school, and on to the management aspects. Simple lectures or review of typical cases using small-group teaching methods sufficed. However, the shift in priorities to teaching professionalism requires the use of more innovative and participative teaching methods.

The Trusts are mandated by the GMC and COPMED to give every F1 doctor one hour a week of bleep-free formal education designed for F1s only. This has to include professionalism. This is equivalent to seven days a year and is sometimes delivered in blocks rather than as discrete hours each week. They are also required to have two additional hours of education relevant to them in protected, bleep-free time, presumably within their clinical teams. For F2s, the expectation is a minimum of three hours' formal, bleep-free and relevant education each week.

In designing the teaching and learning programme for the Foundation programme we should take into account the curriculum and some theory and evidence about learning in medicine. Theories about adult learning abound, but most agree that learning is best when:

- Trainees are motivated and actively involved
- Learning is relevant
- Aims and objectives are clear
- A variety of learning methods are used
- Trainees are able to reflect on their experience
- Trainees get feedback on how they are doing
- Learning is fun

Some theories suggest that individuals have preferred learning styles although the evidence base for this is a bit thin. Honey and Mumford identified four main styles – Activist, Theorist, Reflector and Pragmatist (see page 100). Other models rely on the way in which people prefer to process information, such as the visual–aural–kinaesthetic model. Visual learners, for example, benefit from seeing notes or pictures when being taught, so learning on a ward round without visual aids may not suit them. Aural learners are presumably good at absorbing information mentioned on ward rounds. These are people who are good at languages and can always remember your name even if they have been told it just once. Kinaesthetic learners are likely to be good at learning in practical situations such as ALS courses and in learning practical skills on the job. They find it difficult to sit for long periods and learn in lectures.

In reality, many learners adopt mixed styles or adapt their learning style to the task in hand. It also seems that learning that occurs through a variety of methods is deeper. What is most important is that learners are given a variety of opportunities for learning so that you can cover the needs of a variety of learners and that the information or skills are learnt by each individual in more than one way.

The evidence also suggests that skills are best learnt when active practice is a part of the learning method (e.g. use of video in communication skills or simulation for practical skills). Doing paper-based cases may help trainees to some extent, but it is the application of knowledge and skills in the workplace that seems to be an issue for many of our trainees. For example, on ward rounds and on our Medical Admissions Unit, I repeatedly see patients with shock being under-treated and the severity of their condition not recognised despite the fact that the trainees have done an ALERT and ILS course so I know that they have been taught this material in a practical session. We need better means of translating learning to clinical practice in a way that enables the patient to be kept safe but allows us to feed back and monitor our trainees' performance.

Finally, remember the Chinese proverb about teaching and learning: 'Give a man a fish and he has one meal, teach him to fish and he will never go hungry'. There are clear parallels in the way in which you interact with your trainees. It is all too easy to teach the right answer to a limited clinical problem rather than concentrating on general principles. (See Chapter 5 for further discussion of a practical example of how to teach a general principle rather than an isolated fact.)

So, acknowledging this theory and the curriculum, a typical teaching programme for F1 might look like Figure 7.1. There is a continuous spiral of on-the-job learning opportunities (also called opportunistic or experiential learning), supplemented by weekly clinical teaching (this covers the diagnosis and management of common conditions) and longer sessions covering the professionalism agenda and which offer the chance for deeper learning. This is supported by regular educational supervision meetings. This programme addresses some of the criteria for maximising learning – it has mixed opportunities and methods, its aims and objectives are clear because it addresses the curriculum and therefore it should be relevant to the trainees' needs. The remaining challenges are to involve trainees, to ensure that, in the busy world of the NHS, the trainees get adequate feedback on how they are doing on an everyday basis so that they can reflect and to make it fun!

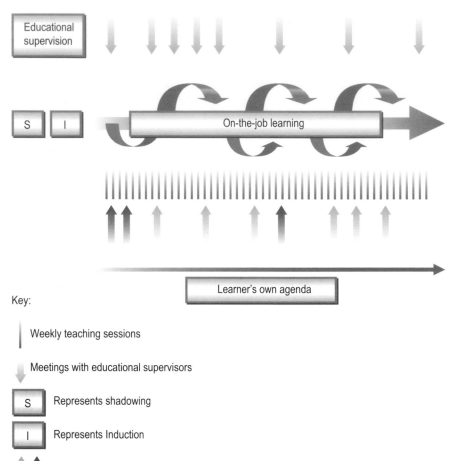

Key:

Weekly teaching sessions

Meetings with educational supervisors

S   Represents shadowing

I   Represents Induction

Represent episodes of formal teaching such as generic skills or ALS course

Fig. 7.1   Representation of teaching and learning opportunities in a Foundation programme.

Learning opportunities offered in the Foundation programme might include:

On-the-job learning

This is described in more detail below because it is probably the most critical part of the scheme.

Small-group learning, such as case studies, mini-lectures, illustrative patients, data interpretation, journal clubs, protocol and guideline development, significant event analysis

The traditional weekly lunchtime hour of teaching definitely has its place. Trainees should, however, have the opportunity to input into the curriculum design and the shape of the sessions.

One-to-one teaching, such as educational supervision and case-based discussion

Trainees will get one-to-one teaching with consultants. Educational supervision should be regarded as having a teaching element, especially in the areas of the trainee managing their own learning and in the effect of the consultant's role modelling of professionalism. Case-based discussion is part of the assessment system for the Foundation trainee but it has formative as well as summative purposes and is probably valued by the trainees more than any other assessment. Trainees only have to do six CbDs a year, but if CbDs were to become a key learning tool rather than mainly summative assessment, there could be no limit on the number that they do each year.

External courses

The resuscitation industry has developed and standardised courses for resuscitation that use a lot of the study leave budget but provide quality assured learning outcomes. This model of educational delivery is being extended to other areas as courses like ALERT are patented and become expensive. There is now a host of courses for dealing with the sick patient. Courses in, for example, cultural diversity and legal issues may well follow. There would seem to be added value in standardised and validated courses replacing a lot of stand-alone teaching sessions continuously reinvented every year in every Trust, as long as the cost does not become prohibitive.

Personal study

The learning opportunities should include time for personal study – time for using CD-Rom and online resources or for personal reflection, practice for exams, reading journals, etc. Trainees report, however, that time for personal study is less in the reduced working week and their commitment to working at home is variable. The chance to include timetabled, trainee-selected modules (akin to the student-selected modules of the undergraduate curriculum) will improve as the increased numbers of Foundation trainees reduce the pressure on timetables. The use of tasters for trainees to gain experience in specialties that they may wish to pursue is described later. Online teaching resources are proliferating and any list given here will quickly become out of date. The materials available at www.bmjlearning.com include systems for creating learning plans and assessing learning needs as well as a wealth of knowledge-based learning about specific diseases.

Audit – both understanding the background and doing it to achieve change

Audit needs to be put into the context of patient safety, which is a major part of the professionalism agenda. It is amazing how much more attractive a teaching session appears to trainees when it has 'patient safety' in the title rather than 'audit and governance'. Trainees should still get the experience of doing audit during their Foundation programme. This works best if they can choose something that is relevant to them and their practice, but hopefully is aligned to issues that are important at Trust or national level, such as documentation by trainees, the use of routine observations on the ward, prescribing errors, NSF targets, etc. Trainees will need support in negotiating

Trust registration systems, in formulating their audit and in ensuring that action is taken to close the audit loop.

Simulated clinical situation

Simulation can teach clinical skills such as resuscitation, examination and managing difficult cases, such as trauma or the acutely ill medical patient. But when used in a sophisticated manner, simulation is also excellent for teaching teamwork. This requires the necessary equipment and environment as well as the input of teachers with sufficient skill in this area. The use of simulators is likely to grow in the future.

Practical skills

When asked to identify their learning needs, trainees rate the development of advanced practical skills very highly. We are not talking here about cannulation and obtaining a blood gas sample which appear in the Foundation programme assessment documents. No, the trainees of today are still trying to disprove the sixth rule of the Fat Man in *The House of God* (New York: Dell, 1978), 'there is no bodily cavity that cannot be reached with a number 14 needle and a good strong arm'. This trainee-led learning need is recognised in the Scottish system, which suggests that there should be a chance to extend practical skills to lumbar puncture and aspiration of body cavities. But, with reduced hours, more non-invasive investigation and increasing specialization of their seniors, the opportunities are getting fewer. So, we need to create new ways of developing trainees' practical skills. Simulation is a key method and practical skills courses are springing up all round the country. However, they tend to be very resource-intensive with a high trainer-to-trainee ratio. We need more and better trainers. It is a rewarding area to teach because the trainees love it. A useful reference for the proper performance of practical skills is Nicola Cooper, Kirsty Forrest and Paul Cramp's *Essential Guide to Acute Care* (Oxford: Blackwell, 2006).

The revised Foundation programme curriculum includes the aspiration to learn more advanced and invasive procedures.

Role modelling

The effect of role models on the development of medical students and junior doctors cannot be underestimated. This has been eloquently described by Jodi Skiles, a senior student from Indiana University School of Medicine ('Teaching professionalism: a medical student's view', *The Clinical Teacher* 2005, 2: 66–71). She describes how, in an era of increased emphasis an professionalism in the formal curriculum, students have become increasingly cynical and sceptical. She highlights the mismatch between the idealised contents of the written curriculum and the behaviour of seniors they observe every day as a potential cause and reminds seniors that 'the example you are setting on a daily basis is reflective of the legacy that you hope to leave in the profession of medicine'. To this we might add the example set by the leaders of the NHS in, for example, the development of a target culture and the way in which many perceive international medical graduates to have been poorly treated.

Teaching professionalism

Teaching professionalism is one of the big challenges of meeting the Foundation programme curriculum and covers areas such as safe prescribing, patient safety, communication and consultation skills, teamwork and time management, recognizing diversity and gaining cultural competence, consent and legal issues, evidence-based medicine, managing your own learning and teaching others. It will involve new teaching methods and skills for many of us as teachers and indeed may mean that we have to look again at our own practice.

There are some resources available for teaching aspects of professionalism, but in general these are not as well developed as, say, the resources and courses for teaching clinical skills or resuscitation. The excellent series of articles from the *BMJ*'s Careers Focus on Competencies for the Foundation programme (accessible through the MMC website www.mmc.nhs.uk/pages/ news, e.g. No. 5, 4 February 2006 on 'Leadership and teamwork') gives some pointers. The Royal College of Physicians has developed an excellent series of small-group teaching sessions ('Laying the foundations for good medical practice'), which comes with all teaching materials, lesson plans and additional resources (go to www.rcplondon.ac.uk and search for 'Laying the foundations'). We have used these materials and found them to be generally excellent and great value.

There is also a centrally developed series of websites with teaching materials related to professionalism (www.healthcareskills.nhs.uk, www.teamworking.nhs.uk, www.ethicsandlaw.nhs.uk, www.patientsafety.nhs.uk). Obviously, there are limits to what can be learnt using this format, but it is a start. A small-group teaching session on safe prescribing has been piloted in London and is likely to be rolled out across the country.

Communication and consultation skills are best taught with the use of video and role play, although there is an NHS website devoted to this area (www.communicationskills.nhs.uk). We have found the Calgary Cambridge framework for teaching consultation skills to be valuable and many students are now familiar with its structure. If you don't know it, we suggest that it may be helpful. It is amazing how just a little theory and a structure for both the anatomy of the consultation and the teaching method facilitate successful learning. This is not the place to summarise the Calgary Cambridge technique, but courses in its methodology are available and the accompanying books (e.g. J. Silverman, S. Kurtz and J. Draper, *Skills for Communicating with Patients* and S. Kurtz, J. Silverman and J. Draper, *Teaching and Learning Communications Skills in Medicine*, both Oxford: Radcliffe, 2004) are excellent. There is also a website giving many details (www.skillscascade.com). Useful reminder cards are available from Jonathan Silverman (js355@medschl.cam.ac.uk). These summarise the essential points of the method.

One limitation of the Calgary Cambridge model is that it is suited mainly to out-patient and GP-type consultations. However, Foundation doctors encounter patients in many scenarios where the content and construct of the interaction is not the same as the consultation model. Indeed, approximately 20% of medical in-patients are probably too confused to follow the model. Some teachers of communication skills focus more on the skills that need to be learnt rather than the model. This should ensure that the skills can be used in any context, whether a short daily interaction on the ward, clerking of patients, interactions in A&E or interactions with carers. One book that takes this approach to the teaching of communication skills is Peter Maguire's *Communication Skills for Doctors* (London: Hodder Arnold, 2000).

GIVING EFFECTIVE FEEDBACK AND ON-THE-JOB TEACHING

Effective feedback underpins on-the-job learning and improving these two facets of our performance as educators would probably lead to the most significant leap forward in trainees' learning. There is not sufficient space in this book to go into great detail, but some guidance and background is given here.

The number of hours at work before a doctor becomes a consultant has been reduced from approximately 30,000 by as much as 50%. It is clear, therefore, that we need to make more of on-the-job learning opportunities such as ward rounds, consultations in GP or out-patient clinics, procedures such as central lines and LPs, theatre and investigative sessions such as endoscopy. Trainees learn better when they have the chance to reflect on their clinical experiences and when mistakes or misconceptions are corrected quickly. Learning is more effective when it is coached than when it occurs by osmosis because clinical experience without feedback can lead to repetition of the error. But in an era of fast patient turn-round, particularly the four-hour trolley wait in Casualty, the erosion of consultant-led teams and frequently changing shifts, the feedback loop to trainees has been eroded. Clinical systems, particularly for admissions, need to be aligned with the learning needs of trainees, particularly when the majority of immediate acute care is still delivered by trainees.

It may be helpful to think of Kolb's learning cycle (Figure 7.2) when undertaking clinical teaching. Kolb suggests that idealised learning consists of four stages – doing something, reflecting on how it has gone, thinking about what you would do differently next time, and planning for that change before doing it again. This is easily translated into what happens in a clinical teaching situation and may help you understand your role better.

Imagine you are half-way through a post-take ward round and a trainee has presented a case of someone who has represented with headache following a brief admission with headache and normal CT and LP and presumptive diagnosis of migraine. On hearing the history you feel that the features are now typical for a post-LP headache, but the trainee's diagnosis is migraine and stress and they have had a bit of a dispute when trying to discharge the patient from Casualty. On questioning and probing, the trainee is stuck on their diagnosis and has not thought about post-LP headache. They appear to be lacking in knowledge (about the causes of headache) and may also have some problems with listening to the patient and seeing things from their point of view. They are not following Kolb's learning cycle and are stuck in the box

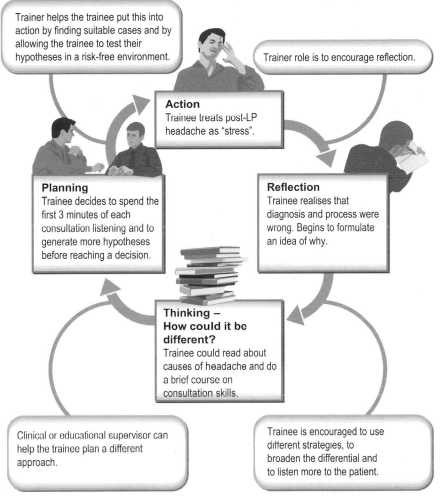

Trainer helps the trainee put this into action by finding suitable cases and by allowing the trainee to test their hypotheses in a risk-free environment.

Trainer role is to encourage reflection.

Action
Trainee treats post-LP headache as "stress".

Planning
Trainee decides to spend the first 3 minutes of each consultation listening and to generate more hypotheses before reaching a decision.

Reflection
Trainee realises that diagnosis and process were wrong. Begins to formulate an idea of why.

Thinking – How could it be different?
Trainee could read about causes of headache and do a brief course on consultation skills.

Clinical or educational supervisor can help the trainee plan a different approach.

Trainee is encouraged to use different strategies, to broaden the differential and to listen more to the patient.

Fig. 7.2 Kolb's learning cycle

of doing without reflecting on what might be going wrong. Your first job is to help them reflect on what has gone wrong and why. If this stage is handled sensitively this should lead to the development of general principles they should focus on in the future. Examples include developing a broader differential, looking for things that don't fit the pattern and taking the patient's view into account. Finally, in the planning stage they may think that to achieve this they need to seek more feedback and more advanced teaching on consultation skills. Using the model below we hope you can take them through this cycle in just a minute!

The one-minute preceptor

A useful model for the development of on the job learning techniques is the 'one-minute preceptor'. For a useful teaching session go to: www.med.uiuc.

edu/facultydev/Clinical Environ or Google it and the site will be found. This model acknowledges that in clinical situations the trainee spends around 10 minutes with the senior on each patient but that nine minutes of this is taken up with the presentation of the case and clarifying the content (e.g. checking drug history), leaving only one minute for active teaching. The model seeks to maximise the use of this one minute in six simple steps:

1. Get the trainee to commit to a diagnosis or management plan
2. Probe their ideas and evidence for the decision
3. Reinforce what was done well
4. Give guidance on errors or omissions
5. Teach a general principle
6. Summarise and conclude

Refer to the online teaching session detailed above for more details, but this is a very powerful technique for maximising the benefits from short opportunities. The technique could also be used as the basis for the longer CbDs that form part of the Foundation programme assessment system.

Other factors known to enhance on-the-job learning

These include:

- 'The single most important factor influencing learning is what the learner already knows. Ascertain that and teach him accordingly' (David Ausubel). In other words, start with where the trainee is.
- Planning – if time is rushed, ask the trainees to direct you to the sickest patients or to the cases where they have the most uncertainty.
- Summarising – at the end of the round or clinic, ask the trainee to summarise what they have learnt and provide your own summary of the main points covered.
- Make sure that you cover generic skills as well as clinical matters – for example, a post-take ward round could focus on the trainee's skills in prioritisation, team working, negotiating skills (how might you have ensured that the patient did get the CT head?), help-seeking behaviour, etc.
- Questioning style – appropriate use of open and closed questions. Open questions allow the trainee to display their knowledge. Start with simple questions and build on the answers. If an incorrect answer is given, don't ignore it but explore why it has been given and correct misconceptions.
- Avoid 'knight's move' questions. These require the trainee to guess the answer to one step before they can answer the second part. They require knight's move thinking to get the right answer. They usually ask about very esoteric subjects, e.g. 'if this patient had a positive LKM antibody, what would the prognosis be?' requires that they know (or can guess) that LKM antibodies are associated with autoimmune liver disease and that they know what the prognosis of this disease is.
- Making best use of opportunities. Spend a few minutes reflecting on how your clinical work is organised and whether the learning opportunities

are maximised – for example, clinic can be passively observed (useful for very inexperienced trainees or to observe seniors' consultation skills in action) or trainees can see a patient and report to you, or the patient can be reviewed by the senior. Each has its place. Theatre has many potential learning opportunities but these are not always maximised. Make a list of opportunities that are appropriate for Foundation-level doctors.

- Teach general principles rather than facts. It is probably more helpful to a trainee to be taught about clinical reasoning than given factual information about a condition. For example, in a patient with pneumonia you could focus on the principles behind the Surviving Sepsis campaign as well as which organism might be responsible and which antibiotic to use.

Further insights into on-the-job learning are included in David Guile's *Informal Learning and the Medical Apprentice*, a booklet due for publication by the Association for the Study of Medical Education. See the ASME website for details and purchase (www.asme.org.uk).

Effective feedback

Effective feedback seeks to promote better insight by the trainee, not to judge or criticise them or provide unasked-for solutions. In order to do that, there are key behaviours to emphasise.

Things to do:

- Build up well-meaning and trust with the trainee. Feedback, particularly challenging feedback, will always be received better and therefore be more effective if the trainee trusts you.
- Choose the right time and place. Offering feedback in the middle of a ward round may not be well received, but four weeks later is no good either.
- Give positive feedback frequently and unreservedly; be fair and supportive rather than critical.
- Always start with the trainee's view of the situation. I have been surprised by what comes out of this. For example, they may well be aware that their communication skills are inadequate but not sure how to change them, and in situations where there is conflict between trainees you may well be surprised when you hear both sides of the story.
- Make your feedback behavioural not subjective. This means giving feedback about something that is directly observable (e.g. 'badgering the nurses') rather than any assumptions you have made about why they did what they did ('she thinks she is above the nurses') or meaningless generalizations ('rude', 'irritating'). As far as possible stick to what you have seen, not what has been reported to you.
- Allow the trainee to come up with solutions to any problems raised. An owned solution is much more likely to be realised.
- Make the feedback balanced: the recipient needs to know which behaviours to keep as well as those to change.
- Offer positive suggestions of alternative courses of action.
- Beware the use of humour – this may well come out as sarcasm.

Don't:

- Be afraid to make feedback unreservedly positive if there are no significant negatives. We tend to qualify even excellent performance with a big 'but'.
- Be censorious.
- Humiliate.
- Use sarcasm.

EDUCATIONAL SUPERVISION

The role of the educational supervisor centres on regular meetings with the trainee. The educational supervisor needs to be aware of the curriculum, the assessment methods, the variety of learning opportunities available and other sources of support available to a trainee. There are potential conflicts of interest between the different roles expected of educational supervisors. Educational supervision has been seen as an essentially formative process that exists for the benefit of the trainee, the general philosophy being to support, nurture, facilitate and guide. However, according to the Operational Framework for implementation of the Foundation programme, at the end you do have some responsibility in signing off their experience and this is where potential conflict can arise. It seems unlikely that this mix of formative and summative roles can ever be resolved, but being aware of the issue may help you to avoid potential problems.

Expectations of educational supervisor

The three main stipulations of the Quality Assurance (QA) framework with respect to educational supervision are that the supervisor should have received appropriate training, that the F1 trainee should meet their educational supervisor in the first week of the job and that they should have a set number of meetings per year. Training for educational supervisors is dealt with below under the heading 'Developing as a Foundation programme educator'. The QA framework suggests that trainees require three meetings for each of their four-month posts (beginning, middle and end), a total of nine a year. In our experience, there will be few trainees who need or want or can get to nine meetings a year. Given that the end of one job is the beginning of another, it might be reasonable to have six or seven meetings – at the start of the year, part-way through first job, end of first job, middle and end of second and end of third, with the option of one in the middle of the third if required. Alternatively, for a trainee who is well organised and doing well, some of these meetings can be with the clinical supervisor rather than the educational supervisor. It will be essential for all trainees to meet someone from the unit they are working on during the first week of each post. On the other hand, a struggling trainee may need periods where they are seen more regularly and you will need to be flexible in accommodating their needs.

The documentation for the Foundation programme is available on the MMC website (www.mmc.nhs.uk). In the first year, trainees were given a satchel with all the curriculum, assessment documentation, etc. included. This has not been repeated and trainees will need to download and print their own copy of the curriculum and assessment tools and the *Rough Guide*. If they are not well organised, they will need encouragement.

One way to conduct an educational review

General approach

The most important thing to remember is that educational supervision is for the trainee so that they are able to reflect on how they are doing, to develop a learning plan and ask for help with career planning and pastoral support. If the outcomes of educational supervision are to be useful, they must be owned by the trainee. Whilst you can cajole or persuade your trainee to make appointments to see you, in the end it is their responsibility.

The skills used to facilitate an educational supervision meeting are suggested in Box 7.3 and some of the skills required are detailed in Box 7.3. The meeting should allow the trainee the opportunity to talk about any issues that are important to them, review their learning since the last meeting, preferably against the learning plan, check their progress in obtaining their assessments and the results, help them come up with a new learning plan and cover any pastoral issues that are relevant and within your skills. The meeting may include careers counselling.

It may be helpful to have a structure to base the sessions on. The structure suggested below builds on the local training in our deanery and our experience of being supervisor and supervisee and gives hints and advice for each phase. However, educational supervision is an organic rather than a formulaic activity. Each trainee is different and each session will be different as trainees' requirements change. You might like to use this structure but adapt it to your circumstances. For example, it is quite hard to make a suitable learning plan without some knowledge of the trainee's career intentions so you may need to move backwards and forwards through the schedule.

The time committed to educational supervision varies enormously, from about 15 minutes to 2 hours. Given the list of functions described above, you will be able to come to your own conclusion on what is appropriate. We like

---

Box 7.3 Skills used to facilitate successful educational supervision
- Planning. Finding out about the trainee beforehand, especially if you have received negative feedback about them
- Choosing an appropriate environment. Avoid interruptions and have suitable seating arrangements
- Communication skills. Use of open and semi-open questions, reflections, echoing
- Non-verbal communication
- Demonstrating empathy. Acknowledging emotions
- Being non-judgemental
- Using effective feedback

to leave at least an hour for each meeting and six hours a year is not that much per trainee. Make sure that you choose an appropriate space in which to conduct educational supervision and that the environment allows you to give them your whole attention.

Start with an open question

In many ways an educational review is like a consultation and it is best to start with the trainee's agenda. 'Is there anything in particular you want to discuss today?' or something similar is a good open question to kick off with. If there is a burning issue that they want to get off their chest, they will not be able to concentrate on the routine aspects of reviewing their portfolio. For example, if a trainee has recently made a major clinical error, this may well be preying on their mind. The use of an open question allows the trainee to set the agenda and I have experienced the response: 'Well, I wasn't going to tell you about this, but . . .'. This led on to a really important discussion of what had gone wrong, why, the trainee's emotional response and their reflections on how to prevent it happening in the future.

Agree an agenda for the meeting

If you have something that you need to share with the trainee, you need to make them aware of this near the beginning as well. Arrive at a shared agenda early on in the meeting: 'So you wanted to discuss the problems you are having with the F2 on your ward. I have your multi-source feedback to share with you, then we can review your portfolio and then discuss your hopes of getting into a surgical rotation. We have about an hour.' You may need to revise the agenda if new issues are raised, but being clear about the trainee's expectations and your limits will help.

Make it clear how much time you have. Trainees will assume that it is not much and tend to rush. If you have longer, let them know.

Discussing the important issues: knowing and setting your boundaries

Having established the agenda, get the big issues out in the open. If none has been identified by the trainee, further enquiry into how the current post is going (the trainee's relationships within it, any workload issues and the learning that they are accessing) may elicit important issues.

Trainees bring all kinds of burning issues to educational supervision. These may be purely work-related (mistakes they have made or perceive they have made, disputes with other members of staff, problems with workload, doubts about career choice, clinical governance issues), they may be at the interface between work and personal life (e.g. stress affecting home life or personal experience affecting work) or they may be purely personal.

The appropriate extent of the pastoral role is difficult to define. Educational supervisors vary in their skills and willingness to become involved with pastoral issues. Your boundaries will be dictated in part by your skills. It is always important to remember that educational supervision is meant to be facilitatory and not directive – help the trainee to reflect and find their own solutions by appropriate questioning and challenging, rather than prescribing the answers. In the context of educational supervision you might be happy to help a trainee reflect on clinical incidents and on their career plans and you might be happy to help them with a certain level of stress. However, if there appears to be a genuine mental health issue, such as depression, it may be best to ensure that you limit your help to where it interacts with work and try to ensure that the trainee is seeking help through their GP or Occupational Health. The educational supervision relationship is limited to helping the trainee to reflect; it is not generally regarded as therapeutic. Trainees will also want different levels of personal support. For some an enquiry into how work is affecting their home life will be welcome, for others this will be seen as intrusive.

Just as in the clinical consultation, you need to build rapport and trust. Patients do not necessarily raise their most significant problems at the beginning of the consultation and likewise trainees will not necessarily do so. Use the same skills that you use in consultations to build rapport with the trainee throughout the meeting.

Review the trainee's portfolio, including assessments and reflections

Review of the trainee's portfolio will lay the ground for them to develop their future learning plan. You should review the learning plan from last time, any assessments and reflections on practice as well as attendance at teaching sessions and the trainee's learning from formal teaching.

The trainee should have a learning plan. Has the trainee met their learning objectives? If not, why, and is it important? Have the learning opportunities in this post been fully utilised? Is the department responding to the trainee's learning needs as much as possible?

One of the most important functions of the educational supervisor is to help the trainee plan their work-based assessments and keep them up to date. These are detailed in Chapter 6, but basically Foundation programme doctors need to obtain two mini-CEXs, two DOPs and two CbDs in each four-month post as well as some multi-source feedback. The multi-source feedback will usually be fed back to the educational supervisor, who then gives it to trainees. The multi-source feedback might be a mini-PAT, TAB or, in Scotland, the Scottish Workplace Assessment tool. If they are falling behind in this schedule, you will need to prompt and cajole them. Remember that with inadequate assessments the trainee will not pass. You may also need to help trainees to reflect on their assessments.

Importantly, the portfolio has a space for reflecting on critical learning events. This should be a part of the portfolio that is confidential to the trainee and shared with their educational supervisor, but not part of the summative assessment. We find that the reflections of trainees on errors or system problems or examples of good practice are often excellent and are an important distinguishing feature of the trainee who has 'got it' as far as professionalism is concerned.

Review any other evidence that the trainee has gathered for their portfolio. This will encourage them to collect more and demonstrate its worth. Types of evidence that they can gather are described in more detail in Chapter 6 but could, for example, include anonymised clerkings or drug charts as evidence for competencies.

In order to be signed off at the end of the Foundation programme, trainees will need to demonstrate that they have attended the prescribed number of teaching sessions. Some sessions are compulsory (e.g. induction and ALS), whereas for regular weekly sessions, there will be a minimum expectation. In our deanery it is 70% of all sessions. You need to help your trainee keep track of their attendance. If they are falling behind, make sure that they are aware of the consequences and facilitate their attendance. Often poor attendance is the result of the written or unwritten rules of the clinical team they are working with so you may need to negotiate with their clinical supervisor to make sure that they can attend. However, it can also reflect the trainee's engagement with the teaching programme so that non-attendance may reflect a negative attitude to the learning agenda.

Careers discussion

Careers will probably be touched on in many educational supervision meetings and should be specifically asked about. Careers guidance has traditionally been poor in the NHS and you may have experienced the very directive approach described in the first level in Box 7.4.

The disadvantages of a directive approach include:

- The possibility of being discriminatory, e.g. advising a woman against a career in surgery
- You may have your own pet likes and dislikes, e.g. would you recommend a career in any of the shortage specialties?
- The trainee needs to own the decisions made if they are to take them forward effectively
- The possibility of being wrong. It is difficult to predict success in a particular career and nothing satisfies someone as much as proving one of their old teachers wrong!

Box 7.4 Skills escalator for careers advice

Careers advertising: This is the form of careers advice that has been traditionally used for doctors in training e.g. 'You're a good type, very bright, good with patients. You should consider a career in cardiology – lots of prospects, good private income, much better than gastroenterology'. This type of (usually unsolicited) advice has its place. It performs the function that all specialties need in advertising and recruiting the best people by getting them interested, but it is not true careers guidance.

Careers advice: The simplest level of help with careers management is careers advice. It functions on the level of provision of information and simple help. Examples might include helping a trainee find out the criteria for applying to a specialty or compiling their CV or interview technique.

Careers guidance: The essential characteristic of guidance is that it allows the trainee to explore a range of options. Questions such as 'Which specialty is best for me?' or 'My applications have all been unsuccessful, what should I do now?' lie in the realm of careers guidance.

Careers counselling: This is a higher level of help with career management that would focus on helping a trainee with serious problems, such as thinking of giving up medicine, significant problems with stress or a disability that affect their career.

Improving careers management is one of the key aims for the Foundation programme. The aim is to equip all trainees with better skills in career management, to improve the training of educational supervisors in giving simple careers advice and to offer higher levels of careers counselling to trainees who are struggling. The full guidance on careers management structures issues is available at www.mmc.nhs.uk/download_files/Career-Management.pdf. Different models are being introduced in each deanery so you need to become familiar with provision within the Trust and beyond.

If you have not had any formal training in careers advice, this will be offered locally as part of each school's plan to develop its faculty. Career management is discussed from the trainee's point of view in Chapter 8 and covers many of the important areas that you need to be aware of. Careers guidance is itself a profession with its own training and comes in varying different levels as detailed in Box 7.4. Educational supervisors will mainly be working at the careers advice/guidance level using a non-directive approach to allow the trainee to explore their options and to help them plan their learning to match their career choice. By the time trainees are having more serious problems you will probably need to discuss with or refer on to someone with higher-level skills such as the clinical tutor, programme director or careers counsellor at the deanery.

There are several stages of careers guidance that may be helpful in your discussions. Keep in your mind the need to allow the trainee to set the agenda and arrive at their own conclusion. Questioning can be challenging, providing that you have enough of a relationship with them, but not confrontational.

The four key stages of careers management are:

1. Self-assessment of skills

In the careers literature a lot is made of the need to match skills to careers. Research into career choice in F2 trainees (including our own, presented in Chapter 8) tends to support a model where trainees try to match themselves to a career where they will 'fit in'. This fit comprises many characteristics, not just the skills or competencies required to do the job. It also relies on their experience of seniors in the specialty, types of patients experienced, degree of generalist or specialist, gender issues, what they want out of a career and many more personal factors. Many careers are rejected on the basis of one negative experience, such as being humiliated by a senior or feeling that an SpR they have observed is under a lot of pressure.

We would also have to admit that the profession's understanding of the skills needed to enter a specialty is not very evidence-based. Trainees should be able to find a niche somewhere within the broad church of nearly any post-Foundation training programme. For example, in my own specialty of gastroenterology the skills needed vary from the holistic approach to dealing with irritable bowel syndrome to the intensivist skills needed in liver transplantation and major GI bleeds, as well as the practical skills in endoscopy. As you can imagine, there is room for many personality types.

There is also inconclusive evidence that psychomotor skills can be evaluated to predict accurately someone's performance later in their career. The tools available for assessing psychomotor skills are not very accurate. In fact, they mostly seem to favour men and particularly those that play a lot of computer games. In other words, they demonstrate skills acquisition and practice rather than an innate or immutable trait. Most people seem to be able to get over a degree of poor coordination if they want to succeed.

Trainees vary in their ability to assess their own skills and match those to the skills needed for the specialty. Trainees also need to identify their weaknesses and any negative factors about a particular career that would make them avoid it, such as high stress, long hours, insufficient stimulation, etc. Their self-assessment can be supported by the use of psychometric tools that allow trainees to match their skills against those required to succeed in each specialty. The Sci45 (more recently, Sci59) and the American version, Medical Specialty Aptitude Test (MSAT), are the most frequently used. MSAT is available free (www.med-ed.virginia.edu/specialties). The Sci45 was developed by the Open University and may be available through your deanery. It evaluates approximately 45 career choices so may give no useful information on specialties that your trainee may be suited to. The Sci45 has since been developed into the Sci59 with more questions and covering about 60 career streams. The Sci45 and 59 have two outputs: they summarise the responses in the form of feedback on twelve key areas – this is probably their most useful function because they help the trainee to focus on their core skills/aptitudes and values; and they offer the best and worst ten career matches to the trainee's responses. The career matches should not be taken literally. In the future the Sci59 may well be available through the BMA or your deanery.

A note of caution needs to be made with respect to these questionnaires – as a gastroenterologist, neither the Sci59 nor MSAT puts gastroenterology in the top ten recommended specialties for me. The Sci59 also recommended neonatology when I specifically replied negatively to questions that asked if I wanted to work with children. They may also be outdated because, today they appear to value research experience as a selection criterion, whereas research will probably be useful only in the academic stream. They also do not take into account the changing role of women in medicine.

These tools are useful for initiating discussion about a trainee's skills rather than in seeking a direct match. There is a danger that, in the changing career structure in which we live, they may reinforce old stereotypes rather than reflect the true skills needed for a specialty. For example, you are unlikely to be recommended to do neurosurgery or an academic career if your responses indicate that you value a family life and wish to work part-time. But surely we should be looking at ways of enabling people who want to work flexibly the chance to follow these careers rather than reinforcing a perception that they are not suitable?

A recent development is the use of Intelligent Career Card Sort (ICCS) (Binding and Loveland: MMC online news articles, 5 November 2005). This is a career exploration tool based on using approximately 120 cards from three domains ('knowing why', 'knowing how' and 'knowing whom') to inform the client's view of their own career. It does not attempt to identify typical careers but seeks to enable the trainee to identify their core characteristics and values to inform career choice. It has been used in only a handful of trainees, mostly with significant career management problems. It is unlikely to be used by an educational supervisor, but it may be a part of the approach from deanery specialists and is being piloted in some deaneries.

Tools such as the Myers–Brigg Type Indicator are also frequently promoted as essential tools for careers advice. However, the MBTI can only be used by someone trained extensively in its use, usually an occupational psychologist. The MBTI can also be expensive, so you will not routinely be expected to use it, as it lies in the realm of more advanced careers counselling and is only likely to be used for trainees with significant career difficulties. It may be offered by the Foundation school or deanery.

It has been suggested by some that the Foundation assessment tools can be used to help a trainee validate their self-assessment of skills. For example, the DOPs tool might superficially appear to be a useful assessment of future practical skills potential. However, these tools have not been developed for this purpose and there is no evidence that they are useful for it so they should be used with caution. For this reason, MMC has always maintained that the scores from the assessment tools will not be used in the post-Foundation selection process.

Perhaps more important than the skills required are the characteristics of a career that will match the lifestyle that the trainee wishes to have. Again, these are discussed in Chapter 8. Examples include the opportunity to pursue research, living in a rural or urban area, working flexibly, etc.

2. Finding out about career opportunities

In this part of careers guidance it may be helpful to check with the trainee which specialties they are thinking of and what experience they have. Given the results of your discussions on what they desire from a career gleaned from the first stage, are there any other careers that appear to be a good match? Do they have experience of these or have they not been considered? Undergraduate education now may be streamlined so that most medical students do not experience a lot of the smaller 'ologies' or have only minimal experience. What experience of their chosen specialties do they have and what additional experience will they need to make a decision? How are they going to get that experience (e.g. through the use of tasters or using contacts and online resources of typical career profiles)? What are the entry criteria? One huge uncertainty in the current climate is the future jobs market. We are moving from a position of being nearly guaranteed a job at the end of the very controlled training to no such guarantee. Many sources of information on specialties, including helpful books, are listed in Chapters 8 and 10.

3. Making a decision

Trainees may make decisions early on, even before entering medical school, or may still be uncertain and changing their mind frequently through F2. They will weigh each factor differently. The ways in which trainees make decisions are outlined in Chapter 8. If they are uncertain about how to make a decision, it can be useful to get them to reflect on a previous successful decision and how they made it. Many will want to keep their options open when applying for a post-Foundation job. Several research studies suggest that up to 30% of F2 trainees will not have made a definite decision. It can also be useful to encourage trainees to have a 'plan B'. Use challenges such as 'Have you thought what you might do if you don't get into your first choice specialty?' or 'What if your first choice doesn't work out?' While it may not be a good idea for a trainee to complete an application form or go into an interview stating that they want this post to keep their options open, or that they are not less than 110% committed to a specialty, this does not mean that the desire to keep options open should be dismissed.

Key questions in making the final decision include whether it will sustain their interest, whether it has the right mix of practical and non-practical skills, how competitive it is and how strong they are as a candidate. It may be useful to challenge the trainee on how they have made their decision: 'You said you had discounted hospital medicine because Dr X was rude to you during your renal attachment. Are all physicians like that?' or 'You weren't keen on medicine because you had seen the medical SpR very stressed one day. Was that just one bad day? How did the other SpRs cope?' or 'Am I right in thinking that you have chosen to go into general practice because you liked Dr Jones so much in the third year? What experience of other GPs do you have?'

4. Making an application

Trainees can derive significant benefit from discussing their application form with you and from interview practice. But they may not realise that this is the remit of the educational supervisor and so may not ask. Obviously, you should not write the application, but you can certainly advise on their drafts. Mock interviews can be used to demonstrate their strengths and weaknesses and the areas that they need to find out more factual information. Base any mock interviews on the person specification for the post rather than your favourite questions as this should reflect the kind of questions they will be asked in real life. Typical questions are suggested in Chapter 8, if you are struggling to come up with some yourself. I have experience of performing mock interviews with many trainees who were struggling with obtaining a training post, including those returning to work and refugee doctors. Without exception they were successful in their next application so the investment of just 1–2 hours of your time will probably be very worthwhile.

Other issues in career guidance include:

Joining up the career guidance and educational supervision

As a trainee's career choice becomes more certain through the Foundation programme, they will need help to plan their learning to demonstrate the attributes required to enter their chosen specialty. The essential and desirable competencies for entry to each training programme will be available through college, MMC or MTAS websites in due course. You should refer to them in helping your trainee plan their learning.

Informational needs for careers guidance

You will need to have a basic understanding of career opportunities to be an effective careers guide and also a working knowledge of where to obtain information that you don't know. Chapter 8 lists a lot more of the information for trainees, including the academic pathway, and Chapter 10 summarises the characteristics of most of the 62 specialties and other options.

Developing a learning plan

Planning learning is critical for trainees to maximise their educational experience, particularly in posts that may not appear to match their career aspirations. The planning will mainly aim to ensure that they fulfil the Foundation programme curriculum, but will also address their needs to obtain the appropriate experience for them to compete successfully for post-Foundation training.

In order for the trainee to plan their learning needs, they will need to follow these steps:

- Review where they are at with their learning – 'What do you know?'
- Define and prioritise their current learning needs – 'What do you need to know?' – or as expressed in the portfolio – 'What specific development needs do I have?'
- Assess the learning opportunities presented by the post they are in and other learning opportunities – 'What are the opportunities to get to know it?'
- Design a plan – 'How I am going to do it?' – or as expressed in the portfolio – 'How will these objectives be addressed?'
- Work out how they will know that they have got there and record when it has been achieved – evaluation and outcome. It will be valuable to agree a means by which they can offer evidence of successful completion of the competency for their portfolio.

As far as possible it would be desirable to express the learning needs through the development of SMART objectives: Specific, Measurable, Achievable, Realistic, Timely (see Chapter 5).

The first step is to help trainees to assess where they are now using a combination of self-assessment and feedback from others. The suggested documentation for the development of the learning plan is in the Foundation portfolio (2005–7 version, p. 12), but this could be regarded as rather superficial and unstructured, allowing only a small space for each of the seven curriculum domains. However, local or other documentation could be used if it serves the purpose better. The Northern deanery has an excellent self-appraisal tool that is available online and can be used by anyone. Go to www.mypimd.ncl.ac.uk and search for 'self-assessment', then click on the document marked 'self-evaluation (salaries)'.

The Northern deanery tool explodes each of the domains into 41 more readily digestible chunks matching the competencies in the curriculum. It asks the trainee to assess their confidence on a five-point scale rather than the three-point scale used in the national portfolio and to prioritise their learning needs for each domain. It has undergone several iterations to get to the present form and has been evaluated fairly extensively by trainees and trainers. We use this tool locally for trainees and get them to fill in a hard copy three times throughout the year. We suggest that they use the same copy and use different coloured pens to track their learning. This helps them to see the areas that they have made progress in and also makes clear which areas the trainee has not advanced in and so helps set the learning plan.

Feedback comes from their assessment tools as well as informally from their peers and colleagues. You may have observed them yourself or you may have feedback from their clinical supervisor. See the section above for guidance on giving feedback. You can also help them reflect on the feedback they have received.

It might be thought strange that we should rely largely on the trainees' self-assessment of their skills to plan their learning. In fact, self-assessment is thought to be a reasonably accurate measure of competence in many areas. It is also probably the most appropriate measure to use in planning learning needs because it has good face value to the trainee and so will motivate their learning. There is clearly going to be a small group of trainees who are not able to evaluate their own level accurately and score themselves consistently too high or too low. If there is a mismatch between the feedback from other sources and the trainee's self-assessment, then sensitive feedback will be needed. It will be difficult but is particularly important. The trainee's learning needs are then essentially defined by the gap between what they need to know/be able to do and where they are at now.

The learning plan can therefore be based on their learning needs and their career aspirations. Applications for post-Foundation training will not rely on having worked in the specialty before, but will require evidence of the skills, attitudes and knowledge needed for the specialty, ongoing interest in and commitment to the specialty and an awareness of what the specialty is like. Career aspirations will therefore have to feed into learning plans.

We have not included examples of completed learning plans in this chapter because the responsibility to develop, document and complete a learning plan belongs to the trainee.

Learning opportunities

It is obviously important for the educational supervisor to help the trainee to make the most of learning opportunities in Foundation programme. Again, this is dealt with in detail in Chapter 5. In guiding your trainee, don't forget to make use of all the learning situations mentioned above. Trainees can get very focused on 'teaching', by which they mean what happens in a classroom. They sometimes need to be reminded that 95% of their work time is spent at the coal face and one of the premises of the Foundation programme is that it will be based in service. Help them get the most out of on-the-job learning opportunities that are relevant to them. Several booklets from the Association of Medical Education (e.g. No. 27, D. Hargreaves, P. Stanley and D. Ward, *Getting the Best out of Your Training*, Edinburgh: ASME, 2000, or the forthcoming updated version, David Guile, *Informal Learning and the Medical Apprentice*) give useful advice.

Particular mention needs to be made of the educational supervisor's role in helping the trainee to plan study leave. In F1, any study leave allowance is likely to be used in compulsory courses and there will be little if any money for self-directed study leave. In F2, the allowance should be the same as it used to be for SHOs – up to 30 days a year and around £650 a year. In most deaneries, part of the nominal 30 days' F2 allowance will be taken up with leave used in F1 (e.g. if you do ALS in F1 this will come out of your F2 allowance). Study leave can be made up of attending courses, private leave for exams and tasters. Officially, the MMC is maintaining that learning in the Foundation programme should be directed towards the generic goals of the Foundation curriculum and that we should be discouraging trainees from taking the first part of specialist exams. However, realistically, trainees have got to do something to give themselves a fighting chance of getting a job post-Foundation and we have already discussed the fact that demonstrating attachment to a specialty and the relevant skills will be criteria for appointment to post-Foundation run-through training. What better way could a trainee demonstrate their suitability to be a physician than to get part 1 MRCP as an F2, or to be a surgeon, attend a STEPS course?

Tasters are a relatively new learning mode for postgraduate medicine, but are familiar in the undergraduate field as student-selected modules. The idea behind them is that they give trainees the chance to experience specialties that they would not otherwise get in their two-year programme. The regulations may vary between Trusts and deaneries, but it would not be unreasonable to request five days of tasters in F2 as part of study leave and your trainee may be able to get some tasters in F1 as well. For example, if a trainee wishes to have a career in paediatrics but is not fortunate enough to get onto a paediatric F2 rotation, they will need to demonstrate interest in and knowledge of paediatrics in their specialty application. They could arrange to spend a week (or five separate days if better for service delivery) doing paediatrics early in F2 to get some experience and also perhaps obtain evidence of their skills using the assessment tools.

It is usually your responsibility to check that a trainee uses their study leave wisely and attends all the compulsory courses before following their own agenda.

Closing the session

Once you have discussed any burning issues, reviewed the portfolio, assessed learning needs, discussed careers and made a learning plan, the session should be closed appropriately. Make sure that there is nothing else that the trainee wishes to discuss and summarise what has taken place. If you have not made a record as you go, get it down on paper or electronically now. Plan the next session and fix a date in both your diaries. I find that if I have a fixed date, it alerts me if they miss it. If no date is made, it is possible to lose track of when a trainee should be seeing you. Make sure you know who the trainee is working with and who to contact with any learning issues that the trainee wants help with. Check with the trainee that they know what they need to do before the next session.

YOUR ROLE IN THE FINAL ASSESSMENT

As discussed above, the trainee will be assessed at the end of the first year as competent to achieve full registration and at the end of the second year to fulfil the F2 competencies, based on the evidence in their portfolio. It is the trainee's responsibility to fill in the evidence summary at the end of F2 to submit to the panel that will sign it off. However, it is your responsibility to check the summary against the evidence and certify that it is a complete and accurate record. This is vital if the competency-based system of performance assessment is to work. More than 96% of trainees will be competent and you will be able to sign off their evidence summary with confidence, but dealing with the very small proportion with performance difficulties will give you a disproportionate amount of work and headache.

Some theoretical issues about the assessment system remain unanswered. The competencies refer only to what should have been learnt, not the standard that will need to be achieved. Clearly, they will not have become fully competent in every area. We are all continuing to learn and develop in some of these areas. So, how competent are they, and in how many competencies do they have to be competent? In the end the trainee needs to satisfy the 'global assessment' that they have done enough towards the competencies. Doesn't this sound like the old signing off system for PRHOs? You had to make a global assessment of whether they had done enough! At least now you have some evidence on which to base your judgement.

In your role as educational supervisor, the time to become concerned about a trainee's development is clearly not at the point when you have to sign off the evidence summary. If you have concerns about the development of one of the trainees you supervise, you should raise this at the earliest possible opportunity with the clinical tutor or programme director and indeed the Foundation school or deanery. We all need support when dealing with a trainee on the cusp of competence. Further guidance on the trainee in difficulty is given below.

SUPPORT YOU NEED FROM YOUR TRUST

With the increasing QA framework and higher standards expected from educational supervisors there needs to be time in your job plan and recognition of the worth of education. In many Trusts this will be extremely pressurised. Education can become a low priority compared to waiting times and balancing the budget. Trusts are, of course, taking a short view of life if they neglect education: the recruitment of future consultants depends in part on their experience as trainees; the better the experience they have, the more likely that they will be favourable to working there. The increase in medical student numbers will also allow the best performing Trusts to obtain new posts as the number of medical students rises from about 5000 to 10,000. You will also need to access training opportunities and get feedback on your educational supervision and teaching. Most Trusts are now starting multi-source feedback systems for consultants that look for evidence of satisfactory clinical performance from patients, trainees, peers and superiors at work. This model should be extended to assess further seniors' relationships with students and trainees and the quality of their educational interventions. Seniors will need incentives to develop their skills and take on greater roles in education, whether through the awarding of discretionary points or by job satisfaction, the award of academic titles and conversion of SPAs to CPAs. In general practice, the education fee acts as a strong incentive to accept trainees, but it is clear that F2 trainees in practice will require more supervision and provide less service benefit than a GP vocational trainee so there will be an incentive for practices to prefer VTS to F2 trainees.

CHALLENGES TO THE MODEL OF EDUCATIONAL SUPERVISION

The model of educational supervision described here, with one supervisor for the whole two years, has many advantages. However, there are potential problems. Not all trainees and supervisors will gel and so there needs to be a mechanism for trainees to change supervisors and for supervisors who recognise a problem to be able to help their supervisee find a more appropriate supervisor. Getting feedback from the clinical coalface to the educational supervisor is also difficult but essential. The best system is probably email contact between clinical and educational supervisors, either just before each meeting or if there is any untoward incident or for positive feedback of high-level performance. It can take a pattern of small, unrelated incidents to occur before it is clear that a trainee is having difficulty. If no one is linking them, then a problem can escalate before it is detected. This will become a greater problem when trainees become more widely dispersed throughout their two-year programme. At present there are relatively few cross-Trust Foundation programmes. People's energy was put into sorting it out within a Trust without adding the complexity of cross-Trust working. Distance will also challenge the model, with some rotations stretching from Cornwall to London and even within a large Trust such as in Scotland or parts of rural England. Holding a meeting with a distant educational supervisor regularly may be difficult.

There is probably also still a considerable training gap between the ideal skills of supervisors and the day-to-day realities of educational supervision.

Developing as a Foundation programme educator and sources of support

In the future it is likely that the standards expected of doctor-teachers will continue to develop. Educational supervisors will be specifically selected, rather than allocated by lucky dip. The development of faculty for specific roles will become more sophisticated. The Foundation programme has seen more central funding directed at the development of faculty and the funding of additional formal posts in education. The clinical tutor role has changed beyond recognition and in many places has been supplanted by the appointment of Directors of Postgraduate Education or similar. Opportunities to pursue a career through the deaneries or Foundation schools are increasing.

Training for a greater role in postgraduate education is summarized in Box 7.5. Much of this will be developed at local level, either by Trusts, Foundation schools or deaneries. Colleges will continue to offer valuable training such as the Physician as Educator programme offered by the RCP London. This course of six days' teaching accompanied by some case study work is offered

---

Box 7.5   Skills required and training for a role in postgraduate education
- Training for educational supervision
- Training in careers advice
- Training for specific micro-skills such as giving feedback
- Training in specific teaching situations such as on-the-job teaching (e.g. ward rounds, out-patients, etc.) or small-group teaching or the teaching of particular skills such as consultation skills
- Evaluating your own teaching and supervision
- Planning your own learning – use of a portfolio or reflective document

---

Box 7.6   Useful contacts for educational supervisors

Within Trust:
Clinical tutor or Trust Foundation programme director
Trust Foundation programme administrator
College tutor
Occupational Health
Medical staffing or Human Resources (may be located in the deanery)

Within deanery or Foundation school:
Director of Foundation school or equivalent
Chief administrator with the school
Careers adviser
Chairs of the specialist training committees
Advisers for overseas doctors (normally one for each specialty)

Externally:
Sources of support for doctors with problems (e.g. addicted doctors, doctors with health problems or a disability; see Chapter 10)
BMA or other trade union body

---

at several sites around the country and offers an excellent basis for developing many of the key skills detailed in Box 7.5.

Academic institutions offer excellent opportunities to develop teaching and education-related skills. Many universities (e.g. Newcastle, Dundee, Hull, Wolverhampton, Cardiff and UCL) offer Certificates, Masters or PhDs in clinical teaching and some of these are available online. Search for one in your locality.

Building up a list of useful contacts (Box 7.6) is important in being able to access specific skills when required.

Other sources of information include online articles, books and pamphlets supplied by the royal colleges (see the publications list on the RCP London website) and journal articles, including frequent summaries in the *BMJ* Careers Focus. Search the *BMJ* or college websites. Particularly recommended are T. Russell, *Effective Feedback Skills*, 2nd edition (London: Kogan Page, 1998); and Trevor Bayley and Michael Drury (eds), *Teaching and Training Techniques for Hospital Doctors* (Oxford: Radcliffe, 1988).

The Northern deanery has developed a self-evaluation tool for clinical educators that can be used to assess your skills in various aspects of education from curriculum design to small-group teaching and plan your learning and development as an educator (go to http://mypimd.ncl.ac.uk and search for 'self evaluation').

OTHER ISSUES FOR SUPPORTING TRAINEES

Bullying

Bullying is a hot issue in medical education and one that is likely to rise in importance. In surveys approximately 10% of NHS staff report bullying and doctors are certainly not immune. Bullying affects not only the individual but the alleged bully and the organization too. Recent court cases have seen payouts of nearly £1 million in cases of bullying in industry.

Bullying means different things to different people, but in occupational circles is defined as 'persistent behaviour likely to erode self-esteem'. It is important to note that this defines bullying from the perspective of the bullied and so whether or not you agree that the behaviour they experience is unreasonable does not matter. This can be particularly important to appreciate having grown up in a system where a certain amount of 'robust' feedback was considered acceptable. Just because you had to put up with it does not make it right. If you know the person who is accused of bullying, it may make it more difficult to deal with as personal views can lead to bias.

Bullying is the action of an individual or group, usually in a position of power over another. Types of behaviour that might be experienced as bullying include:

- Destructive and repeated criticism
- Being shouted or sworn at
- Being given an unreasonable workload that is greater than that of other trainees
- Being ostracised or excluded at work

Trainees may experience bullying from their seniors, including other trainees, from nurses and from managers. We encourage you to take at face value any report by a trainee of bullying and not let yourself be swayed by your view of the trainer or the alleged bully. If you encounter alleged bullying you will probably need to involve others. Your Trust will have a policy on bullying and this should be followed at local level. If you have any doubts as to whether you should act, remember that the best interests of the alleged bully probably lie in your taking early action rather than delaying until the consequences for them are more serious. If a trainee felt that you were bullying them or treating them unfairly you would want to know about it rather than blunder on, wouldn't you?

Doctors in difficulty

Introduction

Dealing with doctors with performance problems is one of the hardest areas of our work. Historically, the profession has struggled to grasp this (at both consultant and trainee level) and it may be partly responsible for some of the problems that the profession has faced. There has been a tendency to ignore problems in the early stages when there might have been time to help, perhaps in the knowledge that they will be rotating to another post soon and it won't be our problem, and then to overreact when the problem cannot be ignored and use disciplinary means rather than supportive and educational ones. The philosophy behind the Foundation programme and the whole continuous assessment model being brought in throughout training is to give us the tools to detect trainees in difficulty at an early stage and offer appropriate support and development to improve their performance.

Problems in performance tend to come under the categories of health (including mental health issues and substance misuse), clinical knowledge, skills and judgement, or professionalism in its broadest sense. This short section is designed to give an introduction to the issue. Further information and training will be needed to deal with any case that you come across. The RCP Physician as Educator course offers further training in this area. Here we look at the initial stages of identifying a problem and its initial assessment. As an educational supervisor you will probably not be dealing with it alone if it is a serious problem or if the trainee does not respond positively when the issue is drawn to their attention.

Recognising there's a problem, gathering evidence and sounding out others' opinions

It can be very difficult to recognise the early stages of poor performance and this is where the central, coordinating role of educational supervisors in closing the feedback loop needs to be developed as described above. Sometimes we are aware that a trainee is not performing at the highest level, but it can be very difficult to put your finger on exactly why, which makes it difficult to raise the issue with the trainee. If you do have concerns about a trainee's performance Box 7.7 gives some hints as to the approach to the problem.

Box 7.7   Stages of dealing with poor performance
- Recognising it
- Gathering evidence/testing others' opinion
- Planning a strategy for approach – What type of problem is it? Is patient safety affected? Who is the best person to deal with it? How to put it to the trainee? Who to monitor? Planning for things that can go wrong
- Talking to the trainee. What is their view, any insight, any explanations, educational and support needs?
- Agreeing a plan. Who needs to be informed?
- Monitoring the plan
- Reviewing progress
- What to do if progress is not satisfactory

In gathering evidence about a trainee's performance you should use multiple sources. The people working directly with the trainee will be able to give verbal reports and their formal assessments may offer a clue. Often, however, the poorly performing trainee has not obtained any assessments, or not enough to be worthwhile. The absence of cause for concern in formal assessments does not invalidate the 'expert opinion' that the trainee is struggling – formal assessments do not tell the whole story and indeed may miss problem trainees who seem competent when observed under the controlled conditions of most of the assessments, but fail to perform all the time.

Planning a strategy

Presuming that you have gathered evidence and there does appear to be a problem, it is worthwhile thinking through the case before approaching the trainee. Ask yourself the following questions.

- How will this look from the trainee's point of view?
- What type of problem does it appear to be – clinical performance, professionalism, health? This will affect the decision of who else to involve
- Is patient safety an issue? If it is, then the options available are different because patient safety will usually take precedence over everything else and you will probably need to involve your clinical or medical director
- Do they appear to have any insight into the problem?
- What has been your own role or that of the department or others in the developing situation? For example, if you are aware that there is a culture of intolerance and poor supervision in the department that the trainee works in, it may not be surprising that they have made errors. If you have been involved in a case or one of your own patients has suffered, you may be angry and this may cloud your ability to deal with the situation effectively

Using these questions you should begin to build up a picture of who would be best to deal with the situation, how to put it to the trainee and the type of solutions or processes that may be suitable.

Finally, before approaching the trainee, plan for things that might go wrong. It is not a good idea to tackle a trainee about a performance problem on a Friday afternoon when they are about to start a weekend on call, unless patient safety is an issue. Make sure that you can offer them independent support afterwards. This could be the clinical tutor or someone in the Foundation school, a trained mentor or a peer support network. Consider the possibility that they will end the discussion not being able to work for the next few days, either through stress or suspension. How will you cover their shifts?

Consider the possibility that things could turn ugly and your need to protect yourself from accusations of bullying, sexism or racism. Consider arranging a three-way meeting so that there is an independent view of what took place.

Talking to the trainee

Like clinical consultations, the initial approach to the trainee is going to shape the outcome. Like a normal consultation, it may be best to agree an agenda at the beginning, using open questions to elicit the trainee's point of view and whether they have any specific concerns. If you have called a special meeting, make it clear why this is and explain to the trainee why other people are involved (if they are). You need to go into the meeting with an open mind about the rights and wrongs of the situation and you need to make that clear to the trainee. If you give them the impression you are judgemental, they are likely to be defensive and/or angry and obstruct the way to a mutually agreed solution.

Openers might include:

'As you know, John, we are here to discuss the incident last Wednesday. Before we start, I wondered whether there were any issues that you wanted to raise as well and I would like to hear from you your views about what happened.'

'Well, Nidal, this is your regular educational review meeting. I see you have your portfolio and we can discuss that in a minute. Before we start I wondered if there is anything that you want to raise? No? Well, I do have something specific that I want to talk about. A couple of people have mentioned one or two incidents recently where cross words have been exchanged on the ward. I want to give you the chance to tell me your version of events.'

Agreeing a plan

The stages after the initial discussion are difficult to define as they depend on a myriad of possibilities. If the trainee has good insight, no previous problems and is well motivated to change, then you may be able to deal with it between you and the trainee, although there will of course need to be a record made in the trainee's portfolio. But few performance issues are this simple. You will almost certainly be wise to discuss the issue with the head of your Foundation programme. If patient safety is at risk, you must involve your medical director (or equivalent in primary care). The key outcome is to agree a plan with the trainee to address the issues raised. For example, if the problem is clinical skills in A&E, the trainee could be directed to discuss all cases that they see with a senior before discharging patients and to complete a reasonable number of formal assessments within a short period until a review decides whether they have enough competence to carry on at their current level. If there is a health problem such as stress, the trainee could be directed to Occupational Health and they may need to be seen regularly to ensure that they are progressing satisfactorily and coping with work. If drugs or alcohol are involved, then this will definitely be out of your hands, even if disclosed to you in the setting of educational supervision.

Monitoring and reviewing progress and further options

You will have to meet regularly and frequently with a trainee who is struggling – as often as every two or four weeks. Look for concrete evidence of progress. If trainees are not keeping up with their agreed plan, you need to find out why and act accordingly. There are many options available for trainees who, despite support and appropriate efforts to encourage their development, continue to fall short of the standards expected. They may be able to undergo a period of retraining and observation in a different role (e.g. as a clinical attachment or observer) to enable them to acquire the relevant skills, knowledge and attitudes. At this stage you will probably be a small part of the equation as other senior staff will need to be involved.

SUMMARY

We hope that this chapter has been helpful. It has reviewed the changed structures of education for the Foundation programme and covered the general areas of educational and clinical supervision and the range of learning opportunities that should be made available to trainees. It has given an introduction to the area of poor performance. Hopefully it will help you identify the areas where you can continue to develop your skills.

Beyond the Foundation programme. Career management for Foundation doctors

8

Jonathan Carter and Mark Welfare

> ❝The biggest mistake that you can make is to believe that you are working for somebody else. Job security is gone. The driving force of a career must come from the individual. Jobs are owned by the company, you own your career.
>
> Learn to enjoy every minute of your life. Be happy now. Don't wait for the something outside of yourself to make you happy in the future. Think how precious is the time you have to spend, whether it's at work or with your family. Every minute should be enjoyed and savoured.❞
>
> Earl Nightingale

INTRODUCTION

Under the new career structure your progression from medical school to senior appointment via the Foundation programme and higher training is meant to be as seamless as Michael Flatley's wardrobe. So in theory you should all have made your mind up during your carefully selected F2 options and be ready to enter the run through specialty or GP training of your choice.

It is currently proposed that there will be 16 or 17 specialty groupings to apply to after the Foundation programme (Box 8.1). For some there will be a short period of specialist training with progression based entirely on satisfactory performance, after which you will be fully qualified. For others, the ST1 and ST2 years will be a common stem and there will need to be a further step of selection to enter a more specialised area in ST3. This step is likely to be 'gated', with the need to pass royal college exams being the gatekeeper. For example, to do gastroenterology, you would need to do the ST1 and ST2 stem of Medicine in General and, having completed the MRCP, apply for a gastroenterology ST3 training post. In specialties such as histopathology, you will progress seamlessly from ST1 to Certificate of Completion of Training with no additional interview steps.

But it won't work out exactly as planned for everyone. So, how do you go about choosing and planning your future career?

Traditionally, medical careers have been thought of as very linear – you finish medical school, do a PRHO job (now the Foundation programme), do

> **Box 8.1 Specialty groupings for post-Foundation applications**
>
> Acute care common stem
> Anaesthesia
> Basic neurosciences
> Chemical pathology
> ENT
> General practice
> Histopathology
> Medical microbiology
> Medicine in general
> Obstetrics and gynaecology
> Ophthalmology
> Oral and maxillofacial surgery
> Paediatrics
> Psychiatry
> Public health
> Radiology
> Surgery in general

SHO and registrar training (now specialty training) and – hey presto! – you have made it and you get a consultant or GP job for the rest of your life.

Two opposing influences mean that things may be much less linear in the future.

First, healthcare in the UK and around the world is changing in ever-faster cycles and both the clinical skills needed and the health service we work in are likely to have changed before you complete your training. Imagine what will happen if the Conservatives are in power rather than Labour. The old adage 'the only thing constant is change' has never been truer. Some examples from recent history include the rapid adoption of coronary artery stenting, which has made many cardiothoracic surgeons surplus to requirements, and the switch to minimally invasive gynaecological surgery, which has meant the closure of many gynae wards. The government has announced their intention to shift 5% of all care from hospital to the community. And if the increased funding of the NHS really does get rid of waiting lists in the way that the government proposes, then private practice is likely to be significantly reduced. So, all of you who had planned to be spending your Friday afternoons as a consultant at the local Nuffield putting in hips or removing adenoids in order to fund your yacht and private education for your kids may need to think again! Similarly, the freedoms associated with Foundation Trusts may have unexpected consequences for careers, and the new training structure may result in the return of senior and junior consultant grades in some form.

Second, the new training scheme is designed to shorten training and make people into 'consultants' quicker. Consultants trained under the new system are unlikely to be the 'finished article' compared to the current position and will require more learning and development in the early stages of their senior career. It seems likely that consultants will move between jobs as they undergo further training post-certification. It is even possible that doctors may be able to retrain in another specialty very quickly as their common learning is recognised and the second training scheme shortened.

The profession is also increasingly recognizing that a Certificate of Completion of Training will not necessarily mean a traditional consultant job in an NHS hospital with a contract and employment rights that current consultants enjoy. The introduction of Independent Treatment Centres (ITCs) may change career structures and in the future it seems likely that people with a Certificate of Completion of Training will enter a variety of jobs including in ITCs and will not just work in traditional consultant or GP senior positions. A level of unemployment is thought by many to be inevitable and even desirable by the Department of Health.

The situation for general practice is equally uncertain. New GP principal positions are becoming increasingly uncommon as existing principals or PCTs employ salaried GPs. American transnationals are just beginning to enter the primary care market but are likely to play a significant role in the future. Some practices now have four principals employing 20 salaried GPs and are beginning to develop along the lines of the American Health Maintenance Organizations (HMOs). Clearly, the main people enjoying the dividends from this large-scale business are the four partners. This changes the balance between risk, autonomy and opportunity that has existed in primary care and there is a danger that many GPs will become hired hands, serving the interest of the practice/business rather than acting as independent professionals

The overall outcome of these two influences is difficult to forecast, but careers are likely to be more mixed or 'portfolio'-based rather than restricted to narrow specialties. Those who are flexible and can exhibit a range of skills are likely to be the most successful. Doctors known to us have followed the following career structures:

- One trained in elderly care, worked as a consultant, then retrained in general practice before working in the local deanery. He then returned to a consultant post specialising in intermediate care
- One trained in general practice before becoming a regional specialist in paediatric gastroenterology
- One trained as a GP, had a career as an associate specialist in emergency care and has now started a business commissioning healthcare
- Another trained as a GP, went back into training, initially as a respiratory physician but then as a cardiologist, and now works as a community cardiologist liaising between primary and secondary care

This chapter should help guide you through your options post-Foundation. It considers a wide range of choices, including having a career break, working abroad and whether to opt for general practice or hospital medicine. More importantly, it aims to help you develop your skills in career management, a skill for life-long career planning from Foundation programme to retirement and beyond.

CAREER MANAGEMENT

At the moment it may well seem that your choice of post-Foundation job will decide your future. In some ways it will, but there will always be unforeseen opportunities and unexpected barriers. There is an old saying: 'When the wind blows, some people build walls and some people build windmills'. Successful career management is an essential skill that will help you harvest the winds of change to develop a successful career. This adaptive approach is exemplified in the Windmills careers guidance approach described below. Careers management should also be put into the context of life management – a career cannot be managed in isolation from the rest of your life. This section will help you think about ways of managing your career and life.

The NHS perceives that doctors have very poor skills in careers management and that careers advice for doctors is also poor. In particular, there is a perception that doctors only seek careers advice when they encounter a crisis of some kind and that around 15% of doctors are being lost to the profession within three years of qualifying, partly because of poor careers advice and management. In response, it has developed a comprehensive, 86-page document (available from the MMC website) which seeks to initiate discussion on careers management and the structures that support it within medicine (see the MMC working group for careers management, *Careers Management: An Approach for Medical Schools, Deaneries, Royal Colleges and Trusts*, London: The Stationery Office, 2005). Laudably, it aims to provide rigorous and systematic careers counselling, enabling trainees to make informed decisions. The document also recognises the importance of linking educational planning and careers management. A concern that we do have is that one of the other main aims is to 'ensure trainees successfully complete training programmes in the minimum time necessary'. From our perspective, careers management should be trainee-centred and focus on what the trainees want and not primarily on the needs of the Department of Health. There is growing evidence that some trainees are concerned that they will not be ready for senior positions, particularly consultancy, if training takes place too quickly. There is also evidence that approximately 30% of trainees are not ready to choose their career after the two-year Foundation programme, which further counsels against too much streamlining.

What are the key elements of successful career management?

There have been surprisingly few studies of what constitutes effective careers management in medicine. Personal experience suggests that chance is a pretty powerful factor and there is even a theory that backs this up (see J. D. Krumboltz and A. S. Levin, *Happenstance Theory: Luck is no Accident. Making the Most of Happenstance in Your Life and Career*, Atascadero CA: Impact Publishers, 2004). So, develop your skills in making use of chance and unexpected opportunities as much as possible, but also consider proactive approaches. One model of careers management suggests that there is a pyramid of cognitive skills for career management, with knowledge of your own skills and the options available at the base, decision-making skills in the middle and

> **Box 8.2   Keys to successful career management**
>
> Knowing yourself
>
> Preparation and planning
>
> Developing generic skills
>
> Developing specific skills, including niche skills
>
> Developing your own opportunities and using chance opportunities – happenstance theory (Krumboltz and Levin, 2004) suggests that there is a specific skill in being able to maximise unexpected opportunities and not just respond randomly to chance happenings
>
> Flexibility
>
> Seeing and seizing new opportunities
>
> Using career support effectively
>
> Managing the work–life–play balance and integrating play with work

meta-cognition and understanding of the way in which you make decisions and control of the way you make decisions at the top.

Some of the skills that you may need to manage your career successfully are shown in Box 8.2 and dealt with in more detail below.

Know yourself

Perhaps one of the hardest skills in any area of work is to know yourself. How do others see you? Are you as effective as you think you are, or do you underestimate your skills? There are formal psychological approaches to assessing your skills and personality, including the Myers–Briggs personality inventory. In terms of career management, it would be very helpful to understand the practical skills you have and many techniques are being trialled to assess whether hand–eye coordination can be used as a predictor for selection into training programmes. So far it appears that techniques of measuring hand–eye coordination generally result in higher scores for men (because they are mainly invented by men?) and are also predicted by heavy use of computer games. This suggests that they do not measure permanent and immutable traits but learnable skills. As it happens, trainees acknowledge this – those who are aware of poor practical skills appear not to be put off applying. They say that they will probably be able to learn the skills with sufficient practice! Other specialties might rely on communications skills or the ability to cope in an emergency. Can you accurately assess your current skills and long-term potential in these areas? Some specialties rely on good eyesight (e.g. pathology and plastic surgery).

There is a current vogue for the use of career-matching questionnaires that seek to match your skills and ambitions with those required in each specialty. These questionnaires can, however, be no more than a guide. They are not a direct match and don't explain clearly what factors made you seemingly so well matched to a specific career. The two main examples are the Medical Specialty Aptitude test (MSAT: www.med-ed.virginia.edu/specialties) and the Sci45 or Sci59, developed by the Open University. As an academic gastroenterologist, one of the authors did the MSAT and gastroenterology came 14th on the list, with aviation medicine (a US specialty), public health, paediatrics and psychiatry topping the list! The Open University kindly made the Sci59 available to us at an early stage. Again, the gastroenterologist appears to have made the wrong choice! Despite scoring 'working with children' low on three separate questions, neonatology was the first career suggested and gastroenterology came 21st. The output of the Sci59 summarises your rating of the main domains assessed which is more helpful than the actual rating list of all specialties. Particular caution should be used in using these questionnaires in the new jobs market – they were developed and validated in the old jobs market and their basis (e.g. their valuation of research skill and interest, or the role of people who want to allow time to be with their children) may become less valid in the new era.

Preparation and planning

This is an essential skill in careers management. You need to plan the development of your skills and gather evidence for them. Many medical students with clear career objectives will have started planning their specialty application in the selection of their SSCs in medical school! The recent upheavals in training have meant that it has been difficult to know what is expected for applications. You need to become familiar with the national job specification for your chosen specialty (available on the MTAS website in due course) and keep yourself well informed about what is needed so that you can build your CV from an early stage. Plan your audit, tasters, optional study leave, etc. to build your knowledge of the specialty and the evidence for your skills and commitment. Generate transferable skills that can be used in any specialty. Find out what the senior job will actually be like. Preparation for the interview is also vital and is addressed below.

Applications skills

The skill of applying for a job is dealt with in detail below. In previous times it was seen as essential to cultivate the seniors responsible for selection and to meet them first – the so-called 'trial by sherry'. Things have changed and now your success will depend on being selected for interview from the structured application form and in your approach to the structured interview.

Being flexible

The aims of the government are to speed up training, making it quicker and more streamlined, with the implication that career planning will be easier and more direct. But there are serious uncertainties in the future. It may well be that the new system will not always produce the effect intended. Workforce planning is unpredictable and there has traditionally been more than one road to Rome. As technology advances the end may not be where we previously thought it was. There also seems to be an unwritten notion that the government wishes to create a degree of medical unemployment, so you will need to keep flexibility in the development and utilization of your skills so that you can switch between specialties. There are also the unpredictable events in your own life that may necessitate the need to change the emphasis of your career development.

Using career support

Doctors have been used to utilizing haphazard and biased careers advice and are actually quite good at doing so appropriately. They have relied on their own resources and skills in most circumstances. The hope is that in the future there will be a smorgasbord of careers support using a variety of techniques and approaches that will allow you to select the most appropriate one for you. There will be a mix of group, online, written and personal approaches. Find out what is for you. Talk to people you respect and who you know are well informed, including your educational supervisor or programme director. Attend your Trust or programme teaching sessions on careers. Your deanery or Foundation school will offer improved careers advice and are likely to organise careers fairs. Keep up to date with the MMC and royal college websites. Consider careers approaches from outside of medicine. Career-minded blogs are also developing, for example on the *BMJ* Careers Focus website. (For some of the relevant websites, see Chapter 10.)

Managing the work–life–play balance

Your time in the Foundation programme may well be the first time that you have had to question whether you have the right balance between the different domains of your life or whether the career you have chosen will give you the right balance in the future.

This chapter draws on the current vogue for life coaching which has some general approaches and lessons that might be useful to consider.

Anita Houghton is a life coach who has written extensively for doctors, including the *BMJ* Careers section, and can be contacted through her website (www.workinglives.co.uk) or email (anita@workinglives.co.uk). She has written two books (*Know Yourself* and *Finding Square Holes*) and runs regular introductory sessions in London. Another sensible and pragmatic approach is the Windmills programme, which is being adapted for Foundation doctors in some deaneries. We particularly like the Windmills idea that work, life and play should not be regarded as mutually exclusive categories and that finding ways to blend them can be one way to a balanced existence. They also have some excellent techniques to help you develop yourself; the materials can be used online (www.windmillsprogramme.com).

Life coaching uses a variety of techniques to help people think about managing their work–life–play balance. To begin to think about how you might manage your life and work, consider these eight domains of existence:

1. Personal development in terms of education and professional development
2. Work – what you achieve and what you get back
3. Finances – security, risk, income, income protection, pension rights, etc.
4. Relationship with significant other and expression of your sexuality in its broadest way

5. Relationships with family and friends
6. Play – what you do in your leisure time, including sport, hobbies and interests
7. Expression of your self, whether through the activities in 'Play' or in terms of spirituality, religious or political beliefs or the arts in their broadest sense
8. Health

How are you going to balance these domains? Different life coaching models use various techniques to help you. At this stage in your career it may even be difficult because it is a time of such rapid change that your anchors and roles are constantly changing. It might be helpful to think ahead to the years of your post-Foundation training or life as a specialist or GP. How will those posts help you to fulfil your dreams in all of these domains?

This simple exercise might help you to think about it:

Step 1: Rank the eight domains above according to which are the most important to you now
Step 2: Score your current satisfaction with each domain from 0 to 10 with 0 being complete dissatisfaction and 10 being complete satisfaction with your current experience
Step 3: Review the scores by ranking. How satisfied are you with the satisfaction scores for your top three ranked domains at the moment?
Step 4: Now think of yourself at 40. You have secured your senior post as a consultant or GP and have been practising for five years. Repeat the exercise of ranking the domains and then scoring them. If you cannot imagine life at 40, think of a role model at work and think of how you would rank the domains and score your satisfaction if you were in their position. How have the changes associated with growing older affected the way you rank the domains? How do the scores look now?
Step 5: Finally, think of yourself at 60, approaching the end of your career. How would you like to look back on your career? This may be difficult, so use an example of a senior consultant or GP or your parents as a working example. Now rank the eight domains and score how satisfied you imagine you would be with your perception of their life.

Another technique to help you plan your career and life is to develop a lifeline. Starting with where you are now, draw a lifeline for the rest of your working life with sections for each decade. Mark the key elements of your projected working and personal life. This will help you see how these two elements are likely to interact and how you may have to adapt each aspect to the other. It may even be helpful for getting you to think about your retirement and how planning your life and career will impact on this. There are many uncertainties and some of you will be more certain than others about the future, but it can be useful to start you thinking.

Are any patterns emerging? Have you recognised any pitfalls you wish to avoid? A colleague told us this urban myth. They had attended a prestigious scientific meeting in the US. The star speaker was not only pre-eminent in the field, but also played saxophone in his own band and the colleague had attended an informal gig he had given. Turning to the person next to him he expressed his admiration for this man who was not only world famous in science but also a skilled musician. The stranger was disdainful: 'What's so great? You probably get to see him more than me. And he's my dad.'

Formal life coaching would ask you to look at the questions posed by this exercise, begin to think about what you wish to do differently and then set yourself a few manageable goals (or SMART objectives). It would also help you to select your future career based on the importance of the domains and which are best matched to particular careers. For example, someone who rates financial gain, security and high status may be most suited to a career that gives access to considerable private practice, whereas someone who values family and friends and has time-consuming hobbies may be advised on a career that gives opportunity for part-time working.

This section is designed only to give you a taste for the concept of achieving an adequate work–life balance. Those interested in the subject should seek more information. The *BMJ Careers Focus* frequently runs articles on life coaching and the work–life balance. You could even try entering 'life coach' into Google and finding your own resources!

CHOOSING YOUR CAREER IN MEDICINE

Now is the time to put these career management skills into practice. For the majority of doctors who still enjoy medicine, even after splitting their glove during a PR, you truly have passed the commitment test. But which career path to follow? Hopefully your experiences in the Foundation programme will go most of the way to confirming or refuting your views on many of the options. What is the next step?

It might be helpful to review briefly the aims of the new career structure. (Further details are given in Chapter 1.)

Two of the main aims of the MMC initiative were to streamline the career pathways for doctors, so reducing the number of trainees who had to switch from their desired pathway because they could not get the SpR job of their choice, and to encourage doctors to train in the so called shortage specialties. So, the carrot is that F2 posts are intended to give you experience in specialties such as genetics, public health or virology. But there is also a stick – by restricting the number of posts for run-through training, you are now forced to make choices early in your career. And if you can't get into the specialty of your choice, the DoH hopes you will choose one of the specialties that has difficulty recruiting.

Another MMC aim is to train more academics. It hopes to make it easier for medical students and junior doctors to gain experience in both research and teaching, particularly in the Foundation programme, and to create structured career opportunities for doctors who want to work as academics. However, academics' career paths will move in a completely separate but parallel direction to the normal training posts and it seems likely that it will be difficult to move into the academic stream in mid-career.

After the Foundation programme you will enter one of approximately 17 specialist training programmes or general practice programmes. You will compete with other F2s for an ST1 year through open and fair competition. As an ST doctor (STD – the abbreviation team has fallen foul of this one!) your specialty will have a curriculum with set learning outcomes. This will be coordinated by the Royal Colleges, the Conference of Postgraduate Medical Deans (COPMED) and the Committee of General Practice Education Directors (COGPED), but will be answerable to the PMETB.

Dissolution of the SHO years – the lost tribe and workforce planning

Workforce planning in the NHS is a dark art practised by ever-decreasing numbers of public health consultants whose job descriptions and management structures have changed every other year during the Labour administration. How can we expect to predict how many consultants Trusts will need in five or more years' time, let alone how many they will be able to afford? Centralised control of numbers in training, combined with independent purchase of the product, is a strange hybrid of Soviet-style planning and free market purchasing. Not surprisingly, therefore, it is an inexact science and it has always been difficult to match numbers of trainees with training opportunities and long-term employment prospects. But the big upheaval of the MMC seems to have exacerbated the problem. SHOs exiting their contracts in 2007 and 2008 are going to clash with F2s applying for specialty training (ST) programmes. It is very difficult to forecast exactly how many trainees will be looking for ST posts at each level. In June 2006 it seemed that there would be only 9500 posts for all levels in ST programmes in England, with no decision made in the other UK countries as yet. However, in October 2006 the number of ST posts was predicted to be 17,000–18,000 with an additional 5000 Fixed Term Specialty Training Appointment (FTSTA) posts, so there should be a reasonable match to the number of people seeking posts. The one certainty is that applications to popular specialty training programmes are going to be extremely competitive between 2007 and 2009, by which time it should have settled down. The number of ST1 posts in the future will we hope be closely matched to the number of F2 posts each year, but has not been decided at the time of writing and it is likely to take 2–3 years to get the system in balance.

The ST programmes vary in length according to specialty. For example, it is at least three years for general practice. For hospital specialties it is likely to vary from four years (acute care) to seven years for dual training in interventional cardiology or some surgical specialties, for example. During this time you will be given a unique training number, similar to the numbers of the old Registrar days. At the end of your time on the Specialty or General Practice Training Programme you will be awarded the Certificate of Completion of Training and be eligible to apply for a job as a consultant or GP or work in an independent treatment centre.

OK, so if all is fair in love and war, and the Foundation programme is designed to make us all equal in terms of competency at the end of F2, how will the application for ST programmes be through 'open and fair competition'?

The original plan was that there would be a national application process starting February each year through the Medical Training Application Service (www.mtas.nhs.uk). The electronic application form would be used for shortlisting followed by a structured interview process which will be decided on at local level, so was likely to vary considerably between locations and specialties. The interview would only tap into the attributes described in the national job description and would function like a mini-OSCE with stations using different techniques to assess the varying competencies required. Applicants would find out whether they have been appointed in April, with a second round of applications in May with decisions in June.

However, in 2007 the MTAS application system was thrown into chaos after uncertainties about the fairness of the shortlisting process and as we write, the whole system is being reviewed. The system for applications in 2008 and beyond is therefore not currently known but it seems likely that it will still be based on a national level electronic application form and local standardised interviewing. Applicants for General Practice (in 2007) had to attend a national assessment centre and complete a written exam for shortlisting and this is likely to continue for the future.

Electronic application systems should have the advantage of reducing the number of applications that have to be made by trainees and processed by Trusts. However there are some potential downsides. The application system is likely to limit some elements of choice. You will only be allowed to apply to two separate specialties and two different 'schools'. The format may well mean that you have little choice in where you actually get work and some ST rotations will involve an enormous amount of travelling. For example, trainees in medicine in the Northern deanery could work anywhere from the west coast of the Lake District to Middlesbrough and up into rural Northumberland. It may well be very difficult to weigh up your choices between a chance to get a post in your first choice specialty against a chance to get a post in the area where you wish to live. The system will be rather inflexible.

You will have to weigh up the balance between applying for the specialty of your choice, the geographical area you wish to live in, your aptitudes and the competitiveness of the specialty.

Unfortunately, there may be tears at some point. If the Cardiology ST programme you were dreaming of begins to slip from your grasp, you may wonder if your heart is really in it after all. What happens then?

Not everyone will get the ST or General Practice programme they want. But if you do fall at the first hurdle there's no need to head off to the Job Centre just yet. MMC has designed the career framework to include FTSTAs. These last a year and allow you to work in the same, or similar, specialties to the one you have set your heart on and to continue getting training in that specialty. These may count towards your CCT if you acquire relevant competencies and they will also allow you to acquire extra skills to apply for the specialty training programme the next year. If you can demonstrate that you have achieved the competencies for, say, ST1, you may, in theory at least, be able to apply for ST2.

The applications for FTSTA posts will be made (in 2007) at the same time as the first round of specialty applications and through the MTAS website. However, it is proposed that the results of these applications will not be made known until after the second round of specialty applications.

FTSTAs will, however, be fixed-term – one year only – and will not provide you unlimited opportunities to continue applying for specialty training posts.

The most that you will be able to do in each specialty will be two years. You will then be able to apply for an FTSTA in another specialty and change career track.

The proportion of ST posts to FTSTA posts is unknown, but is likely to change in the coming years. If a large proportion of doctors end up spending two or more years in FTSTA posts while waiting for an appropriate training post, the whole point of the revisions will have been defeated.

At the end of two years in a specialty FTSTA, if you have not got into the specialty training post of your choice, you will be eligible to apply for a 'career post' in that specialty, something nearly equivalent to the old staff grade. This will effectively be a dead-end post for most with just two years of post-Foundation training and you will be condemned to spend the rest of your life in a drudge service post with little promise of any further training or career development. These career grade posts will not be equivalent to a consultant-level appointment and it is extremely unlikely that doctors in this role will be able to practise truly independently. Salary and access to promotion and senior positions in management are also likely to be severely restricted. You should avoid these posts like the plague unless there is an overwhelming reason why you do not wish to proceed through a full Specialist Training or General Practice programme.

In addition to the opportunities to apply for a Specialist Training programme or an FTSTA post, it is likely that there will still be unofficial jobs with unofficial job titles in which you can gain experience. Again, this may not count towards your CCT, but it will enable you to gain training to help you compete in your applications to the official training programmes. Examples are likely to include jobs designed primarily to deliver service such as 'Trust doctor' posts and those designed to fill other gaps, such as teaching or making up the numbers to have a satisfactory on-call rota in the middle grades. For example, there are many teaching or research fellowships that give you a chance to improve your CV or delay your final career choice. These posts are likely to be less attractive in the future and MMC hopes that the FTSTA posts will be the main 'holding pen' for people who have not been able to enter specialty training.

In theory, a doctor who has received training and experience in any post, can apply to be on the Specialist Register provided they can satisfy the PMETB that they have fulfilled the required competencies. As we write, it is alleged that someone has been given a CCT by the PMETB despite having failed the exit examinations for their Royal College on a number of occasions. This is causing a lot of conflict within the profession. This route to CCT is known as Article 14. In general, the rate of successful application under Article 14 is very low and it would be unwise to rely on it as a route to a CCT. Article 11 applies for doctors wishing to get on the General Practice Register who do not have a CCT.

CAREER OPTIONS – HOW DO DOCTORS CHOOSE?

What kind of doctor do you want to be? People decide on their careers at different stages. Some begin when they're barely out of the uterus; others leave it until a bit later to start showing signs of what they may grow up to be. Approximately 30% of F2 doctors will still be uncertain about their future. Others may not be able to progress in their first choice career and so previous certainty will have to be thought through again.

We have conducted a research study on how F2 doctors make their choices locally and the results are very interesting. Some understanding of this process may be helpful for you to see how your own thoughts have built up and how you could develop your career ideas.

We found that there are four main themes influencing career choice in F2 doctors:

1. The experience you have of the specialties as an undergraduate and Foundation doctor. This is very important and is related directly to trainees' experience of the workplace. Doctors weigh up such things as the types of patients encountered, the level of practical work, the degree of generalist or specialist skills involved, how sick the patients are and the level of distress that they experience, the amount of patient contact and the degree of autonomy they can expect. Also important are the role models that you meet during your experience, the type of feedback you receive and the work environment such as hours, acceptance by colleagues and whether you fit in, the level and functioning of teamwork in a specialty and the way you are treated by your colleagues when doing an attachment.

2. Your internal subjective experience (emotions) and personality. This relates to how a post makes you feel and is also shaped by your personality and whether the internal experience of working in the specialty matches your needs. Your self-confidence and the degree of excitement you need and the level provided by the job are important, as is the interest that you think it will sustain for you. Some doctors wish to be more challenged than others and require greater stimulation to retain their interest. Levels of tolerance of worry about their patients or their own careers vary between people. For some doctors it is important to feel that they have achieved something concrete in their daily work (e.g. hip replacement), others are able to live with smaller or less immediate gains (e.g. working with substance abusers). Some doctors need to have a high degree of diagnostic certainty, whereas others can live with uncertainty.

3. Other external influences, such as perceived career opportunities and the job market. Under this heading we found that factors unrelated to work were important in influencing career decisions. For example, the job market, pay, social status, the influence of career guidance, the influence of the career on your leisure activities and lifestyle, and in particular the opportunities for flexible working are all important. For example, specializing in a tertiary service such as liver transplantation means that you will need to live and work in just one of the six or so centres that offer this service, whereas a desire to work part-time will be more likely to be fulfilled in specialties where continuity of care is less important (e.g. laboratory medicine, acute care or general practice).

4. The timelines around decision-making and your own decision-making processes can also influence the career you end up in. Trainees make their decisions in varying ways. The main considerations here were whether trainees were certain or not about their career, whether they wanted to remain a generalist or specialise at an early stage, and whether they were basing their decision on a positive or negative influence or a least-worst option. For most, the final decision is made on positive criteria, but for some a negative (e.g. too many exams) will make up their minds. For many trainees in our study, the most important aspect of the step after F2 was that they could keep their options open and continue to explore the possibilities – they did not have sufficient information to make a final choice so the next step would be something where they could gain further general experience. Some jobs were perceived as being better than others for keeping options open and allowed the final choice to be delayed. This was particularly true of medical SHO jobs, which were perceived as providing training and experience relevant to many specialties. In the future this will not be necessary because other specialties will have run-through programmes (e.g. radiology) or possible because there will be few ST posts and switching between specialties may not be easy. For those who wish to keep their options open, the choice may be between FTSTA posts and applying to a specialty they are uncertain about and changing at a later stage.

In the end, F2 doctors appear to base their decision largely on choosing a specialty that achieves the greatest degree of congruence between their perceptions of themselves and their perceptions of the specialty in its broadest sense – for example, whether you match the 'type' required to do the job (or at least currently doing it) and the relationship between the options available in their chosen career and your optimal lifestyle.

Many of the influences on career choice that we found are reflected in career choice questionnaires such as the Sci45/Sci59 or MSAT.

Career choice for doctors who wish to work flexibly

Working part-time, whether you are a man or woman, poses significant questions for career development. Women have traditionally gravitated to certain careers in medicine in the UK and there is little doubt that there is not a level playing field for women in some specialties. Careers advice, and in particular the Sci45, Sci59 and MSAT, tend to reflect past experience and opportunities and the current status quo. They will lead women (or men who express a wish to work part-time) towards some careers (e.g. paediatrics or GP) and away from others (e.g. surgery or academic medicine). However, 'times they are a-changing'. In an era where more than 50% of graduates are women, it is likely that career structures and job patterns will have to change to meet the needs of women rather than women change career preference to suit the career structure. Specialties that are not available to women will be weakened by the fact that they will reduce the pool of candidates and will not therefore be able to select the best. In addition, it is likely that more men will want to work part-time or just 40 hours a week with few unsocial hours in the future. So, if your Sci59 does not include cardiothoracic surgery in your top five but you wish to do it, don't be discouraged. It may still be a struggle and you may face discrimination, but when you get there it is likely to look different from how it looks now.

Gaps in trainees' knowledge may affect choice

Trainees – and consultants and GPs for that matter – have very little understanding of the full range of options open to them. For example, did you know that there are 62 recognised specialties in the UK and even more subspecialties, many of which are keen to be promoted as full specialties? How many of the 62 can you name and, even more importantly, do you have any idea what some of them do? Many of these have only a handful of consultants, but there could be a career in one of them for you. You may find Anita D. Taylor's *How to Choose a Medical Specialty* (Philadelphia: WB Saunders, 2003) or Chris Ward and Simon Eccles' *So You Want to be a Brain Surgeon* (London: Oxford University Press, 1997) useful. In Chapter 10 we present our own potted guide to the 62 registered specialties, major subspecialties and the GP and working abroad options, as well as the contact details for the relevant training bodies. If you are uncertain about the way ahead, take a look. You may be surprised at the range of options available.

Few trainees have a clear picture of the daily lives of the seniors in the jobs that they aspire to. Most of their perception about future careers relates to the time when trainees are in contact with the GP/consultant (i.e. twice-weekly ward rounds or occasional out-patients or procedure/theatre sessions). Trainees have little understanding of what seniors do the rest of the time. Another thing to watch out for is the effect on your perspective of a specialty of being in transition from student to doctor. Your experience of the first and second posts in your Foundation programme may have been affected by the difficulties of coping with the new role of being a doctor. If you were put off the specialty because of this, you might like to reflect on what your experience would have been like if you had done the rotation in a different order. Similarly, don't let your experience (good or bad) of one senior doctor make your mind up. They may not be representative.

In our local research programme on career choice in F2, we found that job availability was rarely a major factor in helping doctors to decide their future careers. This seems surprising given that future employment is so important, but in the past there was a more or less social contract between doctors in training and the government. There was, if anything, a slight gap in favour of the trainees between the numbers of consultants/GPs needed and the number trained. There were some well-publicised problems in planning, such as the overestimation of the numbers in respiratory medicine and obstetrics in the last five years, but generally, once you had an SpR job, you were more or less guaranteed a consultant job. Things have changed and so an assessment of the career prospects, and in particular your own prospects, is essential now.

Information on specific careers is available from a number of sources beyond your own experience. The *BMJ* Careers section carries a lot of useful information and the online version has a search facility so that you can check published articles (www.bmjcareers.com). You can also ask a question via their advice zone (www.bmjcareersadvicezone.synergynewmedia.co.uk). There is a plan in the national career management policy to have a central NHS online medical careers advice centre and a book of medical careers, but neither of these had been published at the time of writing. The Royal Colleges provide data on the number of vacancies advertised each year in their specialties and how many remained vacant. Most have reasonably accurate workforce predictions. The PMETB also has a central repository of information (www.pmetb.org.uk). See the MMC website or Chapter 10 for contact details.

A full list of recognised specialties and career options is given in Chapter 10. Here we give a brief guide to the general occupational categories that you might follow.

Hospital consultant

Consultant posts vary enormously in the skills required and the work involved. Job plans are generally divided into clinical sessions (out-patients, ward rounds, on-call, operating lists, procedures and clinical administration) which make up 75% of the job plan, and supporting sessions, including CPD, teaching, service development, etc., which make up the other 25%. As their career progresses, many consultants take on additional responsibilities for management or leadership roles in clinical governance or education. Opportunities for research are likely to be few in standard NHS positions in the future.

Academic posts

'Academic' as a title conjures up many different images. For some, 'academic' will have the pejorative meaning 'it's all academic now', implying that it doesn't matter. The view of academics among NHS doctors varies enormously from very positive to 'ought to get a proper job'. What does academic mean to you and do you know what academic doctors do? In general, academics are university-employed doctors who have considerable responsibility in three areas:

1. Teaching undergraduates
2. Managing undergraduate education
3. Research

The educational role

You will be familiar with the professors who have taught you as an undergraduate, but you may not be aware of the titles 'senior lecturer' and 'reader', which are also consultant-level academic posts. Of course, you do not have to have an academic post to teach undergraduates and much teaching is delivered by NHS consultants and GPs. Academics also have a lot of responsibility for supporting undergraduate education in other ways, such as curriculum design, setting and marking assessments and exams, being personal tutors, helping students in difficulty, etc.

The research role

The main drive to improving the academic career pathway is not for teaching but for research. The Medical Research Council and others wish to ensure that the UK continues to develop high quality medical researchers who will be world leaders in their field. Medical research is seen as a major part of maintaining Britain's economic competitiveness. The UK's research funding streams will therefore be directed much more narrowly at those who are likely to become world leaders in their field. Opportunities for non-academics to obtain research funding are likely to dwindle as bureaucracy increases and the criteria are tightened. Investigator-initiated clinical research has become considerably more difficult in recent years with more steps to obtain approval and greater responsibilities and penalties. Inevitably, therefore, much of the research that is being pursued is in laboratory animals and in the test tube so you should be prepared for the laboratory being your main workplace.

The academic career pathway

The academic career pathway has been completely revised with the advent of MMC and is described in detail in Chapter 2. The general theme is that academics will be selected at an early stage for specific training and will follow a specific training programme from Foundation programme to senior appointment. If you have done an academic post in the Foundation programme you will be well placed to obtain one of the academic post-Foundation posts. However, if you have done a standard Foundation programme job, there should still be some room for getting on the academic training ladder at this stage. You will probably need to work very hard on your CV and competencies to be successful in the competition for an academic post. It is becoming increasingly clear that there will be some division between academics who chiefly have responsibilities in education and those whose main remit is research. It is very difficult to ride both horses at once, especially in today's competitive market. There may be separate advertisements for research and education posts.

The qualities required for an academic training are easy to recognise. Cognitive ability is chief among these, particularly for those pursuing the research trajectory. For the educational side, a variety of skills, including teaching, is required.

General practice

The new contract in general practice has changed things considerably for GPs. They are no longer expected to cover their patients at night and so you can now be a GP and work as many or as few sessions a week as you want. You can even just do night shifts as Primary Care Trusts (PCTs) make separate arrangements to cover out-of-hours care. Many GPs now work as salaried doctors, either for the PCT or for a practice. Salaries for GP principals have increased considerably in the first few years of the contract, especially if they meet all their targets. However, some GPs have effectively lost autonomy and financial clout, working for large practices with one principal partner who hires workers to do most of the clinical work while harvesting a considerable salary for themself. Nevertheless, general practice has become much more attractive and competition for training posts is likely to be stiff. Ask yourself this question: if you can complete your training in three years, earn £100,000 for four days' work, choose how many days a week you work and never have to do any weekend or night work in general practice, why would you wish to pursue a hospital post with another 6–7 years' training and shift work, similar salary and a lifetime on call, with a high chance that you will be resident in many specialties? In fact, why don't I apply for retraining as a GP? There is also the possibility of becoming a GP with a special interest. So, you can have the best of both worlds – a generalist with special skills which should help maintain your interest and reduce the amount of time that you spend looking in kids' ears and throats!

Working abroad

Working in Western Australia was a wonderful experience for one of the authors and the period immediately post-Foundation is as good a time as any to have a career break. The training and medicine are very similar to those in the UK and you never know, you may like it enough to stay a little longer. A quick look through the back pages of the *BMJ* Careers section shows that there are myriad opportunities for working abroad as a junior doctor. Parts of the Commonwealth such as New Zealand, Australia and Canada need doctors, particularly in rural areas, or areas where the population is growing rapidly. Australia in particular is seeking to recruit thousands of doctors and even organises an annual recruiting conference, the 'Australia Needs Skills Expo' (www.immi.gov.au/skillexpos/index.htm).

The opportunities in English-speaking countries may, however, have been created in part by the number of doctors from those countries coming to the UK. It remains to be seen whether the recent changes in the immigration law, which will favour EEA graduates over Commonwealth graduates, will mean that they have to stay at home. If it does, the opportunities for travel may be reduced.

If you go abroad with the intention of taking a break and coming back to rejoin the training programme in the UK, you would be wise to gather as much evidence as possible about your competencies, preferably using the official MMC documentation, such as the assessments and logbooks that will be used in the UK. This will ensure that you maximise the chance of getting your experience recognised when you return.

Other working abroad options include volunteering, working on cruise ships in the Caribbean, working at ski resorts in Europe and taking part in expeditions. Most of the large volunteering organisations (e.g. VSO and Médecins Sans Frontièrers) require more experience than you will have acquired in the Foundation programme. Make sure that you are properly qualified for any voluntary roles that you take on – being a volunteer does not exempt you from the principles of *Good Medical Practice*. You should ensure that you have adequate insurance cover.

Decision time

At some point in F2 you will have to make a choice about which job to apply for next. Remember that this is not your final decision, just one more step on

8

> **Box 8.3   Questions to ask in pursuing a particular career**
>
> Will I fit in and if I don't, does it matter?
>
> Will I be able to sustain my interest?
>
> Will it have the right level of emotional impact on me, in terms of excitement, distress and positive reward?
>
> Do I have the skills required for this career?
>
> Will the general stress level be right for me?
>
> Will it have the right balance of generalist and specialist skills to suit me?
>
> Will it match my other life goals?
>
> Do I have enough knowledge or experience to make a definite positive choice for this and confidently reject other possibilities? If not, how will I get more knowledge/experience?
>
> Do I need to keep my options open?
>
> What are the job prospects like in general and realistically for me?
>
> Are there any risks to this career choice and how should I weigh them?
>
> What do I need to do to maximise my chances of success in this career?
>
> If I don't get this post, what is my 'plan B'?

the pathway and you will always have room for manoeuvre in the future. Both the PMETB and the MMC are making it clear that there will be mechanisms for trainees to switch between specialty training programmes and have some of the common learning from their previous training recognised towards their new specialty. So, if you complete ST1–3 in the General Medicine stem but then decide that you wish to do General Practice, or vice versa, you are likely to be able to enter at ST2 or even ST3 if you can show that you have acquired the relevant competencies.

So, you have equipped yourself with a deeper understanding of your skills and aptitudes using career planning tools and studied the form on the specialties that you are interested in. Once you have come up with some alternatives, we can frame some simple questions to help you decide if you have chosen the right career (Box 8.3). If you have a clear favourite, you might like to try these questions.

If you are struggling to come up with a clear favourite, you might like to compile a list of factors that will positively and negatively influence your choice of career. This can then form the basis of discussion with your educational supervisor or careers adviser.

The application

How are candidates chosen?

Career progression will essentially be based on acquired competencies, skills and your perceived aptitude for a specialty. Assessors don't pick out applications willy-nilly. Just like the Foundation applications, they have a scoring system, a quantitative assessment of the application based on the person specification for the post. Unsuccessful applicants have a right to find out why they were not selected and the choice needs to be defendable in court if required. Scoring systems enable the selection panel to say, 'You scored poorly in the questions assessing management skills, or communication skills'. Remember the catchphrase: 'Points mean prizes'.

Each question on the application form or each part of the interview process can be likened to a round of an amateur boxing bout. You have just a few short moments to score as many points as possible. Instead of scoring with punches to the head from the closed glove, you have to get key words or phrases that the assessors are looking for into your answers.

There will be points for two key areas:

Evidence of your suitability according to the job description
The suitability criteria will be divided into essential and desirable criteria. Essential criteria will reflect factors such as having a medical degree, being registered and in good standing with the GMC, and having successfully completed the Foundation programme. The desirable criteria for specialty training will vary, but don't forget that the purpose of the Foundation programme is to produce generic trainees, fit to do any specialty training post with good skills in professionalism and especially in acute care. It is likely, therefore, that you will be asked to show evidence of your ability to learn from error, to understand patient safety, to manage relevant acute presentations for that specialty, to manage your own learning, etc. You will not be expected to show evidence of your knowledge of the management of obscure specialty conditions or to possess skills beyond those that can be achieved in the Foundation programme. It is your generic skills, self-knowledge and potential that count.

Evidence of your commitment to and knowledge of the specialty
Under this heading you will have to show that you have an understanding of the skills that are needed in the specialty and how you 'fit' with the needs of the specialty. In terms of 'commitment' you will have to show that you have had a sustained interest in the specialty, perhaps even going as far back as third-year undergraduate, and that you have sought opportunities to find out more, such as through tasters or speaking to relevant clinicians. Once you are clear about your choice of career, make every attempt to find out and build evidence of your commitment. Join the trainee part of the specialist society, concentrate your audit and research areas in this area, gather extra evidence of your skills in this area, etc.

Building your CV

Maintaining a curriculum vitae is a part of good careers management because it helps you focus on your strengths and weaknesses and therefore should allow you to plan the acquisition of skills over time. In Chapter 5 we looked at the use of educational supervision to aid your learning and how that learning should be geared towards the gaps in your competencies. A CV is also useful as an aide-memoire for all the wonderful achievements you have gained throughout your distinguished career so far and will save you time because you can copy and paste bits to the application form. It takes longer than expected, so start to plan early. You often forget the odd award or achievement that you have never mentioned before.

What makes your application form stand out?

It's all well and good getting the competencies that are required. But how are you going to convince the panel of assessors that you have them? The art of application writing for the Foundation programme was addressed in detail in Chapter 2 and the general principles apply to the post-Foundation applications as well. At the time of writing the actual application form from 2006 was being reassessed and from 2007 it is likely that applications will consist of a specific application form and a CV, followed by the interview process. So at the time of writing the actual questions are not known. These are the key tips in filling your application form:

- Make sure that you answer the questions in a way that reflects the person specification and answers the question set. For example, if a job specification says that research skills are unimportant but evidence of practical skills is essential for a post in surgery, you will not get any points for mentioning your PhD which discovered a new gene involved in colon cancer, but you will get plenty of points for having passed the surgical STEPS course. If a question asks you to detail a particular skill and how you would use it in the specialty, make sure that you answer both parts of the question.
- Presentation and style. The best candidate in the world could still score poorly if their information is not presented in the right way and if the selection panel is not led to the best bits. Scoring applications is a long-winded and tedious task. Make sure that you keep the assessors interested and use buzz-words to attract their attention and score easy points. See our style guide in Chapter 2.
- Don't use the same achievement to illustrate all the criteria – a maximum of two uses for one achievement should be used.
- It is wise to show your application to as many seniors as you can, to your colleagues (not those applying for the same job) and people outside medicine, such as your parents. You want it to be as well-rounded and refined as possible, particularly if lay assessors are participating in the selection process.
- Don't lie (see Chapter 2).
- Complete the application yourself (see Chapter 2).
- Avoid jokes and cynicism.
- Use concrete examples of your practice to answer the questions. One difference between the Foundation application and the post-Foundation application is the experience that you have. Foundation applications rely on undergraduate performance and because you had no clinical responsibility, they have a certain theoretical feel to them. Post-Foundation applications will rely heavily on your showing how you actually perform in the workplace.

The application form for specialty posts is not available at the time of writing, but Chapter 2 should help you focus on what is required. Remember: this is a cross between a paper-based beauty contest and an amateur boxing match.

Possible questions for specialty and general practice training applications can be related to the following areas:

- Eligibility
- Qualifications and academic achievements
- Non-academic achievements
- Good medical practice
- Teamwork
- Leadership
- Evidence of your appropriateness for the specialty chosen
- Evidence of your commitment to the specialty

One of the key principles that is likely to be utilised in selection in the future is 'behavioural indicators', based on psychological constructs and models. One of the key tenets of behavioural indicators is that 'past behaviour predicts future behaviour'. Therefore you are likely to be asked about how you have approached situations in real life rather than being given abstract problems to respond to. An example of positive and negative examples of behavioural indicators for continuous professional development is given in Box 8.4.

Eligibility

The application form may include a section where you have to demonstrate your eligibility to apply for a post-Foundation post. This will normally mean that you are successfully completing your two-year Foundation and that there are no outstanding fitness to practice or disciplinary issues hanging over you. Things may be more complicated if you are an overseas graduate, if you have had to interrupt your Foundation programme for health reasons or if you decided to go abroad instead of F2 and obtain your competencies overseas. Take advice locally at an early stage if any of these factors apply to you.

Qualifications and academic achievements

This section is where a BMedSci or other intercalated degree will come into its own, particularly if you got a publication out of it. A first class honours degree or a distinction always stands out on your application form like an

Box 8.4 Behavioural indicators for continuous professional development	
High	**Low**
Portfolio demonstrates commitment to personal development	Portfolio demonstrates limited commitment
Learns from clinical experience	Limited ability to learn from experience
Seeks opportunities for learning	Does not take opportunities
Utilises constructive criticism	Ignores constructive feedback
Able to reflect and act on reflections	Lacks self-awareness

attractive sore thumb but most of us wish that we had thought about that from first year medical school. Given the new currency of academic standing at medical school, mention that you were in the top 25% or 50% if you were.

Postgraduate academic achievements are highly relevant. Interestingly, membership exams are no longer essential because of the way the Foundation programme is designed as a stepping stone to specialist training. Having said that, they are worthwhile pursuing if you have decided your career choice. There's a lot to be said for getting your membership early. Having attempted part 1 of MRCP or MRCS is evidence of your commitment to the specialty even if you don't pass, and if you do pass it will be evidence that you have acquired many of the knowledge-based competencies relevant to that specialty. You will have to do them in the end anyway. You could also consider acquiring other qualifications relevant to a specialty, such as the Diploma of Child Health for paediatrics. One advantage of attempting college exams early on is that the first part is often theoretical and may test pathology, physiology and other basic sciences. The longer you leave it after qualification, the harder it will be because you rarely use theoretical knowledge in clinical work.

Alternatively, consider working towards other academic qualifications during your Foundation programme, such as a university certificate or a Masters in medical education or research methods. People interested in public health could consider a Masters in epidemiology. Increasingly, universities are offering work-based qualifications that do not require much theoretical work but are based on your everyday practice. They come under a title like 'Certificate of Clinical Competence' and achieving one should not be too difficult and significantly enhances your ability to demonstrate your competence.

Many post-Foundation posts will require evidence of life support skills as an essential criterion. You need to manage your study leave during the Foundation programme so that you achieve the life support skills necessary to complete the Foundation programme but also to compete for post-Foundation jobs. For example, you can't be expected to participate in the paediatric resus. team without being signed up for paediatric life support (PLS), and if you are applying for a surgical rotation then training in advanced trauma and life support (ATLS) is desirable. It is also very useful to have these courses completed as the standards for the Clinical Negligence Scheme for Trusts (CNST) mean that you should not be undertaking resuscitation unless you are adequately trained. Similarly, if you want to work with children, you need training in child protection.

If your five years at medical school have exhausted your scientific interest and you want to pursue your artistic side, doing arts-related academic work, including A-levels or Highers, can stand you in good stead as long as you can relate it to the skills you need as a doctor in the relevant specialty.

Be careful when answering any supplementary sections to the achievements section. When the question asks you to 'Outline the significance of these achievements', they don't want to read what you needed to do. They're effectively asking, 'How will this prize make you more employable as a doctor?'

For the 90% of you who didn't achieve an outstanding award, you can still pull something out of the bag. Be creative and write about the merit that you obtained for a distant essay or student-selected component in a relevant subject.

All kinds of courses and qualifications are available round the country or online. It will enhance your application considerably if you have achieved something other than passing the Foundation assessments in the last two years. Keep an eye on the *BMJ* ads section which carries hundreds of courses every week, or search the website of your chosen specialty college or local university. Ask colleagues about suitable courses. You may have to fund these yourself as study leave is likely to be taken up by statutory courses. Many trainees are reluctant to invest in their training, but in the competitive jobs market that we are entering it will give you an advantage. The NHS is unlikely to fund all your training needs. Think of it as an investment which will be repaid many times over if you are successful in your chosen career.

Non-academic achievement

It is not clear if the post-Foundation application will include a question on non-academic achievement. Given that you have spent two years working, it would seem more relevant to ask about your work-related achievements and competencies and this would certainly fit with the principles of behavioural indicators. For most people it will be easy to think of non-academic achievement. Music, sport, reading, travel – you've probably done it. But that means that everyone else has as well. If the question is asked in the application process, remember to pick out the 'employable' characteristics that that achievement brought you, and make it as recent as possible.

Good Medical Practice

You will almost certainly be asked to demonstrate evidence that you follow the GMC's bible, *Good Medical Practice*, in a similar manner to the Foundation programme application form. As you have now been working for two years, the answers will need to be rather different from those that you gave for your Foundation programme application and demonstrate that you really follow this in clinical practice.

Good clinical care

On the face of it, this is an easy section to complete. You could write about an interesting patient you cared for, but you need to take it to the next level in a way that demonstrates your insight and reflection.

Example

You clerked a 66-year-old man who had recently had an MI and was admitted with malaise, fatigue and difficulty getting out of a chair. He says he felt as if his muscles were aching all over. You checked a creatine kinase which was found to be 22,000. You then stopped his statin. You presented the case at a lunchtime meeting and filled out a Yellow Card adverse drug form and sent it to the Committee on Safety of Medicines. In terms of this patient's care you feel the conundrum now is how to control his cholesterol as it was 5.8 after stopping the statin, and there is a lack of evidence on the efficacy of the other cholesterol-lowering medication.

So through this case you have demonstrated:

1. Good examination skills and history-taking – i.e. you are able to reach a diagnosis (and it wasn't an easy one) by paying attention to what the patient told you and thinking laterally
2. Appropriate investigations ordered in a timely manner
3. Appropriate management, but not just leaving it at that; able to reflect that this was an adverse drug reaction and consider the management of this man's dyslipidaemia.
4. Patient safety – you were able to complete the loop you needed to feed back to the CSM and share the case with colleagues

It's just an example, but something along those lines would be appropriate.

Maintaining good medical practice

Continuous professional development, patient safety and audit are the keys here. It is your chance to demonstrate your awareness of clinical governance and the 'no blame culture' of a successful safety system. A common question in past interviews was to ask you to explain what you understand by clinical governance – both authors were asked it, 15 years apart. It's amazing how difficult it is to understand such terms before you start work. Of course, we remembered the definition and churned it out (like everyone else did), but we never fully understood it until we got stuck into a few audits. In the future the questions will focus more on what you have actually done in these areas rather than what you know about the theory.

For example, remember that completing the circle with audit is vital for patient safety. In other words, feeding back to the relevant group, making appropriate changes, trying out new way of doing things and repeating the audit is vital. This is where an audit becomes beautiful (if such a thing is possible) – when they are simple and actually lead to a change in practice. If you can get your audit published in the journal *Quality and Safety in Healthcare*, for example, even better.

Example

'During my Intermediate Care rotation I was able to design and implement an audit that looked at drug compliance in an elderly care population that had recently been discharged. The audit looked at how many medications patients were on, and included an interview about their medication, when they took them and why they took them. The results showed that 100% compliance was achieved in about half the patients interviewed, a finding that was concordant with the national average. We introduced a new system at the Intermediate Care Unit which included a concordance checklist whereby we made sure that patients knew what they were taking. We also introduced a medicines booklet in large print where we could write the patients' medication and when they were taking them, and communicate why they were taking them and possible side effects.'

This illustrates the 'behavioural indicators' or 'points means prizes' principle very well through the use of buzz-words which are bound to score points, just like a right hook to the head. 'Concordance' shows awareness of the partnership between patient and doctor.

Teaching and training, appraising and assessing

This is an attractive principle so it will be popular to write about. Interviewers love candidates who want to teach, because it's a desirable quality for a GP or consultant.

Take advantage of any opportunities to teach medical students or F1 doctors. A Certificate of Medical Education is a tricky thing to get because of the time involved, but you could demonstrate that you have been to a teaching skills day organised by the Trust, deanery or medical school. These are usually free and cover areas such as teaching in different environments (e.g. in small groups or on ward rounds) or the teaching of particular skills (such as clinical examination or communication).

Example

'During my medical post I organised a practice OSCE for third-year medical students. The work before this involved being a mentor to four third-year students who shadowed me and I taught them during the 12 weeks of their clinical skills course. I especially enjoyed teaching history-taking and remembering the cardinal symptoms for each group of diseases. The OSCE involved using mark sheets similar to the real thing. I was able to learn with the third years by teaching them and asking for feedback.'

Relationships with patients

Things relevant here could include your reflections on your consultation skills, perhaps aided by a video review using the Calgary Cambridge model, or the consent/assent issues you have faced as a Foundation doctor. Only a few procedures performed by Foundation doctors require written consent, but like lumbar punctures or chest drains require verbal consent, and not everyone is good at documenting what they have told the patient.

Example

'I instigated, designed and implemented an audit looking into documentation of consent for chest drain insertion during a Respiratory Medicine post. The audit was retrospective and looked at whether consent was documented and what risks were conveyed to the patient. Only 60% of doctors documented what could be called "satisfactory" consent, regardless of whether they had talked about it or not with the patient. I presented this audit to the medical directorate and it was made Trust policy to document that the main risks of chest drain insertion and other ward-based procedures had been discussed with the patient. This audit highlighted the importance of documentation from a medico-legal point of view and focusing on making the patients' care the first priority.'

Working with colleagues

An interesting angle here is communication between primary and secondary care or between different teams in a hospital. GPs are left in the dark much of the time when patients are discharged. When you start doing discharge letters or do a GP attachment you will appreciate this. Sometimes the discharge won't be done for a few weeks. You find out that the patient has been readmitted during that period, and everyone is knocking down your door to find out what happened the last time the patient was in hospital. The other example is the classic 'repeat U&E in a week on discharge', and by the time you've done the letter four weeks have elapsed. It's not a fool-proof system, and if you've audited the system, it provides an interesting talking point.

Example

'I designed and implemented an audit that looked at discharge letters to GPs. It was based on the gold standard that all discharge letters should be completed within 24 hours of discharge from hospital. Of 200 discharges audited, only 60% of letters achieved this target; and 10% were done one week after discharge, making this potentially unsafe for patients who needed bloods checking in a few days. As an adjunct to the audit, a questionnaire was sent to GPs asking them what they thought of the electronic discharge system from secondary care. Only 40% of GPs were fully satisfied with the information received. Criticisms included lack of clinical information (e.g. blood tests), lack of mention of follow-up and mentioning what tests had been ordered and needed chasing.

I was able to feed back this information to the medical directorate who amended the format of the electronic discharge summary to cover these important bits of information. Practical suggestions were also offered, including completing the discharge letter at the same time as writing the script, and liaising with the nurses during the 'board rounds' to make sure we knew who was going home in the next few days so we could write the letter in advance.

This audit drew attention to the importance of continuity of care between hospital and general practice and some of the pitfalls in transferring information between colleagues. It also highlighted the importance of good clinical note-taking, a fundamental aspect of a high standard of patient care.'

Teamwork is another aspect of working with colleagues that is difficult to demonstrate. It is also discussed below.

Probity

Probably the toughest section to write about, but probably the least popular, so here's a chance for your uniqueness to shine. Themes might include financial probity (e.g. not putting someone in a residential home you have a financial interest in, not making bogus expense claims), the importance of being honest in all communications with patients and any difficulties that you have had (e.g. avoiding answers to difficult questions from a patient when you have known they have cancer but can't tell them until an appropriate time; not overstating the effectiveness of treatment when trying to persuade a patient to take it) and issues that might arise from observing a lack of probity in a colleague and being uncertain what to do about it.

If you do something along these lines for probity, you'll be one of a few and a breath of fresh air as far as application form reading goes, so don't cast this one aside.

Health

This section of *Good Medical Practice* is unlikely to be chosen by many, so here's another chance for you to make a break for it. It may be more straightforward than it initially seems. It's probably not ideal to write about a needlestick injury you sustained, but if you've done an audit on the reporting of needlestick injuries, it would be a great thing to talk about in an interview. It's a little bit different, and not everyone knows about the procedure and 'bleed it, wash it, report it'. Similar things could be done about lifting and back care, or the services offered by Occupational Health.

Example

'I designed an audit to look at whether the Trust's needlestick injury policy was being adhered to. This was done by examining Incident Report Forms and Occupational Health records. This was supplemented with a questionnaire to assess doctors' knowledge of what to do following a needlestick injury. The audit found 90% of cases were fully compliant with Trust policy, including timely risk assessment. Where the audit fell down was on documenting the initial steps following a needlestick injury, and in 50% of cases it was unclear whether there had been a "bleed it, wash it, report it" approach. This was confirmed in the results of the questionnaire which showed that 50% of doctors were unaware of how long to perform the tasks for.

I presented the results to the medical directorate and, as a result, Occupational Health now run bi-annual workshops on needlestick injuries. This audit taught me the importance of documentation as a means of accurate communication. It also taught me that information often needs to be repeated throughout the year and reiterated.'

Teamwork and leadership

These linked subjects were covered from the Foundation programme application point of view in Chapter 2. The best thing to write about teamwork might seem to be when you were the team leader. However, there may be a separate question on leadership, so you need to ensure you make different points in each answer. You could show that you have thought about how to make the team work better, for example through the multidisciplinary team (MDT) meetings. You could do something like a brief questionnaire that asks each member of the MDT how much they feel valued, and how useful they find the MDT meetings, and any ideas about how to make them more helpful. An alternative would be to offer some reflections on your role as a team player using information derived from the multi-source feedback or a personality inventory. You could also use a non-medical example of your role as a team player, but it should be recent.

For a leadership question, captaincy of teams and presidency of societies or committees come to mind. Remember, the panel are after reasons why you think that experience is significant to your medical career and are looking past 'because it would make me a good team leader' as an answer; that is implied in the question. If you captained the medics' sports team, say how, as a leader, you had to know how to motivate people when energy levels were low, and you had to act as an inspiration to others by behaving as a professional. The best answers will include reflections on what you learnt about yourself as a leader from a concrete example.

Be aware that doctors are often good at taking the initiative but not that good at following the lead suggested by others. This is the skill of 'followership' and one that can be regarded as important as leadership. For an interesting example of the relationship between leadership and followership, look at the account given by a successful Everest expedition: www. armyoneverest.mod.uk. The essential principle is that a team needs to work together towards common and agreed goals to ensure a safe and effective outcome. On Everest this means not only a successful ascent but also a successful descent. Apparently 1 in 10 climbers on Everest die and 1 in 20 climbers who reach the peak do not make it down successfully. By establishing clear rules and agreements on conduct that all members were prepared to follow, even if it meant that their own aspirations or views were thwarted, this expedition had no fatalities.

Evidence of your appropriateness for the specialty chosen and evidence of your commitment to the specialty

The kind of evidence that they will be looking for here may seem vague, but is essential for a successful application. It is probably one of the questions that will help discriminate between candidates because it allows you a lot of leeway. For a start, there is very little evidence base for the particular skills required for any discipline. We have even heard of a surgical trainee who had got quite far in her training before anyone realised she had very poor eyesight. Locally, we have been trying to draw up a list of essential and desirable qualities for the early years of the General Medicine training programme. However, as physicians perform roles ranging from invasive cardiology to palliative care, the range of skills required is huge and it would be difficult to favour one set of skills over another.

The questions in this section are therefore likely to require a degree of flattery to those reading your submission. Questions are likely to be framed something like: 'What are the qualities needed to be a successful rheumatologist in the twenty-first century and can you demonstrate that you have them?' Suitable replies would read: 'Rheumatologists have to demonstrate the intellect of Einstein because of the wide variety of diagnoses seen, the practical skills of Leonardo da Vinci to aspirate small joints, the diplomacy skills of Paddy Ashdown to work between orthopaedic surgeons and GPs, and the patience of Job and analytic skills of Freud to help patients with chronic fatigue syndrome'! How on earth you could demonstrate that you possessed these skills we will leave you to decide, but you get the picture. The assessors will be looking for skills that reflect their own glory and this is inevitable in this type of question.

The evidence for your commitment to the specialty is easier to gather. This is where your choice of student-selected components from your undergraduate years and where your planning of study leave and other learning opportunities in your Foundation programme will come in handy, as well as evidence from your portfolio or even better the specialty college logbook. This is also where you get payback for staying around when on call and learning some of the less common procedures, like DC cardioversion, lumbar puncture and bone marrow or liver biopsy. You should guide many of your educational activities towards this question if possible. Audits, research, online learning, shadowing, tasters – everything can be usefully harnessed to gather evidence for this area.

Whilst research and publications have been specifically excluded as a desirable, let alone essential, competency for doctors who are not following the academic pathway, you can still use research experience to gain extra points. It is likely that research will retain some degree of status for a long time in certain specialties which have a strong research history, although without major effort publications are trickier to find than a stethoscope on a surgeon. Use research experience to show evidence of your use of evidence-based medicine, written communication skills, analytic skills, ability to work in a team, tenacity in the face of overwhelming bureaucracy, etc. Some research experience in your specialty area would certainly count as evidence of your commitment to the specialty. Some ways in which you might be able to get a publication without undergoing three years' lab work are outlined in Chapter 2, particularly by contributing to the *BMJ* Careers Focus, writing a personal view for the *BMJ* or a letter in response to a journal article. Publishing your audit has been described above. Another approach is to email the editor of a journal and ask if they need an article review or a leader article.

References

The background to references is described in Chapter 2. The switch to electronic applications which are assessed anonymously has significantly reduced the importance of references. Apocryphal stories suggest that you used to need certain professors batting for you to obtain a job and that rival consultants would veto each other. But the days of such extreme patronage are long gone. You do need references, but who writes them is not critical and what they say does not matter that much, unless it is very critical. It is almost certain that your referee will have to complete a structured reference tailored to the job specification but that also asks about your sick leave record and any disciplinary actions taken against you.

APPROACH TO THE INTERVIEW

The application form will be used for shortlisting, and final selection will be based on a structured interview of a minimum of 30 minutes. The approach to the interviews should be similar to application forms. There will be a series of questions or scenarios designed to assess your competencies or aptitude in specific areas. From the guidance notes currently available, you will have considerable latitude to present any evidence you wish to demonstrate that you have the relevant skills, behaviours and knowledge relevant to your chosen specialty. In most interviews, candidates will face the same scenarios so that they can all be directly compared and scored. As in the application form, you know what the assessors are likely to ask and what the answers are. It is your job to get in as many of the buzz-words as possible and convince them that you understand what they mean and that you have the skills. General practice appointment procedures have long experience in designing assessment procedures to assess all aspects of the essential and desirable qualities of a candidate. Sometimes they include a test of knowledge in the form of a written exam.

In the future, interviews are likely to use OSCE-style stations assessing communication skills and ethics as well as using more traditional interview questions to assess understanding of the specialty and how much the candidate has thought about the end point of their training. For medicine, for example, the questions could assess your competence in explaining something to a patient or ask how you might deal with an ethical or legal problem, similar in format to the PACES part of the MRCP exam. The question may ask you to deal with a specific problem or how you dealt with a recent real-life problem. Real-life problems seem to be a much better assessment of what you actually do (behavioural assessment) than whether you can come up with a perfect answer to a set problem.

Like all skills, you can improve your performance by practising interview skills. Just like consultation skills, repetition bears fruit and it is always going to be easier to answer a question that you have heard before than having to think on your feet. You should seek out opportunities for practice interviews with your educational supervisor or another trusted senior. Practise with your peers, each coming up with a question that seeks to assess an aspect of the essential and desirable competencies from the job description.

For a start, try these:

- Give an example of a difficult situation you faced recently and what you learnt from it
- Give an example of your skills as a team leader from the recent past and what you learnt about yourself
- What skills do you have that will make you a good physician/surgeon/GP, etc.?
- What might the effects of competency-based training be on the future of this specialty? This tests whether you have familiarized yourself with the likely changes to your specialty from one of the recent policy initiatives. ('Technology' or 'the EWTD' can be substituted for 'competency-based training')
- Talk us through your Foundation portfolio and show how it demonstrates your approach to continuous professional development
- Use your Foundation portfolio to demonstrate the knowledge, skills and behaviours you have that are relevant to this specialty

You may be asked to use role play to assess your skills in explaining a diagnosis or test to a lay person:

- Please explain the procedure for inserting a chest drain to this patient
- Please explain a diagnosis of bowel cancer to this patient
- This mother's child has just had a febrile convulsion. Please explain this to her

You can think up many more examples yourselves or ask your seniors.

Techniques to use in interviews
- Think before replying. There is no harm in spending 10–30 seconds thinking of your answer in an interview. A brief pause will allow you to think of more than one alternative and will also allow you to give some structure to your answer.
- Use signposting to lead your assessor through your answer. If you start your reply with: 'There are three elements that I would like to bring into my answer' or 'When faced with an ethical problem like this it is helpful to look at it from the four ethical standpoints' or 'In approaching this clinical problem it would be important to deal first with resuscitation using the ABC system and then go on to take a full history and examination', the assessors will know you have a sound approach to the problem. They will now be looking for the extra points that you hope to pick up.
- Answer the questions truthfully and say what you would actually do – the assessors can always detect a fake. If there is a clinical skills question, take your history as you would in real life; don't dress it up. Remember the general principles of consultation skills if you have to take a history or provide an explanation.
- In reply to any question about generic skills, use a real-life example, but demonstrate that you learnt a general point from the event.
- Don't be afraid to demonstrate any weakness or discuss an error. If you are asked to talk about a difficult incident or a mistake you have made, the assessors want to know if you can learn from experience; they are not trying to trip you up. You will get more marks for showing that, no matter how bad an error you made, you dealt with it honestly and openly, were able to learn from it and took appropriate action to ensure that it would not be repeated. It is simply not believable to state that you have never made an error or faced a difficult communication situation. If you do, the assessors will take this as evidence of a lack of insight.
- Don't be put off by the assessors' attitude. They will probably seem largely indifferent and will give you little feedback. This does not mean that you are bombing. Just like exams, they are trained to be neutral so they do not favour one candidate over another. If they repeat your answer (echoing) it does not necessarily mean that you have got it wrong – they may well be seeking elaboration or checking whether you are certain that you are right. If you are, don't be deflected from your answer.
- Get there in plenty of time. You should aim to be there at least 30 minutes, and preferably more, before the interview. If you are going to a big hospital or somewhere you have not been before, allow another 30 minutes at least to find it, park and walk from the car park to the place

where the interview will be held. You cannot arrive too early for an interview. You don't want to arrive at the last minute distracted by your worries about being late and still sweating with high levels of adrenaline swilling around your body. If you are late, it will be within their rights to refuse to interview you and anyway, you will have created a very bad impression and will be too distracted to answer the questions properly. If you are going to be late, phone and let them know why. If the interview is far away, consider travelling there the night before as the UK's transport infrastructure is notoriously unreliable.

- Dress – this is important chiefly in that it can create a negative impression rather than there being one essential style. Don't look as if you were in a rush to get there. You don't necessarily need to invest in a new outfit that you will only wear once. Men should be smart, have clean shoes and wear a tie and a reasonably conservative suit or jacket, unless you are applying for a very casually dressed specialty. A bow tie and velvet jacket mark you out as an eccentric, so consider whether that is the impression that is likely to get you appointed. For women, dress respectfully and smartly. Midriffs and unusual piercings should not be seen.

Things to avoid
- If asked at the end of the interview if you have any questions, it is best to stick to some very neutral ones. Asking how you have done looks weak; asking what is in it for you sounds arrogant. Suitable responses include: 'No thanks. I think all my questions had been answered in my preparation for this interview', or something similar. Don't ask about pay and conditions. These are not the interviewers' responsibility and make you sound mercenary. If you want to know about these, ask Human Resources after the interview.
- Don't ask for any special favours (e.g. a telephone interview or interview on another day) unless it is a matter of life and death. In the past interviewers would sometimes arrange to see people on a different day if there was a reason why they could not attend an interview. However, with the need to make decisions defendable it is essential that all candidates are asked the same questions, by the same people and with the chance to directly compare the candidates. You are extremely unlikely to be interviewed on a different day. So, at an early stage, inform your work colleagues when you are likely to have an interview, make sure that secretaries know to cancel clinics and that you have someone you can swap on-calls with. Don't plan your dream honeymoon during the period when interviews are likely to take place. Do plan ahead so that you will be available at relatively short notice.
- Don't get into an argument. If you disagree with the assessors or if you think they have made a discriminatory remark or treated you unfairly, then complete the interview, make a contemporaneous note and, if you feel strongly about it, inform the employing authority, make a formal written complaint or appeal the decision (if it goes against you).
- Avoid the subject of religion in both the application form and interview. Doctors feel strongly about religion – some feel that only people with

faith can practise medicine properly, others feel just as strongly that medicine is a humanist construct and religion introduces bias and prejudice. You will not know what your assessors' views are, but they are likely to be subliminal and will remain unexpressed. Saying that you wish to do a particular specialty because of your faith could well raise suspicion in an atheist, but equally it would be unwise to criticise religion. You should never be asked anything about your faith by the assessors.

You have now completed the application process and, if you have been successful, once you have accepted a post it is both polite and ethical to stick to it. Once accepted you cannot change your mind in order to apply for a better post, a post in another part of the country or in another specialty. This will probably end in your being reported to the GMC. If you want to transfer to another deanery or school, you will have to start the post you have been accepted for and then ask for a transfer.

WHEN YOU ARE UNSURE IF MEDICINE IS FOR YOU

For a small number of newly qualified doctors, clinical medicine will not live up to expectations and they will be uncertain about the way ahead or will have made a definite decision to leave medicine or pursue other options. If you have doubts, if possible finish the first Foundation year and get registered with the GMC as a medical practitioner. Many people who leave medicine return later, or consider returning, and it will be easier to reactivate your registration rather than try to register for the first time if you do have a change of heart. Before you finalise your decision, it may be helpful to think about why you did not enjoy the Foundation programme. Was it having to deal with patients and their suffering, the pressure of work, the unsocial hours, the NHS, factors outside medicine such as family life, or could it just have been the one or two firms you worked on? Were you bullied? There can be a considerable mismatch between an individual and a team so working with a different team may give you a very different experience of medicine. Alternatively, there may have been personal circumstances that affected your view, such as ill health or the illness of a parent or close friend.

Understanding the reasons for wanting to leave will help you decide your future options. If you are thinking of leaving medicine altogether, then you would almost certainly benefit from independent careers counselling from someone with higher-level career counselling skills and probably someone who is not directly involved in your training so that they are completely independent. This could come from the deanery or Foundation school or a private career counselling service. Seek advice early if you are thinking of leaving. There is no shame in this and certainly no blame. As we have said, approximately 15% of trainees are not practising three years after graduation so you are not alone. Well-trained careers advisers will help you look at all of your options and will suggest options that you may not have thought of.

If you are uncertain about your future in medicine, you can consider working part-time or having a career break initially or thinking about whether any of the many options discussed above would be more attractive. If patient care does not suit you, consider a medical post with no or limited patient care such as pathology or certain parts of radiology. In the end, if you do choose to leave clinical medicine, you have a choice of future careers that use your medical education or starting completely afresh.

Using your training in an alternative career

It is very natural to feel that you wish to use your five years' training so far in earning a living if you are not sure about a return to clinical work. Fortunately, many options are available to you. These include taking a course to convert to medical journalism or law or pursuing something that interests you such as medical history, humanities or ethics. You could also build on your training in Western medicine and pursue training and a career in one of the other healing arts, such as homeopathy. Medical education also offers opportunities to be more creative in your working life. Working in the pharmaceutical industry may be a possibility, although some experience after Foundation programme would be useful. The *BMJ* Careers Focus section has many examples of people who have used their training to go in a different direction.

Choosing a career outside medicine

In choosing a career outside medicine, you will be making a brave choice. You may well find that you meet resistance and negative reactions from your friends, colleagues and family. Careers advice may well be directed at persuading you to carry on with a medical career in some form. Don't let people put you off if you are certain that you do not wish to continue. Seek a truly independent adviser, someone with training in mentoring (a non-directive technique used to help people make decisions) or perhaps someone outside medicine, such as a life coach. An understanding of the reasons why you wish to leave is essential. At this stage, it may not be possible to see a clear way ahead. If the experience has been distressing, it may well be very hard to disentangle the various elements of the problem and it may be desirable and unavoidable to delay a decision on your own future. Remember that your four or five years in medical school will not have been wasted. You will have learnt many skills and gained much knowledge that is relevant to any future career. Alternative careers pursued by people known to us include attempting to succeed in the national skiing team and retraining in interior design as well as becoming a full-time parent.

WHAT IF YOU DO NOT GET THE TRAINING POST YOU WANT?

It is highly likely that many trainees will not succeed in obtaining the post that they want in the first years of run-through training. It was always thus, but with one point of application to training posts for the whole of the next year, it will seem much worse than in the days pre-MMC. At least pre-MMC you would have had the chance to apply for a job that was advertised next week. Now, if you miss out in the two rounds of the formal applications, you have to wait a whole year to reapply. Your options include applying for the FTSTA posts described above, going abroad for a year or two to obtain more experience, doing something else to improve your chances next year such as research or teaching fellow posts or expedition work, or having time off. The need to repay your student loan may mean that not working is not an option. Reappraising your chances of succeeding in your first choice specialty is very important. Consider the ratio of applicants to posts and whether there are any other specialties that will fulfil your desires but are less competitive. For example, if gastroenterology or cardiology appeals because of the technical aspects of the specialty (e.g. endoscopy or cardiac catheterisation), then consider radiology because there will be plenty of opportunity to do procedures. If it is the acute admissions in medicine that appeal, consider pursuing the new specialty of acute medicine which is just developing and should have lots of new consultant posts in the future as all Trusts move towards having three acute care physicians to take care of their admissions units. If you don't succeed in your first application, make sure that you use your waiting time to best advantage and build your skills.

SUMMARY

This chapter has reviewed some of the skills that you can develop to manage your career successfully and match it with your other aspirations. It has looked at how Foundation doctors choose their careers and given further information on the types of careers available. It has looked at your application and the interview process. In all of these areas, there are practical exercises that you can do and sources of further information. The chapter then looked at options if medicine does not seem to be right for you. Good luck in your job hunting.

The next chapter looks at your responsibilities as a doctor and in particular at risks to your registration and your health, and how to prevent stress and burn-out.

When medicine is difficult

Mark Welfare

9

> ❝Success or failure depends more upon attitude than upon capacity.❞
>
> William James

INTRODUCTION

This chapter deals with your responsibilities as a doctor and in particular looks at risks to your registration and your health, and how to prevent stress and burn-out. It uses examples from each of the seven sections of the GMC's *Good Medical Practice* to increase your understanding of your responsibilities and covers the tricky issues of self-care, managing your performance and what to do if you do fall from grace and become a 'doctor in difficulty'. It also briefly describes the multitude of disciplinary, complaints and legal systems that doctors can face and what to do when other people's behaviour makes your working life intolerable.

One or two of you will know someone who went 'off the rails' as a medical student. Starting work may be even more stressful. Most of you will get over the problems, but if they persist and you are struggling, or if you find that medicine is not for you, you may need more than a shoulder to lean on. Hopefully this chapter will help you find your way.

To set the scene, take our 'Lifestyle and professionalism challenge' and you can add ten years to your life and reduce your chance of becoming best friends with the GMC Regional Misconduct Adviser.

THE LIFESTYLE AND PROFESSIONALISM CHALLENGE

How often do you think about changing your eating or smoking habits, exercise pattern and early morning ritual of shower, shave and s(h)elf-assessment form? Not often we suspect. It's only when you have a reality check that things start to change and you shift your whole perspective on life (e.g. if one of your friends is diagnosed with type 2 diabetes).

You have watched *Honey We're Killing the Kids* so you know that it can work. Complex analysis of your eating habits, use of legal and illegal drugs, exercise pattern and attitudes to work and your team members by a highly trained life coach can help you develop a Zen existence and add ten years to your life. Do you think it's realistic? We do, but as you are not on television, we can't afford a life coach.

Now that the government is adding five years to your working life before you can draw your pension, you have to take a long hard look at yourself and figure out how you are going to complete this crazy steeplechase of a career while maintaining stability. So go on, take the challenge and formulate a personally tailored recovery plan for the rest of your life. In the best traditions of glossy magazines, answer the questions below and add up your scores to find out how you are doing:

The Lifestyle and Professionalism Challenge

1. In preparation for work every day:

   a) You rise at 5.45 am, complete the draft of your audit project, then read *Nature Genetics* before a high-fibre breakfast cereal and freshly squeezed juice. You arrive at work an hour early to ensure adequate handover and check your patients before the ward round.

   b) You rise at 7.30, take a quick shower, have brown toast with real butter, walk the 30 minutes to work for exercise, arriving 15 minutes before start time.

   c) You rise as late as possible, down three cups of strong black coffee to clear your head after a rather heavy night and then drive from the doctors' residence to the hospital car park to save the 400 m walk. You have learnt a sneaky way into the hospital so that your late arrival is not witnessed by consultants looking out of their office windows.

2. It's been a bad day at the office. Several unexpected results popped up on the ward round, Mrs Jones' relatives have now filed a formal complaint about the MRSA septicaemia from the cannula that you put in and your favourite patient has taken a turn for the worse. When you get home from work do you:

   a) Ring your mum to discuss your feelings of disempowerment and existential *angst* before relaxing in a herbal bath with a papaya and granola smoothie and take in *Newsnight*'s review of NHS funding.

   b) Go straight to the gym and double your normal exercise regime in the sure knowledge that a pizza and a couple of pints of lager are going to be needed tonight whilst you watch *Big Brother* and go over things with your mates.

   c) Stop off at your dealer's on the way home to score some dope knowing that you are going to need a lot of relaxation tonight. Spend evening alone at home on a chatline with Priscilla from Las Vegas, whose voice is disturbingly deep but you've already paid the subscription, so in for a penny, in for a pound.

3. Your idea of a good evening out is:

   a) The opening of the latest Chekhov at the regional theatre then returning to your friend's flat to discuss the performance over a decaf soya latte.

   b) Trying out the new fish restaurant which is reputed to have a great wine list.

   c) Meeting up with mates and downing six pints before a vindaloo and a spot of robotics on the dance floor of the local night spot. You know your dance moves went out in the 1980s, but – hey – you're trying to bring them back into fashion. If you get home before 2.00 am it's been a failure.

4. At the weekend:

   a) You help out at the kids' camp run by the local place of worship and spend Sunday night studying for part 1 of the membership exams.

   b) On Saturday morning you play for your local sports team before watching TV and relaxing. On Sunday you enjoy the delights of spring in the local nature reserve before popping round to your parents to mow their lawns and share an evening dinner with them and the rest of your large family.

   c) You play for the darts team on Friday and wake halfway through Saturday afternoon just in time for the cup final. On Sunday you flick through your address book to see if anyone is free, but no one is in so you spend the day cleaning your flat and watching extreme sport on the TV. At 10.00 pm you pick up your books to start working for the part 1 exam in three weeks' time but by 11.00 you are asleep.

5. You life plan includes:

   a) Getting the membership of your chosen college within three years of graduating, being appointed to one of the new academic run-through training posts, being published in *Nature Genetics* and being a professor by 40.

   b) Getting experience abroad after the Foundation programme, getting an AS level in Arabic and having three kids. Would be nice to live in the country.

   c) What are you talking about, a life plan? Well, I will obviously be a consultant with a large private practice and good wine cellar. But that's ages away. Now I'm just having fun.

6. Pensions:

   a) I will have an A+ merit award so no problem there.

   b) I have started buying added years; they seem good value.

   c) They are for old people, aren't they?

7. You find some shotty lymph glands in your neck after an upper respiratory tract illness. Do you:

   a) Go online to find out the newest chemotherapy regime for stage 3 non-Hodgkin's lymphoma and book yourself into the professor of haematology's clinic.

   b) Ignore them, but plan to visit your GP if they are still there in four weeks' time having looked up the lymphoma referral guidance to GPs on the National Electronic Library for Health (Nellie) website.

   c) Prescribe yourself some antibiotics from the hospital pharmacy, making sure that they cover syphilis, just in case (even though you've only ever contracted electronic viruses from Priscilla).

8. Mr Smith has been on the ward for six weeks since admission with a UTI. He remains mildly confused and is unlikely to go home. He has been 'medically fit for discharge' for four weeks. In the multidisciplinary team meeting on your elderly care attachment, the social worker reports that no progress has been made in choosing a residential home because she was on leave for a week, the family have been in the Caribbean for two weeks and yesterday he had one loose stool so no home will take him until he has three negative stools for *C. diff.*

She also tentatively suggests that the medical team should consider an anti-depressant because he has become withdrawn. Do you:

a) Say that if a bed has not been found for him by Monday he is to be discharged home because this is costing the NHS a lot of money. Back this up with evidence that delayed discharge is associated with a high incidence of hospital-acquired infection and excess deaths.

b) Listen, assess the patient's needs and suggest that an inter-professional team is convened to review the discharge planning procedures on the ward. 'There are lessons to be learnt for all of us from this difficult case.'

c) Point out to the social worker that the patient is obviously depressed because he has been kept on an acute ward for four weeks too long and that if she had got her finger out, he would have been discharged weeks ago. You storm out of the room, grabbing the last doughnut on the way.

Now count up the number of a's, b's and c's in your replies.

Mostly a

Summary: You are highly organized, well motivated and will succeed in your chosen career. You treat your brain as a temple and are totally committed to practice. On the minus side, you don't take much exercise and are in danger of burning out from all that wholesomeness. Can you relate to your patients with all their foibles and faults?

Self-care: With that lack of exercise you are at risk of obesity and diabetes. Could die of hypochondriasis.

Personal issues: Will you ever meet someone you can live with? With all that perfection, how will you cope when something goes wrong? You may rub up your colleagues the wrong way if you're too critical.

Careers advice: This kind of headstrong behaviour may draw you to surgery. Alternatively go into laboratory research or hospital management.

Mostly b

Summary: You are a well-rounded individual who has a good balance between play and work and keeps fit. You have a good support network.

Self-care: When jogging, watch out for buses. More likely to suffer shin splints than die early.

Personal issues: You should be able to cope with most of the ups and downs of life.

Careers advice: GP might seem the obvious choice, but why not go for a hospital career and work flexibly? You sound like you will make an excellent teacher and an inspiration to others on how to practise and live the right way.

Mostly c

Summary: You are having a hedonistic youth. Good luck for now.

Self-care: Do you want to end up on the liver ward with the sad dipsomaniacs? Get a GP. Take precautions.

Personal issues: What has your multi-source feedback been like? Performance issues could be around the corner. It's a cut-throat world out there, so getting a specialty training post could be tough unless you start planning.

Careers advice: You obviously have the attention span of a gnat. Acute care might suit you if you can get your act together.

Well, it's not exactly scientific and, in the spirit of magazine questionnaires, relies on a few stereotypes. In reality you will probably have wanted to pick pieces from each of the answers, but hopefully it has raised your awareness of the health and lifestyle issues that might impact on your performance as a doctor. What then, in plain language, are the greatest risks to your health or your registration?

RISKS TO YOUR REGISTRATION, OR HOW TO LIVE UP TO *GOOD MEDICAL PRACTICE*

Chapter 3 introduced the GMC and gave an historical account of its role and the development of *Good Medical Practice* and *Duties of a Doctor*. Here we go through *Good Medical Practice* in more detail and give some examples of good practice and the risks that you are most likely to face.

Good clinical care

Good clinical care is the central business of a doctor and so we should not be surprised that if you are found wanting in this area you will be hauled up for it. The key areas that you must be aware of are the need to make a full and appropriate assessment of each and every patient, to document your findings clearly and accurately, to recognise your limitations and to make appropriate referrals when your expertise is exceeded. In your future career, the need to delegate appropriately is also important, but with the spread of nurse specialists and 'medical care practitioners', as an F2 you may be delegating tasks to others. It might be helpful for you to consider whether delegation of responsibilities to you by your seniors is appropriate. Are you being asked to do something that you are not competent in, or transferring a competence to a new situation where your skills might be inadequate? If in doubt, ask. The last thing you want is for your consultant to find you with a grey cannula in someone's jugular vein after your SpR told you this method was all the rage in Latvia.

We will also consider your responses to medical error. Error should be regarded as a normal part of the complex interactions involved in medical practice, but the way you deal with it is vital.

Consider the following examples and how serious you think they are:

Example 1
A patient made a complaint against an F2 doctor in Casualty when they attended with abdominal pain. A UTI was diagnosed on history alone and no examination was performed. The next day the patient was admitted with a perforated appendix.

Example 2
A doctor faced an enquiry following a complaint made by a patient's family about poor clinical care during a GP attachment in F2. The patient had leg pain, chest pain and shortness of breath. The doctor diagnosed a muscle strain when in fact the patient had a DVT. The patient subsequently

died. There was no documented examination in the notes at the time and the doctor had not recorded the pulse and blood pressure.

Example 3

An F1 doctor provided a prescription of benzodiazepine for a friend's girlfriend who was terrified of flying. She did not meet the 'patient' or examine her and did not inform the GP. The patient had a paradoxical reaction to the tablets and had to be removed from the flight.

Example 4

An F2 working in Casualty was investigated after the death of a patient from a methadone overdose. The patient had attended Casualty saying that they had lost their methadone prescription from their GP and the surgery was now closed. The doctor knew of the guidance on prescribing to addicts but had not stuck to them and had issued a script. The patient had never actually used methadone and died of an overdose.

These examples show a range of aspects of poor medical care, from inadequate diagnosis to unsafe prescribing. For more examples of the standard of care expected of medical practitioners you should see the casebook of the Medical Protection Society (www.medicalprotection.org).

You should be reassured that you are not going to be admonished or struck off for a simple clinical error or for not spotting a rare disease or even for one serious and significant error. Reading the case notes of the GMC we see doctors who are guilty of making a long series of mistakes, often compounded by lack of insight and attitudinal problems such as rudeness or altering medical records. Most doctors removed from the Medical Register have fallen down on more than one of the categories of *Good Medical Practice* and the fact that the doctors have not expressed regret or insight into the seriousness of their errors is often a deciding factor in their removal. (See the latter part of this chapter for further details of the GMC's procedures.)

As an educational supervisor, I am frequently faced with Foundation doctors who have made an error. Error is natural and in many ways inevitable in the messy world of medicine. So making an error is not necessarily a worry in a trainee. It is their response that is one of the most important determinants that distinguishes between the doctor who understands professionalism and the one with problems. Most medical error arises not from a single person's error but from a lack of systems to prevent it. This is the Swiss cheese model. For an error to occur, several holes need to be aligned. The more barriers that are erected, the less likely it is that an error will be made. Ideal systems mean that one person's slip could never lead to patient harm because of the overlapping security of a system of checks. So, if you do make an error, be consoled by the fact that it is likely to result from a combination of factors and not be entirely your fault.

There are a number of things that you should do if an error is made, either by yourself or others. The first thing is to record the error in the patient's notes. The patient needs to be informed as soon as possible. For minor errors, such as wrong drug administration with no harmful effects, it might be appropriate for the person responsible to inform the patient. For more serious incidents, it may well be more appropriate for a senior to inform the patient, so tell your senior immediately if you are aware of a serious error. Informing a patient about a serious problem could be a very emotionally charged experience if you are feeling guilty and upset. It might also make it difficult to remain open and honest and not get defensive.

Once the patient has been informed and the notes written, the incident has to be reported. Local reporting systems vary, but someone will probably have to fill in a local reporting form (Incident Report form) which goes to a Trust manager. This is usually the end of your responsibility and the manager will investigate and make appropriate changes to the systems if they are needed. The NHS has belatedly got serious about learning from error. The government has set up the National Patient Safety Agency (NPSA) (www.npsa.nhs. uk) to investigate common errors and introduce changes on a nationwide basis so that lessons can be quickly disseminated. Recent changes introduced by the NPSA are the standardization of the crash call number throughout the NHS, improving the storage of potassium chloride to prevent accidental death, changes around the administration of intrathecal chemotherapy and the 'Clean Your Hands' campaign. See Box 9.1 for guidance on what to do or not do if you make an error. Anyone working in the NHS, including Foundation doctors, can make a report to the NPSA.

Remember that in these days of transparency and probity, medical error is not a witch-hunt. We are, at least theoretically, living in a no-blame culture, and that is what Incident Report forms exist for. The hospital management are not looking at the doctor only, but at the systems and policies already in place and how they can be revised to prevent the same mistake recurring.

One of the authors once turned up late for a night shift for reasons beyond his control. Pathologically late, in fact. Anyway, an Incident Report form was filled out and as a result, switchboard now has a contact number for every junior doctor so that they can be contacted if a similar situation arises. After filling countless forms for patients who have fallen out of bed, you may have thought that incident reporting never led to any change. Now you know that, used wisely, it can lead to important change!

Box 9.1   Response to error

Good response	Bad response
Tells patient immediately, explains	Avoids patient or lies to them
Documents the error	Tries to hide it
Takes responsibility	Blames it on others
Reflects on error in portfolio	Portfolio empty
Finds out how to avoid it again	No analysis of what went wrong
Appropriate emotional response	Not concerned
Uses hospital reporting system	Does not know about reporting systems

> **Box 9.2   Ways of demonstrating that you have kept up to date**
> *Participation in clinical governance procedures*
>
> - Audit – complete an audit in a subject area relevant to your future career ambitions. Write it up, concentrate on what changed as a result of your findings, or if nothing changed, why not
> - Keep a record of clinical incident forms that you have completed and the outcome
> - Keep a record of Yellow Cards (for adverse drug reactions) that you have submitted. These are a much underused resource and a valuable feedback tool
>
> *Use of study leave*
>
> - If you want to do paediatrics, use study leave to do a paediatric resuscitation course or a course on child protection
> - If you want to do acute medicine, take a medical procedures course
> - If you want to do surgery, take a basic surgical skills course
> - Take some online courses such as those found on the *BMJ* website or at doctors. org. Make sure you print off the certificate of completion. Any evidence that shows initiative is good evidence for your portfolio

Maintaining good practice

You have only just qualified, so you have recently demonstrated that your knowledge and skills are of the level needed. To pass your Foundation programme you will need to demonstrate your development and the acquisition of new skills and knowledge using the tools discussed in Chapter 6. If you are well organised, this should not be a problem and it would be difficult at this stage in your career to face an issue with your registration in this category if you have kept your Foundation portfolio up to date.

This is a category where as a Foundation doctor you have a chance to get your head and shoulders above your colleagues and should not be cause of problems. You should use this category to develop material to put in your application for post-Foundation jobs. (This is also covered in Chapters 5, 6 and 8.) Box 9.2 gives some examples of evidence that you could gather to demonstrate that you have actively maintained good medical practice.

Teaching and training

You will have a role in teaching and training medical students, and with your peers may also be involved in the education of students from other health professions (e.g. nursing). You will also be involved in the assessment of your peers through multi-source feedback. Teaching and training are rarely problem areas for doctors, although there is an increasing tendency for students and trainees to make a complaint against those who abuse their power, so even in your position it is best to be aware of a few simple rules of behaviour. The rules are the same as you would expect your seniors to stick to when dealing with medical students and junior doctors (Box 9.3). The most

Box 9.3 Simple rules for teaching, or 'do as thou would be done by'

- Be punctual
- Be polite
- Respect learners
- Don't humiliate or embarrass
- Avoid any casual comments that display prejudice or could be seen as prejudicial
- Make sure you are informed about where students are at and what the learning outcomes are for the session. It's no good teaching them all about different types of hip replacement if they have come to learn how to examine the hip
- Use a questioning style that allows the students to express what they do know
- Don't swear
- Model excellent behaviour, e.g. towards patients

Box 9.4 Creative ideas for improving and evidencing your teaching and training

- Work with the nurse in charge on your ward to develop the observational skills of healthcare assistants
- Evaluate the teaching that you give medical students or even the directorate using a simple feedback pro forma
- In F2, undertake a Certificate in Medical Education or equivalent
- Keep a reflective diary of teaching you have delivered
- Play an active part in influencing your Foundation teaching programme
- Read relevant journal articles. Try the BMJ Education section or the journals Clinical Teacher or Medical Education
- Develop your understanding of contemporary educational issues through background reading
- Join the Association for the Study of Medical Education or the new Academy of Medical Educators

important thing to remember is not to abuse your position of authority over those below you, particularly in relation to sexual advances or relationships.

In general, the teaching and training section is another area to develop your skills and gather evidence for your post-Foundation job application rather than something that will trip you up. Examples of things that you could do to improve your teaching and 'buff' your CV for future applications are given in Box 9.4.

Relationships with patients

Your key responsibilities here include respecting patients' autonomy with respect to consent for examination and treatment, respecting their lifestyle and points of view, maintaining confidentiality and matters related to intimate examinations and not crossing the doctor/patient divide. Problems in this domain are a frequent source of disciplinary problems for trainees and seniors alike.

Example 1

A 65-year-old woman was admitted to hospital with back pain. The male trainee asked to examine her breasts. She assented but later complained to other staff. No chaperone was offered. She did not understand why it was important to examine the breasts when she was complaining of back pain.

Lessons: Guidance from the GMC (www.gmc-uk.org/guidance/archive/intimate_examinations_2001.pdf) suggests that patients should always be offered a chaperone for examination and that if they decline, this should be noted, as should the identity of the chaperone. It is wise to explain why you want to perform an intimate examination. Don't make assumptions about who might be upset by this or what constitutes an intimate examination. Men can be perturbed by examination as much as women, young as much as old, and same-sex examinations are not entirely problem-free. One of the oldest medical jokes asks: 'Why does the doctor get you to get undressed behind the curtain when he is going to see you naked?' However ironic this might seem, it does fit the GMC's guidance that you should allow the patient to undress in privacy and do not help the patient get undressed unless invited to do so. Always cover the patient appropriately during the examination using drapes. Be sensitive to cultural differences, and if the patient does not have English as a first language, arrange a time when you can explain your intention using an interpreter. Use of family members as interpreters and chaperones poses many problems. Don't be afraid to defer an intimate examination if no appropriate chaperone is available, unless it is absolutely essential in a life-threatening situation. The situation in primary care presents real challenges. Surgeons will no doubt berate GPs for not having done a PR examination when referring people with colorectal problems. But when looked at from a primary care perspective, it is much more understandable. GPs rarely have a chaperone even within the practice and if patients have been seen alone in their own home it is probably very wise not to perform a PR.

Example 2

A patient was a routine admission for corrective surgery for bunions. You are seeing them in the pre-admission clinic and notice that they have not completed their consent form, which would usually have been done by the consultant in clinic. In trying to be helpful, you explain as best as possible to the patient and take their written consent. Subsequent to the operation they develop a DVT and end up with a chronically swollen leg and sue the Trust. An internal investigation shows that the consent process was deficient as the risk of DVT had not been explained and the case is settled out of court. The hospital investigation reminds the consultant, the theatre team and you that only consultants or other staff who are qualified to carry out the procedure should seek consent for surgical procedures.

Lessons: The GMC guidance on consent has very clear definitions of who should obtain consent for a treatment or procedure. Normally, this should be the doctor providing the treatment, to ensure that the person obtaining consent has a 'comprehensive understanding of the procedure or treatment, how it is carried out, and the risks attached to it'. The GMC makes provision for delegation of the consent process, but it is unlikely that a Foundation doctor would qualify as having sufficient knowledge of surgical procedures to be able to obtain consent. In the Northern Foundation school we have a very clear rule that F1 doctors should never be asked to obtain consent for procedures that they cannot do themselves and it would be very sensible for F2 doctors to follow this as well. Observing a senior taking consent is a good way to go about things at this stage.

Example 3

An 88-year-old woman is being investigated on the ward for suspected liver metastases, but you don't yet have any proof. You have a general discussion with the patient and her daughter about the way ahead. Afterwards the daughter tackles you in the corridor while her mother is at ultrasound and insists that you must not tell her mother the diagnosis if it is cancer. You have a lengthy discussion about the rights and wrongs of this, but unbeknown to you the patient has returned from ultrasound and hears every word. The patient complains that you have broken confidentiality and trust by discussing matters with her daughter without obtaining any kind of consent.

Lessons: Your duty of care is primarily to the patient, not to the family. You should always seek the express consent of the patient to talk to their family. The patient's age does not absolve you of that responsibility. Make it good practice never to talk to a patient or carer in the corridor or waiting room. Go into the office or treatment room. If possible, don't talk to patients behind the curtains as the rest of the ward being able to hear is an invasion of their confidentiality and privacy. (You will know what I mean the next time you do a Mini Mental State Examination and the rest of the patients in the bay think you're hosting a game show.) The GMC gives detailed advice on confidentiality and regards breaches as very serious. See the guidance on confidentiality on the GMC website. Disclosure without consent can be justified under certain circumstances, primarily in the public interest such as when a crime has been committed, but you are unlikely to be responsible for these decisions.

Example 4

A 75-year-old man with Alzheimer's disease is admitted with a significant upper GI bleed. He needs urgent endoscopy. His abbreviated mental test score is 3 out of 10 and he is not able to understand your explanation of endoscopy and its risks and benefits. You find out from his wife that he normally has a fairly good quality of life in the residential home.

Who gives consent for this procedure? Is it:

- The patient's wife?
- The patient's daughter?
- The patient?

Lessons: Again, the GMC has guidance for patients who lack capacity, that is, the ability to take-in, understand, recall and weigh up the risks and benefits of a procedure. The patient's prior wishes, if any, need to be followed and it is good practice to include the family and the rest of the clinical team in the decision-making process, but in the end it is the senior doctor's decision. So, the answer is actually: no one can consent for a patient who lacks capacity. The consultant responsible for this patient can decide if a procedure or intervention is appropriate and in that patient's best interests, and go ahead with it if necessary. For patients who lack capacity, there is a specific NHS consent form: Form 4. This should be completed by the team referring the patient for a procedure or operation and by the person performing the procedure.

Many breaches of confidentiality are unwitting – conversations when you think no one is listening, leaving computer screens visible to others, giving information when you thought consent had been given but had not. If you get a request from an outside agency for information, be particularly careful in what you divulge. For example, Citizens' Advice agencies, insurance companies, employers or the police may all request information. Always check that the consent forms from other agencies refer to release of medical information to them. Sometimes they are just a very general consent form for that agency to be able to release their data to others, not for you to release medical information. If you start a blog or write articles for medical newspapers, be exceptionally careful what you say. You do not have to give a person's name and address to make them 'identifiable', which is the test of the law. Giving a 'humorous' account of a recent visit to your surgery from a local priest with sexual health problems, for example, could easily lead to the patient feeling that they can be identified. (That reminds me to ask, why is it that most writers in the free medical newspapers are disaffected reprobates? Does no one happy in their job want to express themselves in those publications?)

Releasing information about a patient to the police is another potential problem area. You can be sure that criminals will be the first to know and to exercise their rights, so be scrupulous in your dealings with the police if you wish to avoid a complaint. You are under no immediate obligation to reveal clinical details of a patient's condition to the police, or when they are going to be released from hospital. You may get firsthand experience of this 'pressure to divulge' if you do A&E (e.g. when dealing with road traffic accidents or assaults). There is a statutory duty under the Road Traffic Act 1998 to reveal a patient's address and name to the police if they are suspected of being responsible for a crime under the Act, but not any clinical information such as details of injury, time to discharge, etc. Get in touch with your senior if the going gets tough. Remember, it's not you making the confession.

Working with colleagues

This is an area where doctors frequently fall foul of disciplinary systems and also one that will make your working life very hard if you do not get on with colleagues. This works both ways and we need to consider the possibility that your colleagues may not be as cooperative as you would wish.

Example 1

An F1 doctor approached the family of a patient cared for by another team about the standard of care that they perceived their relative had received.

They did not document the discussion in the notes, nor did they inform the responsible consultant about their concerns or the concerns of the family. The family subsequently made a complaint against the consultant responsible, quoting the opinion of the trainee that they had spoken to.

Lessons: Similar cases have led to a reprimand from the GMC and could certainly lead to internal disciplinary procedures. One of the obligations for a doctor is to keep colleagues informed and not do anything that could undermine the relationship between a patient and any of their doctors. If you have concerns about the standard of care received by a patient, raise them with the consultant responsible for that patient. If this does not work, raise them with the medical director or a consultant you do trust. Do not make the clinical competencies of your colleagues or other doctors the subject of gossip. Don't talk to others in a way that you would not wish to be spoken of yourself.

Example 2

It's the end of the first month and you are increasingly frustrated by what appear to be incredible inefficiencies on the ward. You spend 90% of the day on your one ward yet as soon as you leave it seems that your bleep goes off with a nurse asking for a minor job to be done. When it happens for the fourth time in an hour you shout down the phone at the nurse, tell her you have just left and will be back soon and slam the phone down. You know straight away that this was unprofessional, but you are really irritated and hope that your display of temper will stop people bleeping you unnecessarily. When you return to the ward half an hour later, the nurse responsible has gone off duty. You notice the change in mood of the nurses and it's not for the better! Suddenly no one is available to set up a trolley for that CVP line, there is no one on the ward who can do male catheterizations and a lot of the patients seem to need pr exams to check they are not impacted. You are worried about your forthcoming multi-source feedback, which suggests that at least one nurse should be asked to give their opinion on you.

Lessons: Medicine is a tough profession and there will undoubtedly be times when you are frustrated and angry, but that's not an excuse to lose it. Never shout. And if the worst happens and you do lose your rag, apologise immediately and directly to the person you offended. A prompt apology is an effective apology. A late apology is much less meaningful and may be too late to stop the story of your behaviour going round the hospital. Just like looking after children, if you lose your cool, you have lost their respect. Once a shouter, always a shouter in the eyes of those who have witnessed or heard about your tirade.

Working with colleagues – the red tide phenomenon

The red tide phenomenon is known to psychologists who help footballers and police drivers to control their behaviour – think of David Beckham kicking out against Argentina in the 1998 World Cup or Gazza in the FA Cup final. The red tide is the mounting frustration and anger that spin out into loss of control and aggression. Most anger results from a belief or perception that something unfair or unjust is happening to you over which you have no influence. Recognizing this will enable you to take three steps to prevent and deal with frustrating situations:

Recognition

Recognise your emotions and your physiological response. Be aware of mounting anger and its corollary in adrenergic output – sweating, tachycardia, increasing respiratory rate and muscle tension (e.g. jaw clenching, neck and shoulder stiffness). Once your emotions and physiological response get this far, it may be difficult to scale them back. Try to recognise them early on in their development.

Cognitions

Think about where your anger has come from and your role in the situation. Think of win–win scenarios which leave you and the other party feeling that you have made progress.

Actions

There are a number of actions that you can take when you first recognize the signs of the red tide rising. Walk away, politely put the phone down, terminate the interview if it is with a patient. Breathe deeply or clench and unclench your fists. Suggest some positives, for example, put up a board in the doctor's office with 'Countdown to Friday' on it, or cartoons/newspaper clippings about the world's fattest cat. Looking forward to annual leave always chills you out. Nurses' jobs lists are quite a good idea, where nurses can document, for example, that Mrs Cannybody needs a new cannula, so you can do it and put your initials next to the completed task.

Working with colleagues: diversity issues

Diversity issues are currently not as high on the agenda of the NHS as they should be. Discrimination affects doctors (and other health workers) and patients alike. The law states that employers and health professionals should not discriminate on the grounds of race, sexuality or disability. But ask yourself how many disabled junior doctors or openly gay or lesbian doctors you know. Your undergraduate training in this area is likely to be slim.

The NHS has many examples of so-called institutional racism that are not being addressed and have got worse recently. Until 2006, we depended on non-EU overseas doctors for 25% or more of our SHO posts. Then in one fell swoop the government announced that, with only a few months' notice, non-EU doctors would be appointed to posts only when there was no suitable EU candidate. Instead of being able to compete on a level playing field (at least on paper), all non-EU candidates were sent to the back of the queue. As most of the non-EU applicants are from South Asia or Africa, this inevitably means that mainly white EU candidates are being preferred over mainly black or Asian candidates despite the fact that doctors from South Asia or much of Africa are educated in English, whereas a Greek, Spanish, Latvian or Polish doctor does not have to demonstrate their language competence. Even UK-qualified doctors who are citizens of another country will be sent to the end of the queue for post-Foundation appointments. This is not very positive in encouraging equal treatment and the creation of a new tier of service posts (FTSTA) that run parallel with numbered training posts is also likely to lead to discrimination. At present many claims for discrimination related to the failure to recognise the training of overseas doctors in non-standard posts are going through the courts. The BMA have even had to pay out large sums in compensation because they were found guilty of not adequately defending an overseas doctor's claim of equivalent training.

It seems ironic that throughout medical school we are taught pattern recognition of patient presentations that could reinforce stereotypes. For example:

- Farmers with swollen testicles – think brucellosis
- Jaundiced sewage workers – think leptospirosis
- Refugees – think high risk for TB

This method simply makes it easier for us to digest huge chunks of knowledge and is not meant to discriminate, but it can reinforce stereotypes. The trick in real life is to assume nothing, otherwise you could end up looking foolish.

This book cannot deal with diversity issues in depth and readers are referred to resources such as those provided by the GMC (www.gmc-org/guidance/library/valuing_diversity.asp). Some areas where you could reflect on your attitudes and behaviour and see whether you are really as open-minded as you think are suggested in Box 9.5.

Probity

Many people say that they do not understand what probity means in the context of registration. But probity is one of the main issues that cause doctors

---

Box 9.5   Some challenges to your attitudes

- In assessing your peers using MSF, are you sure that you judge all colleagues the same irrespective of whether they reflect your own background, personality and likes and dislikes?
- A 62-year-old Caucasian has an MI and you refer him to the cardiac exercise rehabilitation clinic. Would you have referred a 62-year-old who dresses in traditional Pakistani style and has English as a second language?
- Do you agree that obese patients should not be offered hip replacement? Is this evidence-based medicine or prejudice? Are you concerned about surgical complications or the longevity of the joint? Search www.library.nhs.uk for the evidence-based answer. In summary, there is very little evidence that obese patients suffer more complications or have shorter joint life than non-obese and in fact young age at operation predicts the need for early replacement most accurately
- In the gastroenterology clinic, you see a 25-year-old with probable IBS. The GP print-out of past medical history mentions two terminations of pregnancy. Does this alter your attitude to the woman?

to lose their registration rights. The GMC is clear that doctors should be expected to be 'honest and trustworthy'. This seems a very straightforward expectation and one aspect of professionalism that is easy to comprehend and define.

Would you recognise if the following examples fulfilled this stipulation and what would you think would be the consequences for the doctor?

Example 1

An F2 doctor with an exemplary health record was unexpectedly ill and required two weeks' sick leave. A chance encounter through cross-Trust referral discovered that while on the sick he was doing a locum in a nearby ITU. Subsequent investigation discovered that he had taken study leave on three occasions but had not attended the course.

Example 2

Using routine monitoring techniques, the IT department discovered that a newly qualified F1 doctor had been accessing porn sites from the Trust network during night duty despite the Trust's policy on appropriate usage. The F1 had signed a contract saying that he understood the policy.

Example 3

An SpR had a high reputation with consultants for having reviewed all the overnight admissions with carefully dated and timed entries in the notes. However, the nursing staff on MAU reported that she was never seen in the night and could frequently not be contacted. Subsequent investigation revealed that she turned up 30 minutes before the consultant at 7.30 am and made entries timed for the time of the patient's admission, not when she had seen them.

Example 4

An F1 doctor had 15 day case admissions to clerk every Wednesday for minor surgery. There was no time to take a full history and perform an examination, but they perceived that this was required by the anaesthetist so they documented a 'normal' cardiovascular and respiratory examination in all of them in order to get the job done.

Example 5

In applying for their Foundation post, a medical student claimed that they worked in a soup kitchen every Friday night and had played first team hockey for the university. They were selected as part of the 10% audit of Foundation applications. It was soon discovered that they had not played hockey since first year and they were forced to admit that they had only attended the soup kitchen on a couple of occasions.

We are sure that you will recognise that all of these cases involve a degree of dishonesty. Some may seem to be relatively minor, but all could lead to instant dismissal from your job and could result in a report to the GMC and, in example 1, a criminal trial for fraud. In 2006 a junior doctor was removed from the register for falsifying their qualifications on an application form. So next time, think before you state that you are an avid Shakespeare fan based on going to a performance of *Macbeth* when you were 15!

The GMC is also explicit in its advice about other aspects of probity, such as accepting gifts from patients. It is not considered appropriate to accept all but the most minor gifts, including services, and you must not borrow from patients or suggest donations to specific funds from which you could benefit. So best start digging deep into your own funds for that new stethoscope and don't ever consider accepting your patient's offer of a free MOT and service for your old banger.

Probity is fairly straightforward: when acting as doctor you must be honest and trustworthy. Don't be tempted to cut corners; don't do anything that could be seen as taking advantage of a patient; don't make false claims in applications; and never falsify clinical documentation. You may well be found out and lose your livelihood for ever.

HEALTH AND STRESS

Health issues are one of the major sources of problems for all doctors and it can be difficult to recognise that there is a problem, to negotiate the system and to work out the best way ahead for you.

In F1, self-limiting illnesses can be a problem if they take longer to recover than the absence allowed to achieve full registration. In this situation you may have to sit part, or all, of your F1 year again in order to fulfil the learning outcomes.

More serious illness may threaten your job and your career or even your life. Illness frequently interacts with performance issues – poor health, especially mental health, can cause poor performance, and poor performance can quickly impact on health, particularly if you become the subject of an investigation.

Doctors tend not to be good at dealing with their own health and many adopt a 'won't happen to me' attitude. This section deals with the interaction between illness, particularly stress, and your job. It is not intended to offer comprehensive advice on dealing with serious illness (e.g. severe depression or cancer) or physical handicap that impairs your ability to work in an unmodified job. In Chapter 10 you will find contact information and we hope that this will get the ball rolling if you're prevaricating about seeking help.

Your main duty as a doctor is to manage your health so that it does not affect the care of your patients. Some of the frequent issues include:

- Stress or mental health issues and their impact on performance
- Addiction or substance abuse and its impact on performance
- The impact of chronic illness (e.g. arthritis, MS, depression or cancer) on your career
- Transmissible disease (e.g. hepatitis B, hepatitis C or HIV/AIDS)

We will look at health issues in more detail through the use of some case histories.

Stress

It's one of the GMC's *Duties of a Doctor* to make sure you're in tip-top condition to look after patients – it's what Hippocrates would want you to do. So don't put things off in the hope they'll sort themselves out. If you're struggling at work with stress, take steps to get it sorted now. That is one of the reasons why there are so many support services for doctors, from your educational supervisor or mentor to the psychological support services offered by Occupational Health services, the BMA or voluntary agencies. It's extraordinary how few doctors think of stress as a medical problem that can be fixed, much as a bone or obstructed coronary can be. Many tend to accept things and effectively become one of Pavlov's dogs.

A useful resource is *Stress and the Medical Profession* (London: BMA, 1992).

Chapter 4 looked at the stresses associated with starting the Foundation programme and some suggestions were offered on how to deal with them. It introduced the idea that a degree of stress is normal but that it needs to be managed. But it's not always easy. If you are feeling stressed or down, don't imagine you're alone. There have been so many tragic tales of suicides in young doctors who have worked themselves into the ground, literally. You are never alone, no matter how bad it seems. Forget all the 'Physician, heal thyself' malarkey. This is the 21st century and times have changed. The minute you tell someone you have a problem at work, whether it's stress, difficult relationships, drugs, booze or whatever, you will begin to feel the weight come off your shoulders. There are times when you really need to think of yourself and treat yourself as you would one of your patients. Box 9.6 suggests ways of recognizing stress in yourself and Box 9.7 suggests means of help.

The following example looks at the interaction between stress and your role as a doctor.

Example

> Jim was never sure that medicine was right for him and went into it only because he had the right A-levels and his teachers suggested that this was the best career. He did not have any other concrete ideas. He struggled for the first two years as an undergraduate and had to sit his stage 2 exams

When medicine is difficult

Box 9.6   Recognizing stress – symptoms that may indicate high levels of stress

- Poor sleep
- Irritability at work or at home
- Excessive dissatisfaction with work
- Loss of interest in things
- Loss of libido
- Excessive alcohol or drug consumption
- Errors at work

Box 9.7   Resources for dealing with stress

- Friends and family
- Your GP – you should always have a GP, even when moving round the country
- Educational supervisor
- Clinical tutor or head of Foundation programme in the Trust
- Mentor – either official or unofficial
- Director of the Foundation school or deanery representative
- Occupational Health in the Trust – offers confidential advice and support by either a nurse or doctor and often has the option of referral to a psychologist
- Phone lines and other confidential services such as those offered by the BMA, Addicted doctors service or the Samaritans

twice, but when he had more patient contact he felt that there was a strong possibility that medicine would be OK. He had been treated with medication for depression on two occasions and his sister had severe postnatal depression treated by ECT.

Jim has not settled well in his F1 post. The first post in surgery was reasonably straightforward, even if unsupported, but working on the dialysis ward in medicine has been very hard. Most of the patients have a poor quality of life and there have been several deaths of young patients. There have been two recent cases where he made minor mistakes, although there were no serious consequences for the patients. However, his consultant has made it clear that these incidents have been noted.

Jim has found that things are getting on top of him and has started having difficulty in sleeping, feels low in mood and has no energy for any social activities. Next week he has a three-day on-call weekend and feels that he really cannot get through it.

What are Jim's responsibilities to his patients and himself at this stage?

Responsibilities to patients: The real danger here is that stress and mental health issues will impact on clinical performance and lead to a major clinical error. Clearly, Jim has a responsibility to identify the fact that his performance is affected and arrange to leave work before such an event occurs. How can he do this?

Responsibilities to self: If you are not well, you have a high level of responsibility to yourself to make sure that your health does not suffer. How should you go about this? You have a number of possibilities to make sure that your health is protected.

If you feel that you are not fit for work, then three people can sign you off. For short periods (five days), you can self-certify; for longer periods your responsible doctor (usually your GP, but it could be a psychiatrist or other specialist) can certify you as unfit to work; finally your Occupational Health department can evaluate you and agree that you are not fit to work and make appropriate arrangements for you to be treated and assessed as fit to return to work.

If you are fit to work but need help to carry on, there are several options. You can apply to your programme director or Foundation school director to work flexibly on the grounds of ill health. Flexible working involves a period of working part-time, either in your regular post or in a supernumerary post. Recently, the opportunities to work flexibly have reduced because of financial stringency in the NHS but illness is still a valid reason to request flexible working. You will have extra time to achieve the same Foundation curriculum outcomes and will still get the chance to go on to higher training. More importantly, your health will be safeguarded.

In planning your future career, it may be helpful to think of a planned career break or diversion if stress is a problem. For example, plan a six-month trip or something that you will enjoy after your Foundation programme. Knowing that a stressful post will end and that you will have time off to recover and reflect on your future career may help you maintain a positive outlook and get to the end of the post.

Jim is unsure of the way ahead and speaks to the clinical tutor in his Trust. The clinical tutor helps him negotiate a short period of sick leave to ensure that he does not have to do a 13-day unbroken stint. The clinical tutor also reaffirms the need for Jim to seek regular support to help him recover and to be appropriately monitored for his depression, use of medication and suicide risk. They agree that the Trust occupational psychologist is a suitable means of support, in addition to the GP.

The clinical tutor helps Jim to explore his feelings about medicine and review the positives and the negatives. Jim decides that he wishes to finish the first year of the Foundation programme and review things towards the end of that period. Together, they come up with some alternatives if Jim decides not to enter the second year of the Foundation programme, including taking a six-month career break or pursuing a part-time course in tropical medicine whilst finding out more about a career in fine art photography, which is Jim's secret desire. They meet regularly until the end of the Foundation programme when Jim decides that he will take the career break and negotiates a deferred stand-alone F2 position for the subsequent year.

Addiction and substance misuse

Example

Jemima has an excellent academic record and is looking forward to a career in infectious diseases. As a student she had a caution for drunk and disorderly when she was picked up by police wandering the streets at 2.00 am and got into an argument with them. She and her flatmates also had a disciplinary meeting with the Dean in year 5 when their neighbours complained to the university because of persistent noise into the early hours. Like 50% of students, Jemima has used cannabis and taken ecstasy, but recently she has been using cocaine, including at the ward Christmas party. She is unaware that people have been commenting on her demeanour at the party. She turns up to the late shift (starting at midnight) one night having drunk a couple of pints of lager earlier in the evening, thinking the effect will have worn off by the time she starts work. The sister on A&E reports her for coming to work smelling of alcohol.

Jemima is called to a meeting with the medical director and informed that she has been accused of misuse of alcohol. She enlists the help of her defence union, who vigorously defends her. The internal enquiry finds it difficult to prove that she had consumed alcohol before work in the absence of biochemical evidence, and it comes down to her word against one nurse's. She is given a warning and the matter is closed, but the incident remains on her record.

Lessons: This has been a narrow escape. Don't drink before going to work even if it is a very late shift. The Trust could have reported her to the GMC or dismissed her. She should seek help for her drug and alcohol use. There are many suggested resources in Chapter 10. Alcohol problems are related to approximately 25% of performance cases identified by doctors' peers, and many of the cases that come before the GMC include dependency as a contributory factor. This kind of behaviour in a young person may seem like high jinks but it is a strong predictor of later, more serious problems. Most doctors with alcohol problems start their drinking career early on and things get worse so having problems at this stage in your career does not bode well.

Severe or chronic illness

Doctors with chronic health problems or disability are poorly catered for in many parts of the NHS and frequently experience negative attitudes from their peers and seniors. Doctors aren't expected by their colleagues to be ill. The insistence that doctors have to do a standard year after graduation to become fully registered is a potential bar to disabled graduates. If you have to do the same job as everyone else but cannot run to a cardiac arrest, it is difficult to get fully registered, but a disabled doctor may bring many supplementary talents to the practice of medicine.

Example

Matthew is an F2 doctor who develops painful fleeting polyarthropathy. After a period of self-treatment with over-the-counter NSAIDs, he develops pleuritic chest pain and requires admission. A rheumatologist diagnoses rheumatoid arthritis. This is devastating news as Matthew wishes to pursue a career in surgery. It takes three months to get back to work and requires treatment with second-line therapy which needs regular monitoring. In this period Matthew misses the deadline to apply for the national run-through training posts and so does not have a job after July. Although the visible swelling and redness have gone, he feels excessively tired and is not able to concentrate for more than eight hours a day. He struggles to make it through the longer shifts. On occasion he has to ask a colleague to hold his bleep so that he can have a rest, but they have not been very helpful. He thinks they talk about him behind his back and feels excluded from the social scene.

What are Matthew's options now?

It can be very hard to accept that you have a long-term condition that is likely to recur and may cause disability. Matthew may benefit from talking to his educational supervisor, although many educational supervisors will not have had experience of dealing with doctors with a chronic illness. Other resources that may be of help are the programme or Foundation school director, a mentor or an occupational health specialist. In some deaneries there is someone with specific responsibility for doctors with health problems. Issues that Matthew will face include: financial, selecting the right career path, keeping training going and interactions between health and work. It can prove helpful to contact colleagues who have faced similar issues – several organizations put doctors with health problems in touch with other doctors who have faced similar problems. The doctor's support line (0870 7650001) offers confidential advice from volunteers with health and stress problems. The BMA careers service also offers support to doctors with health problems (020 7383 6303 or 6238, www.bmjcareers.com where there is a Web resource for doctors with disability – go to 'Medical careers and education'). The recently launched BMA 'Doctors for Doctors' service is described as an enhancement of the BMA counselling service (08459 200169). The BMJ Careers chronic illness matching scheme (web.bma.org.uk/public/chill.nsf) is a popular scheme that allows doctors with a chronic illness or disability to communicate with other doctors who have a similar illness or disability, or who are currently working in a similar job. The MMC national director has indicated that trainees with well-founded personal reasons for working part-time should be able to access appropriate opportunities through their Foundation school.

Helping a colleague or friend who develops a health problem

As a profession we can be very unforgiving of 'weaknesses' in our colleagues and this compounds the difficulties they may face in making psychological and physical adjustments to their illness. Maybe this is because we don't want to have to think that something similar might happen to us. Doctors really aren't invincible. If you encounter a doctor with a chronic health problem, put yourself in their shoes and be sympathetic.

Make sure that you keep absolutely confidential any medical facts that you glean about a colleague's condition if you have to treat them.

Transmissible disease

Example

A general surgeon discovered that his child had HIV infection following a series of hospital admissions with infections. The surgeon took no action with regard to his own health and carried on operating. An anonymous caller informed the Trust of the child's health status.

The man was initially referred to Occupational Health but initially did not attend. He declined HIV testing and was referred to the GMC.

Lesson: If you have any cause to suspect that you have acquired a transmissible infection, you must seek advice on your work practices from an occupational health physician or other suitably qualified doctor. You have a clear duty to act to protect the patients and you should not rely on your own assessment of the risk. It is your right to refuse to have an HIV test in these circumstances, although the GMC states that in the event of an outbreak, they would expect a doctor to comply with a request for testing. It may be very difficult for an occupational health physician to give you sound advice if you don't have appropriate testing. See the GMC's guidance library for further details.

Taking care of yourself: diet, exercise and weight

What you eat is recognised by all major authorities – other than NHS chefs – as being important to health and satisfaction with life. You are what you eat. Well, if you spend a week on call in an average NHS hospital, you will end up as a potato chip. The average spend on a day's food for an NHS patient is around £1.75 and it shows. Canteen food is designed to give good value to the incredibly poorly paid ancillary staff. In fact, in many hospital canteens you can find people who have no connection to the hospital enjoying a cheap, subsidised meal. So the hospital diet is unlikely to suit the average young doctor, most of whom probably consider themselves not far behind Jamie Oliver in cooking fresh food and are more likely to buy their food from Marks & Spencer rather than one of the cheaper supermarkets where there are no brand names. In studies of cancer risk and premature death, high levels of fruit and vegetable consumption seem to be the most consistently protective factors. So, as your hospital diet is likely to be high in fat and starch and low in vegetables and fruit, especially out of hours, you will have to work hard to achieve the recommended five portions a day.

Exercise is recognised as a major factor in preventing excessive stress and in protecting against obesity, the major predictor of metabolic syndrome and the development of type 2 diabetes, hypertension, dyslipidaemia and heart disease. If you have fallen out of the habit of exercise, it's a good idea to get back into it now before things get out of hand. It might shock you to find out that the mean BMI at diagnosis of type 2 diabetes is 27! To calculate your BMI, see one of the many internet calculators. In addition to BMI, we now recognise waist size as an important factor in predicting the metabolic syndrome, particularly in those with a BMI between 25 and 35. For Caucasian men a waist of ≥94 cm (37 inches) conveys increased risk and 102 cm (40 inches) conveys substantially increased risk. For Caucasian women the measurements are 80 cm (32 inches) and 88 cm (35 inches) respectively. For people of South Asian origin the waist size at which risk begins is lower.

Example
> A youthful 40-year-old gastroenterologist heard a talk on risk factors for diabetes and was shocked to discover that being overweight (BMI 25–29), not just obese (BMI ≥ 30), was a major risk. He calculated his own BMI as 27 and not wanting to lose his toes or become impotent at a young age, decided to do something about it. Regular brisk walks and reduced carbohydrate consumption at lunch and evening meals enabled him to get his BMI down to 25 in six months. In the maintenance phase he struggled a bit to keep up with the exercise regime and bought a dog so that he had to walk for half an hour every day.

Lesson: In talking about exercise, we do not necessarily mean joining a gym, wearing Lycra and getting sweaty. Past experience suggests that this is a way to lose £s not lbs! It is probably better to take a 30-minute brisk walk every day rather than 30 minutes of brisk exercise three times a week; it may also be better on your joints. Calorie restriction plays a part. We tend to get 40% or so of calories from carbohydrate, so reducing our carb intake is a relatively easy way to cut down on calories.

Health-seeking behaviour – diagnosis and prescribing for yourself, your family and friends

Historically, doctors have often diagnosed and treated themselves and their families. Many did not have a GP. A study of American doctors found that they had even treated family members for cancer and performed high-risk surgery (e.g. aortic valve replacement) on them. But self-diagnosis or diagnosing your family carries many risks. One of the authors had the experience of misdiagnosing his father's melanoma as a seborrhoeic wart. Fortunately, he followed the golden rule of not diagnosing family members and told him he must see his GP who also thought it was a seborrhoeic wart but referred him to a dermatology clinic where it was successfully excised. If I had been tempted to move beyond my expertise and told him it was definitely not a melanoma, I would be bitterly regretting it now. Similarly, if my children are ill I am guided by my wife's opinion on whether they need to see the GP rather than my own.

You may be asked by members of staff to give an opinion on their health. I have been asked by nurses to take a blood sample because they are tired and want to check they are not anaemic. This may be flattering to you as a newly qualified doctor but it is not professional and falls short of the GMC's stipulation that you must make a full assessment of every patient based on history and examination. Politely decline, pointing out the GMC's guidance if necessary, and suggest they visit their GP.

You should be aware that recent guidance from the GMC suggests that treatment of self and family should be done in an emergency situation only; otherwise it is considered unprofessional. Be aware that inappropriate prescribing for yourself and family could lead to your registration being challenged. If you do have to prescribe for yourself, make sure your GP is informed.

In summary, make sure that you are registered with a local GP and see them with your health problems, even if you think you can diagnose and treat yourself. In particular, don't diagnose or treat friends, family and workmates.

DISCIPLINARY PROCEDURES FOR FOUNDATION DOCTORS – A SUMMARY

Numerous bodies and systems have their sticky fingers in the issue of dealing with problems in medical care. One of the big injustices is that patients and others could potentially use up to seven grievance procedures against a doctor if they wish (Box 9.8), whereas doctors have virtually no way of dealing with a paranoid, malicious or barmy complainant. Sadly, the way to approach patient care can be 'How am I going to stop this patient or their relatives suing me or complaining about me?' instead of 'How can I help this patient?' We will briefly describe the disciplinary systems in common use throughout the NHS, starting with the least serious.

> **Box 9.8   The seven procedures that can be taken against a doctor**
> 1. Informal complaint
> 2. Formal complaint
> 3. Request for independent review
> 4. Health service ombudsman
> 5. Civil action for damages
> 6. GMC
> 7. Criminal allegation, such as assault

Informal complaints

Many doctors will find themselves the subject of an informal complaint at some stage in the Foundation programme. This could come from a patient or a member of staff. Most of these are related to attitude and communication.

Example 1

After a particularly hard night on call, Geoff has to obtain venous access from an elderly patient. He forgets to swab the skin, does not introduce himself and fails to get the drip in despite three attempts. The patient tells the nurse in charge about the incident and she asks to speak to him the next day.

Example 2

As a member of the hospital at night team, Ahmed was bleeped by a nurse to review a patient on the surgical wards whose blood pressure has dropped and has some bleeding from their mastectomy wound. Ahmed believes that it is the responsibility of the surgical registrar to review post-op complications but the nurse says she has contacted him and he has asked that you be bleeped. Ahmed tells the nurse he will get there when he can. He is not able to go straight away and when he goes 1½ hours later he finds that the nurse has filed a clinical incident report form because of the difficulty in getting a doctor to see a patient in what she felt was a relevant period.

Lessons: Both scenarios involve tasks that the doctor in question does not really want to do, whether because of fatigue or because they did not see it as within their remit. Remember that you have a duty of care towards the patient. In example 1 remember that a patient will recall a rude doctor for life. In example 2, the best thing to do would be to get on with it, remain pleasant with the patient and try to see things from the nurse's point of view after she has filled in the incident form. There may be an error with the system in the second scenario. Perhaps it was in the surgical registrar's remit to review post-op complications, or maybe your surgical job is incorrectly banded. Your first duty is patient safety, so whether or not it is your job, see the patient and make an appropriate plan. Leave any argument about who should be doing it until the morning. Then, if a reasonable approach to the surgical SpR does not meet a positive response, you can fight fire with fire and fill out an incident form yourself, documenting the events. That way, a long-term solution can be found.

Formal complaints

Formal complaints are dealt with by a manager who investigates the problem and then drafts a reply to the patient for the Chief Executive to sign. Junior doctors are rarely the main subject of formal complaints, which are often related to a whole series of issues rather than a single incident. Perhaps the public understand that trainees are inexperienced and allow them some latitude. It seems to take quite a lot to get people to put pen to paper. However, if you do feature in a complaint, do not take it personally.

Most formal complaints involving doctors are related to attitude and communication, often mixed with unresolved grief or guilt on the part of the complainant. However, although you may rarely be the subject of a complaint, you have a major part in preventing them through your role as the intermediary between the patient/carers and the consultant, and in the way complaints are dealt with. You may well be asked by an investigating manager about the incidents and your written notes will form the basis of the investigation. This is why it is vital that your notes are both accurate and legible. If you know that a patient has made a complaint, do not treat them differently by doing more tests, for example, or avoiding them. Be polite, thorough and make doubly sure that you document progress accurately.

Example 1

> A 45-year-old single man was due to be admitted for a liver biopsy for alcoholic liver disease. He phones on the morning of the biopsy obviously the worse for wear and says that he is not coming into hospital and does not want any follow-up. Six weeks later he is found dead. His family make a formal complaint through the hospital PALS system that his 'treatment' was cancelled by the hospital and that if had been admitted he would have survived.

Outcome: Fortunately, the F1 doctor on the team documented in the notes his phone call with the patient and the Trust is able to explain to the family that the patient had cancelled the appointment himself.

Lesson: Always document discussions with a patient, whether these are face to face or on the phone – documented incidents allow an investigation to evaluate exactly what happened and allegations to be defended. Remember: good notes make a good defence in court; bad notes make a bad defence; no notes and you have NO defence.

Example 2

> An 82-year-old widower with metastatic prostate cancer is admitted to a general medical ward for pain relief. Three months previously he had completed a round-the-world cruise and he had been walking 5 miles a day. He has now lost weight and is in severe pain. He is started on

morphine but this does not control his pain. After two weeks in hospital he is put on a syringe driver. His only son lives at the opposite end of the country and visits for the first time after two weeks, by which time his father is barely conscious and dies 48 hours later. From the moment the son sees his father he is very hostile to the ward staff, unable to understand how his dad could have deteriorated so fast and seemingly suggesting that the morphine has been responsible for his decline. He does not get the opportunity to talk to a consultant before his father's death. Two weeks later there is a written complaint that his father's medical care has been mishandled and picking up on many details of ward care, such as his father not being shaved, dust in the corners of the room and the attitude of the trainee who certified him in the middle of the night and was not able to give satisfactory answers to all his questions.

Issues arising: This is a classic complaint where a relative has not visited as quickly as they might, is horrified by the deterioration in the patient's condition and expresses their confusion, guilt and feelings about the impending death through anger to those caring for the patient. Much could be done by the staff to prevent this situation and to deal with it when it starts to become a problem. One key issue from many complaints that I see is the lack of clarity about diagnosis and prognosis in people who are dying, especially when the situation is changing rapidly. The rapid change in this man's condition (from healthy world traveller even at 82, to palliation in three months) signifies a potential problem from the start. Was the father communicating with his son? Did the father and the son understand the deteriorating situation, and were they continually apprised of each change? Did they understand the reason for admission and what it implied? If you feel that a patient is not keeping their family informed of their condition, it may well pay to explore why. Many patients wish to protect their family from bad news or may not feel that they should trouble their children who have busy lives of their own.

Once the son arrives and starts expressing his anger, several things could be done. The first is to contact the consultant and get them involved straight away. Consultants will naturally vary in their skills and interest in dealing with these situations, but in general their involvement is likely to help the relative understand the problem. They should have seen this situation several times before so will be more familiar with it. Furthermore, their seniority normally ensures that the angry patient or relative will listen to them more than to a junior doctor. Make sure that the consultant documents his discussions with the son in the notes.

As the trainee in the thick of it there are a number of other agencies that you can involve. The Patient Advice and Liaison Service (PALS) in your hospital does what it says on the label – it advises and liaises in a friendly manner and acts in many ways as an advocate for the patient/carer. Suggest at an early stage if a patient or carer seems unable to accept what you are telling them, PALS will be able to help. You might also like to involve your palliative care service at this stage. Palliative care is there to deal with difficult adjustment or grieving as much as with difficult symptom control. This is exactly the type of case where their involvement will be useful.

When medicine is difficult

Civil actions through the courts

Civil actions through the courts are not as common as in the USA, but they are increasing. They are, however, very rarely a cause of concern for junior doctors as the person being sued is usually the consultant and the situation is usually dealt with by the Trust's legal team. In general, you will be highly unlikely to be involved in a civil action. However, your notes and documentation might well be the factor that enables the action to be defended successfully, so it is vital that your notes are up to date, legible, signed and dated. It is helpful to print your name, or even use a stamp with your name on it, next to all entries in the notes because civil actions may take some years to come to light, by which time no one will recognise your distinctive handwriting.

Reporting to the GMC

There are few things to make a doctor's heart tick faster than a letter on the mat from the GMC. One in early August is OK – it will contain your registration certificate. But at any other time of the year it is a worry. The following is designed to make you aware of the things that might cause referral and, if it does happen, to help you through it. If you do get a letter from the GMC stating that you have been referred, try not to panic. The vast majority of referrals do not end up with a conviction. But there is no doubt that, even for a totally spurious case, referral to the GMC will seem like the worst possible thing that has ever happened to you. And it can be a long wait to get the all-clear.

The GMC may become interested in your fitness to practice for a number of reasons such as misconduct, deficient performance, a criminal conviction or caution, and physical or mental health. Examples include but are not restricted to:

- Serious or repeated mistakes in examination, diagnosis, treatment, procedures or prescribing
- Failure to examine properly or respond reasonably to patients' needs
- Fraud or dishonesty
- Serious breaches of confidentiality
- Treating patients without adequate explanation or consent
- Sexual advances to patients
- Misuse of drugs or alcohol

Patients may report you, your employer may or the courts may if you get a conviction for anything at all. Happily, the GMC indicates that convictions for parking offences will normally be dealt with quickly and will not affect your registration. But be aware that any conviction (e.g. drink driving or possession of drugs) or caution (e.g. for drunk and disorderly) will mean that the GMC will be notified.

There is also a proposal that medical students should be registered with the GMC and that they should be subject to performance procedures similar to doctors. Increasingly, poor attitudes to medicine are weaned out at an early stage in medical school. Examples include probity (e.g. plagiarism), substance misuse and criminal convictions. This may seem harsh, given the cultural history of student medical societies, cheese and wine evenings, and the annual Medsoc Dentsoc yard of ale challenge. But it's a positive step in becoming more accountable for ourselves and re-establishing trust between medicine and the public. So, think twice before putting that traffic cone on your head during your next night out!

How does the GMC start to investigate an allegation against you? As of 2006 the whole system is being opened up to debate and things may well change in the future. However, the current situation is the following. Initially, any referral will be investigated and then assessed by two assessors and a decision made on whether there is a case to answer under fitness to practice procedures. They may make further enquiries from your employer. The vast majority of investigations by the GMC end up with no action being taken against the doctor's registration. This does not mean that the doctor has necessarily behaved impeccably, just that the behaviour did not meet the criteria for affecting registration or that the case was unproven. The GMC also has the option of issuing a warning. This is normally carried on your record for five years and further complaints could initiate further enquiry. The GMC also has a category of 'Undertakings' when they find deficiency that is not sufficient to affect registration. An Undertaking is an enforceable agreement between you and the GMC that you will undertake certain actions or restrictions such as retraining or not handling certain types of cases.

If the assessors find that there is a case to answer and you dispute the findings or facts, a hearing will take place. If found guilty, three actions are available to the GMC: limitations on your practice, suspension or erasure. Erasure is usually permanent.

We have discussed above some typical cases that might give rise to an appearance before the GMC in the sections on 'Good clinical care', 'Working with colleagues', 'Probity' and 'Health and stress'. As indicated at the beginning of this chapter, admonishment from the GMC usually comes because of a series of serious failings and is unlikely to arise from a single incident unless it is extremely serious and clearly negligent.

Criminal actions through the courts

Prior to 1990 there were very few cases of doctors being prosecuted through the criminal courts for medical misadventure. However, like all employees, we are responsible for our actions and there have been some recent high-profile cases where doctors were held accountable in the courts rather than through professional channels.

Think of two prominent prosecutions in England. In the first, a man was prosecuted when he accidentally drove onto a railway when over-tired, causing a fatal train crash. In the second, two subcontractors working on the railway were prosecuted for using a carriage with inadequate brakes. Four men were killed in the resulting accident.

The courts and the general public increasingly see death resulting from medical misadventure in the same way. Possible charges against doctors include assault for treatment against a patient's will or manslaughter for medical misadventure (e.g. wrong drug administration or the wrong kidney removed). These prosecutions are running at just 4–6 a year so unless you do something extremely wrong, you are unlikely to be the subject of criminal charges.

SUMMARY

This chapter has reviewed some of the health and disciplinary issues that you may face as a Foundation doctor. We hope it has given you insight into some of the common pitfalls and will allow you to avoid them or to deal with them if you are unfortunate enough to experience them. It has briefly detailed the types of disciplinary and performance issues that can arise for Foundation doctors. You are not alone and there is always a solution to every problem. Many sources of help are listed in Chapter 10.

Miscellany: specialty guide and other useful information

MEDICAL OATHS

The following medical oaths are offered to stimulate your thoughts about your role as a doctor. The Hippocratic Oath is the foundation of medical oaths and set the scene for many centuries but unsurprisingly, given its age, has some rather outdated notions. Many of its themes, such as confidentiality and respect for life, can be traced through to the modern-day versions and are reflected in the GMC guidance.

The Hippocratic Oath

❝ 'I swear by Æsculapius, Hygeia, and Panacea, and I take to witness all the gods, all the goddesses, to keep according to my ability and my judgement, the following Oath.

To consider dear to me as my parents him who taught me this art;
to live in common with him and if necessary to share my goods with him;

To look upon his children as my own brothers, to teach them this art if they so desire without fee or written promise;
to impart to my sons and the sons of the master who taught me and the disciples who have enrolled themselves and have agreed to the rules of the profession, but to these alone the precepts and the instruction. I will prescribe regimens for the good of my patients according to my ability and my judgement and never do harm to anyone.

To please no one will I prescribe a deadly drug nor give advice which may cause his death.
Nor will I give a woman a pessary to procure abortion.
But I will preserve the purity of my life and my art.
I will not cut for stone, even for patients in whom the disease is manifest; I will leave this operation to be performed by practitioners, specialists in this art.

In every house where I come I will enter only for the good of my patients, keeping myself far from all intentional ill-doing and all seduction and especially from the pleasures of love with women or with men, be they free or slaves.

All that may come to my knowledge in the exercise of my profession or in daily commerce with men, which ought not to be spread abroad, I will keep secret and will never reveal.

If I keep this oath faithfully, may I enjoy my life and practise my art, respected by all men and in all times; but if I swerve from it or violate it, may the reverse be my lot.'

(Source: en.wikipedia.org)

The Geneva Declaration

1948 saw the establishment of the Geneva Declaration after the atrocities committed by Nazi doctors during the Second World War. The Declaration seems much more in tune with the 21st century than the Hippocratic Oath and involves treating people equally, regardless of colour or creed, and avoiding any practise that could contravene humanity:

'At the time of being admitted as a member of the medical profession:
I solemnly pledge myself to consecrate my life to the service of humanity;
I will give to my teachers the respect and gratitude which is their due;
I will practise my profession with conscience and dignity; the health of my patient will be my first consideration;
I will maintain by all the means in my power, the honour and the noble traditions of the medical profession; my colleagues will be my brothers;
I will not permit considerations of religion, nationality, race, party politics or social standing to intervene between my duty and my patient;
I will maintain the utmost respect for human life from the time of conception, even under threat, I will not use my medical knowledge contrary to the laws of humanity;
I make these promises solemnly, freely and upon my honour.'

(Source: www.cirp.org/library/ethics/geneva)

The Oath of Lasagna

In 1964 Dr Louis Lasagna brought out an oath that emphasises the need to treat patients as human beings and not as 'textbook' cases:

'I swear to fulfil, to the best of my ability and judgement, this covenant:
I will respect the hard-won scientific gains of those physicians in whose steps I walk, and gladly share such knowledge as is mine with those who are to follow.
I will apply, for the benefit of the sick, all measures [that] are required, avoiding those twin traps of over-treatment and therapeutic nihilism.
I will remember that there is art to medicine as well as science, and that warmth, sympathy, and understanding may outweigh the surgeon's knife or the chemist's drug.
I will not be ashamed to say 'I know not,' nor will I fail to call in my colleagues when the skills of another are needed for a patient's recovery.
I will respect the privacy of my patients, for their problems are not disclosed to me that the world may know.
Most especially must I tread with care in matters of life and death. If it is given me to save a life, all thanks. But it may also be within my power to take a life; this awesome responsibility must be faced with great

humbleness and awareness of my own frailty. Above all, I must not play at God.

I will remember that I do not treat a fever chart, a cancerous growth, but a sick human being, whose illness may affect the person's family and economic stability. My responsibility includes these related problems, if I am to care adequately for the sick.

I will prevent disease whenever I can, for prevention is preferable to cure.

I will remember that I remain a member of society, with special obligations to all my fellow human beings, those sound of mind and body as well as the infirm.

If I do not violate this oath, may I enjoy life and art, respected while I live and remembered with affection thereafter. May I always act so as to preserve the finest traditions of my calling and may I long experience the joy of healing those who seek my help.'

(Source: www.pbs.org/wgbh/nova/doctors/oath_modern.html)

What are medical oaths for?

Having read the oaths, how do you feel about them? The Geneva Declaration seems to demand almost super-human qualities. We like the Lasagna Oath best – it fits with the modern notion of medicine as a special calling but in the end as a job of work, and acknowledges the balance between doing your best and not striving to preserve life under any circumstances. It also recognises the primacy of knowledge, which seems to have been forgotten in the current climate. Oaths are only guidance, and it's down to you to be inspired and put your ideals into practice.

HEALTH AND SUPPORT FOR DOCTORS RANGING FROM ADDICTIONS TO LIFESTYLE ISSUES

BMA general contact number: 020 7387 4499
BMA counselling service: 08459 200169. www.bma.org.uk

The BMA is the largest, but not the only, trade union for doctors. It represents its members' interests in discussions at national level, but if you are a member, it will represent you in disciplinary or contractual problems with your employer. It offers many other services, including financial advisers and conveyancing, although these are not necessarily the cheapest or the most independent.

The Medical Forum: www.medicalforum.com
Independent information on career support and guidance.

www.rose.nhs.uk
This website offers International Medical Graduates, including refugee doctors, advice on working in the UK, including details on registration and job hunting as well as conferences and courses.

www.doctorssupport.org
Trains volunteers all over the country for confidential peer support for doctors and students. Volunteers needed.

www.dsn.org.uk
The doctor's support network deals specifically with doctors experiencing stress or mental health problems:

Sick Doctors Trust
0870 4445163; www.sick-doctors-trust.co.uk
Deals specifically with addiction problems, including alcohol.

Samaritans
08457 909090; www.samaritans.org; Text 07725 909090;
    email: Jo@samaritans.org
Confidential, non-judgemental support service 24 hours a day.

Life coaching
www.workinglives.co.uk
Anita Houghton, life coach, anita@workinglives.co.uk

Doctors' Support Line (anonymous peer support)
0870 765 0001

Gay and Lesbian Association of Doctors and Dentists
0870 7655606; www.gladd.org.uk

Medical Women's Federation
020 73877765; www.medicalwomensfederation.co.uk

Women in Surgical Training (WIST)
020 7869 6217; www.rcseng.ac.uk/career/wist

EDUCATION AND NEWS

BMA A–Z of medical education
www.bma.org.uk/ then 'A to Z' in the search facility.

www.doctors.net.uk
This website is developing a series of accredited online learning modules. More than 150 are available. They use a common format and there is a variety of learning methods, such as interactive cases, MCQs and resource lists. Subscription is free if you are registered with the GMC and you get your own email address.

National Association of Clinical Tutors: www.nact.org.uk
Clinical tutors have traditionally taken the lead in postgraduate education within Trusts. This position has been eroded recently with the appointment of directors of education and similar positions. However, every hospital should have a clinical tutor, and the NACT is still a major influence in postgraduate education. Much useful information can be found through this organisation.

The Academy of Medical Royal Colleges: 020 7486 0067; www.aomrc.org.uk
The AoMRC is responsible for the curriculum for the Foundation programme. A new curriculum is planned for 2007 which will address many areas not covered in the previous curriculum and offer more direction in how the objectives can be achieved. See the website for further details.

www.copmed.org.uk
The website of the influential Conference of Postgraduate Medical Deans who influence the direction of postgraduate education.

www.rcplondon.ac.uk
Many teaching materials are found here, including the Foundations for clinical practice teaching materials. Browse the education section or enter 'foundations for good medical practice' in the search facility.

Royal Society of Medicine: Tel: 020 7290 2900; www.rsm.ac.uk

www.miaduk.com
Doctors as teachers, support for your teaching skills.

www.gmc-uk.org (the GMC website)
Has many documents you should be familiar with. Bearing in mind the inclusion of consent in the syllabus for the Foundation programme, there is an excellent guide here, entitled *Seeking patients' consent: the ethical considerations*.

NHS teaching materials can be found at the following websites. They give a general introduction to the subject of their title but the evidence base for learning skills such as communication and teamworking is that they are best learnt in practice rather than from a book or website:

www.clinicalteaching.nhs.uk
www.appraisaluk.info or www.appraisal-skills.nhs.uk
www.healthskills.co.uk
www.teamworking.nhs.uk
www.communicationskills.nhs.uk
www.ethicsandlaw.nhs.uk
www.patientsafety.nhs.uk
www.liberatinglearning.nhs.uk

Other interesting sites include:

www.nationalobesityforum.org.uk
www.webhealth.co.uk
http://news.bbc.co.uk then click on the Health button

The *British Journal of Hospital Medicine* is currently running a series of articles relevant to the Foundation curriculum and can be found in most hospital libraries. Online subscribers can view all past copies at www.hospitalmedicine.co.uk

Many textbooks are available online and with PDA versions. Try searching the publishers' websites or ask at your local medical library, which may well have agreements to access books online. The NHS library website has many online textbooks as well as journals.

MEDICAL BLOGS AND WIKIS

Thousands of doctors around the world are blogging, sounding off about their patients, their employers and life in general in online journals, otherwise known as blogs. By their nature these are often ephemeral so we have not listed the current best medical blogs. Warwick and Newcastle Universities, for example, have an index of their own bloggers. One of our favourites is www.neenaw.co.uk/ a blog by an ambulance controller of bizarre 999 calls. The *BMJ* Careers Focus also have a series of blogs. There seem to be relatively few doctor blogs from the UK so here is your chance for fame and fortune.

Wikis are continuously updated web pages. www.wikiMD.org has many pages devoted to clinical subjects.

NHS ORGANISATIONS

http://www.npsa.nhs.uk/health/resources/ipsel
National patient safety website for educational materials on patient safety. All trainees need to register. Look out for things like intrathecal administration of the wrong cytotoxics or inadvertent potassium administration which killed people and left trainees in court. The concept of a national safety agency is therefore very worthwhile and to be supported.

Modernising Medical Careers: www.mmc.nhs.uk

General Medical Council: 0845 357 3456; www.gmc-uk.org

The GMC has numerous publications designed to guide you through the maze of clinical practice (e.g. *Good Medical Practice*; *Duties of a Doctor*; *Confidentiality: Protecting and Providing Information*). You should be familiar with the main conclusions of these documents as they are the best guide we have to the standards expected of us.

Hospital at Night: www.healthcareworkforce.nhs.uk/hospitalatnight.html

Medical Training Application Service: www.mtas.nhs.uk
The system through which all applications to the Foundation programme and ST programmes will be made.

Postgraduate Medical Education Training Board: www.pmetb.org.uk
The new body for setting and maintaining training standards. Having an increasing role in all aspects and locked in a love/hate relationship with the old boy, the GMC. Both struggling to wrest power from the other while smiling for the cameras.

www.library.nhs.uk
This is the site for Connecting for Health, the ambitious and comprehensive internet access for information for all NHS employees. You need an Athens password but you can easily register and obtain one. It gives access to the chief databases such as Medline and also online textbooks and journals. It continues to develop and has a huge variety of guidelines and clinical evidence with links to Cochrane, etc.

National Institute for Health and Clinical Excellence: www.nice.org.uk
This independent body examines the evidence for treatments and advises the
NHS on their cost-effectiveness. It is designed to end the 'postcode lottery' of
access to treatment.

The Cochrane Collaboration: www.cochrane.org
An international organisation that provides up-to-date information on the
effects of healthcare. It uses systematic review to examine the evidence for
and against treatments and covers many areas of healthcare. Generally speaking a Cochrane review is accepted as the highest quality of evidence on a
treatment.

CAREER MANAGEMENT

The Medical Specialties Aptitude Test: http://www.med-ed.virginia.edu/
specialties/

Ask a question on careers via BMJ:
http://www.bmjcareersadvicezone.synergynewmedia.co.uk/

Windmills career management approach: http://www.windmillsprogramme.
com/

National policy on careers management:
http.//www.mmc.nhs.uk/pages/careers/career-management

BMJ Careers Focus. www.careerfocus.bmj.com Sister journal to the *BMJ* with
a useful series of articles on many aspects of careers.

Chris Ward and Simon Eccles, *So You Want to be a Brain Surgeon* (London:
Oxford University Press, 2001). Gives details of most careers and tips on
workload, training requirements, etc. Perhaps out of date now that training
has been revolutionised.

The Northern deanery has a careers advice website (being updated) with
many useful links: www.info4docs.org

Also see the websites of the various Royal Colleges.

PROTECTION SOCIETIES

Medical Defence Union (MDU): 020 7202 1500; www.the-mdu.com
Medical Protection Society: 0845 605 4000; www.medicalprotection.org
Medical Doctors and Dentists Defence Union of Scotland: 0845 270 2034;
    www.mddus.com

PROGRAMMES FOR PERSONAL DIGITAL ASSISTANTS (PDAs)

www.diagnosaurus.com
This programme helps with differential diagnosis

www.med-ia.ch/medcalc
This programme enables you to calculate medically relevant formulae.

www.collectivemed.com
www.medspa.com
www.skyscape.com
www.pdamd.com
www.doctorsgadgets.com

MISCELLANEOUS OTHER SITES

www.MomMD.com
Website by a mum-doctor

BOOKS

Samuel Shem, *The House of God* (New York: Dell, 1978).
This seminal book about the experience of a resident in the American hospital system of the 1970s touches a lot of raw nerves. Aspects of this experience will be identified by many F1 doctors today, for example the third and seventh rules of the Fat Man ('At a cardiac arrest the first procedure is to take your own pulse' and 'Age and blood urea nitrogen = Lasix dose') and the debate that still rages about whether or not to give someone with jaundice steroids. The book captures the survival aspects of being a junior doctor and has been described as '*Catch-22* with stethoscopes'. Not necessarily politically correct, but it does reflect the *zeitgeist* of being a new doctor.

Michael Balint, *The Doctor, His Patient and the Illness* (London: Churchill Livingstone 1957)
Another seminal book that captured a change in the attitudes and skills of the doctor. It is evidence-based and remains relevant today as an account of the relationship between the doctor and the patient. The book focuses on primary care, but should be seen as relevant to all doctors today.

Nicola Cooper, Kirsty Forrest and Paul Cramp, *Essential Guide to Generic Skills* (Oxford: Blackwell, 2006).
This has useful practical advice on the basics of clinical practice that you will need as a Foundation doctor.

SPECIALTY GUIDE

What follows is a guide to the specialties on offer from the Foundation programme and Modernizing Medical Careers that undoubtedly reflects the authors' biases and may therefore lack objectivity. For further information see bmjcareers.com – an excellent website for finding out about these specialties from doctors who have been there, but beware that it is likely to be as biased as this guide. In our review, each subject is presented under the headings of pros and cons, skills needed, risks in pursuing the specialty and little known facts.

Accident and Emergency, also known as emergency medicine

Pros: Exciting and unpredictable specialty. Vast range of presentations, from the confused granny with the UTI to major multi-vehicle pile-ups – a good hideaway for the adrenaline junkie.

Cons: Prone to abuse – sadly, many people do not understand what an 'accident' or an 'emergency' is. Bed bureaucracy and four-hour waits. Lack of follow-up – once the patient has been shifted you'll never know if the ward doctors laughed at your '? Janeway lesions' spot diagnosis.

Skills: Quiescence under pressure. Ability to multi-task when asked by four different F1 doctors at the same time if they can run something past you.

Risks: Low. There will always be accidents or emergencies.

Little known fact: The Cook County Hospital in Chicago is the busiest A&E in the world and sees around 350 patients a day (www.ccbh.org). Think twice about that back pain you've had for three years before presenting there.

Contact: 020 7404 1999; www.emergencymed.org.uk

Acute medicine

See General internal medicine.

Allergy

Pros: Interaction with varied specialties, e.g. respiratory (asthma), gastro (lactose intolerance) and dermatology. A challenging new specialty. Lots of research opportunities.

Cons: You need to have a passion for allergy – it is after all a subspecialty of a subspecialty.

Skills: You hold the key to turning someone's life around who has anaphylactic reactions.

Risks: Low. Training posts are being added as we write. Good opportunity for private practice too.

Little known fact: The word 'allergy' stems from the Greek for 'strange activity' (www.etymonline.com).

Contact: British Society for Allergy and Clinical Immunology: www.bsaci.org

Anaesthetics

Pros: Cleverer than medicine but with half the paperwork and twice the gas. Eye-opening emergencies, eye-closing routine work and out-patient exposure (e.g. pain clinic). Lots of technical procedures.

Cons: Reliance on your consultant at night for complex 'will we, won't we' calls to transfer to ITU, particularly when starting out. Chronic patience required for chronic pain.

Skills: Increasingly the only people who can put in a central line or get that difficult LP. Need to be comfortable with that number 14 needle and have a strong forearm.

Risks: Low. Sick people will always need their airways protecting.

Little known fact: Where have you heard of sodium thiopental before? It is the mythical 'truth serum' drug, that doesn't actually make you tell the truth. So if your patient tells you that you're rubbish at intubation, don't believe them.

Contact: Royal College of Anaesthetists: www.rcoa.ac.uk; or the Intensive Care Society: 020 7280 4350; www.ics.ac.uk

Audiological medicine

Pros: Satisfying work. Broad range of options, including paediatric audiology and balance problems. Lots of scope for research. Contact with the medics and surgeons, as well as a holistic approach to hearing problems.

Cons: Not well known to the lay doctor, leaving your services prone to poor referrals.

Skills: Virtually the only doctors who can perform Rinne and Weber's tests with the right frequency tuning fork and interpret the results correctly.

Risks: A growing specialty with low risk and huge patient pool.

Little known fact: The telephone was actually the first hearing aid, born out of Alexander Graham Bell's experiments to facilitate communication between the hearing impaired (www.scran.ac.uk).

Contact: British Association of Audiological Physicians: www.baap.org.uk

Cardiology

Pros: Something for everyone, whether you like a practical, hands-on approach (electrophysiology, pacemaker insertion, implantable cardioverter defibrillator insertion, angioplasty), looking after patients with rare congenital heart diseases or academic cardiology. More evidence-based than life itself.

Cons: Very competitive. You seem to need to be able to play golf to do cardiology. Diagnostically a bit dull – in the end much of it is coronary disease.

Skills: Being able to remember the minutiae of every single cardiology drug trial in existence. Able to slow down time so they can see all five components of the JVP, and are not just able to tell whether it is elevated or not like mere mortals.

Risks: Low if you can get on the training scheme, although deaths from heart disease are falling rapidly with reduced smoking and more effective drugs.

Little known fact: I was once told by a cardiologist that 'accessory pathway ablation is the only condition in medicine that is a true cure and will never ever come back again'. Any takers?

Contact: British Cardiac Society: 020 7383 3887; www.bcs.com

Cardiothoracic surgery

Pros: Highly technical, highly demanding job, with big rewards for hard work and commitment. Life-changing operations (e.g. CABG) coupled with curative work (lung cancer resection).

Cons: Life-long commitment required. Competitive. Intense public scrutiny of your success and failure as outcomes are published regularly.

Skills: As if repairing a coronary artery on a still heart wasn't tricky enough, 'beating heart' surgery is performed with only an isolated part of the heart frozen. A bit like trying to eat peas with a fork on a rollercoaster.

Risks: Thoracic component: low. Cardiac component: exercise caution – with the evolution of percutaneous intervention, bypass surgery is not relied upon as much.

Little known fact: As a Foundation doctor, don't forget that pleural effusion is a common cause of SOB after a CABG. Transudate or exudate? Hmmm, got you thinking now?

Contact: Society of Cardiothoracic Surgeons of Great Britain and Ireland: 020 7869 6299; www.scts.org

Chemical pathology and metabolic medicine

Pros: A growing and important specialty as more people are developing metabolic problems (e.g. diabetes, dyslipidaemia, obesity and hypertension). Management skills in running the labs and trying to halt the unstoppable rebel force of spurious troponin T requests.

Cons: Can be a heart-sink specialty when managing patients who can't/won't alter their lifestyle and managing doctors who request tests when they don't know the difference between sensitivity and positive predictive value. Not much limelight – many people will confuse you with a lab technician.

Skills: Knowing, and caring, about the five types of primary hyperlipidaemias. Not tearing your hair out over the overuse of D-dimers.

Risks: Low. Plenty of job opportunity.

Little known fact: The hypercalcaemia of sarcoidosis is actually from vitamin D-producing macrophages found in the non-caseating granulomas.

Contact: Royal College of Pathologists: 020 7451 6700; www.rcpath.org

Child and adolescent psychiatry

Pros: Fascinating dealing with the autistic spectrum disorders and holistic approach to ADHD. Close liaison with social services, forensic psychiatry and general paediatrics.

Cons: Considerable investment in time per patient needed to reap the benefits of treatment. Exposed to a lot of cases of child abuse, requiring a strong heart and mind.

Skills: Connecting with patients who don't know who you are, don't care who you are and don't understand what you are saying.

Risks: Excellent career opportunities, partly because of the stigma associated with child protection work.

Little known fact: The drug given for attention deficit hyperactivity disorder is, paradoxically, a stimulant related to amphetamine.

Contact: Royal College of Psychiatrists: 020 7235 2351; www.rcpsych.ac.uk

Clinical cytogenetics and molecular genetics

Pros: Largely lab-based, close work with clinical genetics and inherited diseases in clinical practice (e.g. chromosome typing in leukaemia). Technically demanding and constantly evolving.

Cons: Little patient contact.

Contact: Association of Clinical Cytogeneticists: www.cytogenetics.org.uk; Clinical Molecular Genetics Society: www.cmgs.org

Clinical genetics

Pros: Good opportunity for research. Fascinating clinical presentation of disease, ranging from dysmorphic features to MDT meetings with medical specialties (e.g. neurology, respiratory).

Cons: Few jobs, competitive. The main genetics research centres are few and far between, which may mean you have to move and live close to an urban centre.

Contact: Clinical Genetics Society: www.clingensoc.org; and the British Society of Human Genetics: www.bshg.org.uk

Clinical neurophysiology

Pros: Interesting mix of patients, from neonates with retinal problems, to diagnosing epilepsy and non-epileptic attack disorders, to dealing with myasthenia gravis. Few on-call commitments.

Cons: Lacks the recognition of the more popular specialties. No follow-up of patients past the diagnostic stage.

Risks: Plenty of jobs available due to current low-profile status. To be part of the neurosciences specialty training programme so opportunities may change in the future.

Contact: British Society for Clinical Neurophysiology: www.bscn.org.uk

Clinical oncology

Pros: Varied caseload. Dealing with sick patients and making a difference. Close contact with patients. Multidisciplinary involvement from most specialties. Research opportunities. Differs from medical oncology in that it is primarily radiotherapy-based, whereas medical oncology is (broadly speaking) more chemotherapy-based.

Cons: Dealing with dying and breaking bad news a lot of the time, so you need to be emotionally strong. Little diagnostic element to the specialty – you become the referee rather than referrer. Lots of theoretical exams.

Risks: Low. Unfortunately, the cure for cancer still eludes us.

Little known fact: DXT (the abbreviation for radiotherapy) stands for 'deep x-ray therapy'.

Contact: Royal College of Radiologists: 020 7636 4432; www.rcr.ac.uk

Clinical pharmacology and therapeutics

Pros: Something for everyone – close liaison with NICE, the Committee on Safety of Medicines, Toxicology Units, research into chemotherapy drugs, pharmacokinetics and clinical trials.

Cons: Can run into problems with politics with regard to funding for the best drugs available. Difficulties in helping people who repeatedly overdose.

Risks: A popular specialty.

Little known fact: Intravenous alcohol is a legitimate treatment for methanol (contained in antifreeze and methylated spirit) overdose.

Contact: The Faculty of Pharmaceutical Medicine of the Royal Colleges of Physicians of the United Kingdom: www.fpm.org.uk; and The Association of the British Pharmaceutical Industry (ABPI): www.abpi.org.uk

Clinical radiology

Pros: Diagnostically challenging, and for that reason rewarding. You are quite high up in the intellectual food chain and well-respected by those whose requests you haven't declined too frequently. There can be patient contact and opportunities for highly skilled interventional procedures (e.g. percutaneous transhepatic cholangiogram). The training programme has been totally revamped with three new radiology academies and a system of online learning for those on the programme (www.riti.org).

Cons: Little chance to follow patients through their illnesses (for some, this could be a pro). Having to deal with minions who are really a tennis ball involved in a tense rally between you and the consultant requesting 'unnecessary' investigations.

Skills: Ability to see lymph nodes on a CT scan. Could drive home blindfolded in a snowstorm with their ultrasound skills.

Risk: Uncertain. In the early 2000s there were several hundred unfilled jobs in the UK but the new training scheme is throwing out a lot of CCT holders, and Polish workers could do for radiology what they have done for plumbing in the Home Counties.

Little known fact: A CT abdomen gives radiation exposure equivalent to several hundred CXRs and a cancer risk of one in several thousand.

Contact: Royal College of Radiologists: 020 7636 4432; www.rcr.ac.uk

Dermatology

Pros: Good mix of clinical, surgical and private work. Few on-call commitments. Rewarding (e.g. in helping someone gain confidence after treating their acne).

Cons: Ferociously competitive.

Skills: Intricate knowledge of the differences between emollients, ointments and emulsions. Good visual memory.

Risks: Dermatology is unlikely to change in the foreseeable future.

Little known fact: There are thought to be some 3000 dermatological diagnoses.

Contact: British Association of Dermatology: 020 7383 0266; www.bad.org.uk

Endocrinology and diabetes

Pros: Challenging and varied, ranging from the complications of diabetes and the general medical knowledge required, to the rare and exotic endocrine disorders. Multidisciplinary approach to looking after people with diabetes. Good evidence-based knowledge about general medicine, as people with diabetes tend to have cardiac, renal, ophthalmic and neurological problems. Currently very easy to get into.

Cons: 90% of your workload is persuading overweight people to eat sensibly, lose weight and exercise more. The smell of an infected ulcer is the most pungent of smells, ranking just above melaena in the all-time top five. (While we're here, you may as well have the other four: necrotic foot ulcer; melaena; lung abscess halitosis; vulval intertrigo; a festering alcohol withdrawal.)

Skills: They are the only people who truly understand hyponatraemia.

Risks: What if someone finds a cure for diabetes? Lots of P45s to be issued, but does this seem likely?

Little known fact: Diabetes mellitus means 'honey siphon'. This harks back to the times when tasting urine was part of history and examination – be thankful for urine dipsticks!

Contact: Diabetes UK: www.diabetes.org.uk; and the Society for Endocrinology: www.endocrinology.org

Forensic psychiatry

Pros: Emotionally challenging, fascinating psychopathology. Frequent court appearances and cross-examinations requiring gall and a focused mind. Rewarding in terms of rehabilitation for patients.

Cons: Due to the high-security nature of the job, more paperwork than most specialties. Need to be headstrong and emotionally detached – you'll be dealing with the extremes of the psychiatric and human spectrum.

Risks: Low. Plenty of consultant jobs on the horizon.

Contact: Royal College of Psychiatrists: www.rcpsych.ac.uk

Gastroenterology (including the soon to be full specialty of hepatology)

Pros: Multidisciplinary approach, combining input from radiology, pathology, surgery and a strong nurse input (including nurse endoscopists). Practical stuff (e.g. endoscopy, ERCP, close work with transplant unit depending on where you work). Varied caseload, from youngsters with IBD or IBS, to alcohol related liver disease, to bowel cancer, to emergency bleeders. Diagnostically interesting.

Cons: Competitive. Need to be able to deal with non-medical aspects.

Skills: Have you seen the shape of a colon and the shape of an endoscope?

Risks: Few. Too many incurable long-term conditions.

Little known fact: Bury (Lancs) has a high rate of false positive faecal occult blood (FOB) tests due to the large amount of black pudding consumed there.

Contact: British Society of Gastroenterology: 020 7935 3150; www.bsg.org.uk

General internal medicine, including acute medicine

General internal medicine (GIM) used to be acquired through unselected medical takes during your specialty training, in effect leading to your being dual-qualified. Patients could be referred to your clinic with multiple problems of a 'general' nature that required further tests. Nowadays GIM is often replaced by acute medicine, and there are fewer consultants who practise it.

With the colleges' final stance on GIM still uncertain, this section deals with acute medicine only.

Pros: Varied, surprising, busy, boring and mad, all at the same time. Like A&E but with medical patients (the ones the surgeons have managed to bounce). High patient turnover.

Cons: Patience is a virtue – stressful when bed-blocked and you may well ask why many patients need to be there.

Skills: The ability to know when someone needs to come in. Sounds simple, but it is always easier to admit than discharge. Requires vociferous decision-making skills.

Risks: Acute medicine is one of the newer specialties. Jobs will be available, but expect competition.

Contact: the Society for Acute Medicine: www.acutemedicine.org.uk; Royal College of Physicians (all specialties): 020 7935 1174; www.rcplondon.ac.uk; Royal College of Physicians of Edinburgh: 0131 225 7324; www.rcpe.ac.uk; Royal College of Physicians and Surgeons of Glasgow: 0141 221 6072; www.rcpsg.ac.uk; Royal College of Physicians of Ireland: 00 353 1 6698800; www.rcpi.ie/

General practice

Pros: Another specialty that has undergone a facelift. After dwindling popularity, GP is now back in vogue and is one of the most competitive specialties. Opportunity to work closely with colleagues you get on with. Less stressful than hospital medicine. Attractive salary if you can get a partnership. Suitable for flexible training and developing special interests for your portfolio career. As much or as little on call as you like. Varied caseload – you don't know what's going to come through the door next.

Cons: Lots of politics, red tape and hoop jumping. Driven by targets and guidelines that you must meet to get money. Patients who require lots of patience. Potential for lack of opportunities to get a principal post – many practices are taking on salaried GPs in a distinctly 'assistant' role, with reduced responsibility and smaller salary, and less chance to be autonomous and fulfil your potential.

Skills: Knowing when someone needs to be admitted to hospital. Ability to take a full history and examination in eight minutes.

Risks: Very competitive. You need to have done your homework if you want to progress on to the General Practice training programme. Future jobs may look very different from now.

Contact: Royal College of General Practitioners: 0845 456 4041; www.rcgp.org.uk; The National Recruitment Office for General Practice Training: www.gprecruitment.org.uk

General psychiatry, including liaison, rehabilitation and substance misuse psychiatry

Pros: Varied cases, from acute psychoses and sectioning under the Mental Health Act, to chronic depression and out-patient work. Liaison psychiatry is mainly hospital-based and deals with psychiatric problems in medically/surgically ill patients. Rehabilitation is mainly community-based. Complex social, medical, family and criminal interactions require a holistic approach and lateral thinking.

Cons: As with many specialties, psychiatry has its heart-sink patients, whose social problems are irreparable and often the root of their problems. Get a lot of stick from hospital doctors who don't fully appreciate the dynamic nature of psychiatric diagnoses, the time taken to come to a conclusion and how organic illness masks the facts.

Skills: Being able to take a history in 50 minutes and not feel bad about it.

Risks: Low. There are many unfilled senior posts in the UK and it seems unlikely that the private sector will take over because there is not enough profit in it.

Little known fact: The first electroconvulsive therapy was performed in 1938 on patients who were awake (www.ect.org).

Contact: Royal College of Psychiatrists: www.rcpsych.ac.uk; National Treatment Agency for Substance Misuse: www.nta.nhs.uk/

General surgery

Pros: Able to handle complex surgical patients and critically ill patients with breadth of knowledge about the 'general' surgical subspecialties, including breast, endocrine, upper and lower GI, and vascular. Good hands-on experience for juniors (e.g. lipoma removal, hernia repair, appendicectomy, pilonidal sinus, varicose veins).

Cons: Dying breed, unless planning to work in underdeveloped world. May have to do frequent and busy on-call work.

Skills: Like GPs with a knife.

Risks: Being phased out due to the reduction in training hours and the move towards sub-specialization.

Contact: Royal College of Surgeons of Edinburgh: 0131 527 1600; www.rcsed.ac.uk; Royal College of Surgeons of England: 020 7405 3474; www.rcseng.ac.uk; Royal College of Physicians and Surgeons of Glasgow: 0141 221 6072; www.rcpsglasg.ac.uk; Royal College of Surgeons of Ireland: 00353 1 412 2100; www.rcsi.ie/

There are also many sub-specialties of general surgery:

Vascular surgery

Pros: Highly technically skilled operations. Exciting future prospect of endo-vascular surgery.

Cons: Lots of on-call work and operating during the night when on call.

Skills: Micro-suturing two arteries together is pretty cool.

Risks: If radiologists take over with endovascular devices, career could be brief.

Little known fact: The maggots used to heal leg ulcers come from the larvae of the green blowfly and will set you back about £100 for 200 maggots.

Upper GI surgery

Pros: You'll be at the forefront of innovative, minimally invasive surgery and the ever-evolving skill of removing bigger and bigger organs from smaller and smaller holes. More private 'weight loss' work than you can shake a stick at. Interaction with multidisciplinary team (e.g. staging for upper GI cancers and assessment for bariatric surgery).

Cons: Has been fiercely competitive. On-call commitments. Lots of gallblad-ders if you don't work in a centre offering cancer surgery.

Skills: Try practising eating your meals with long chopsticks through holes in a blanket.

Little known fact: The current record for the quickest laparoscopic cholecys-tectomy is 14 minutes.

Contact: Association of Upper Gastrointestinal Surgeons of Great Britain and Ireland: 020 7304 4773; www.augis.org

Colorectal surgery

Pros: Rewarding, whether resecting a cancer or controlling embarrassing faecal incontinence. Interaction with the multidisciplinary team. Evolving minimally invasive opportunities.

Cons: Competitive.

Skills: See gastroenterology.

Little known fact: The average person passes around 500 cm^3 of flatus a day, roughly dispersed over 14 intervals of passing wind (www.heptune.com).

Obvious fact: Men pass twice as much flatus as women.

Contact: Association of Coloproctology: 020 7973 0307; www.acpgbi.org.uk

Genito-urinary medicine

Pros: Satisfying – diagnosis reached quickly and usually at first consultation with effective results. The challenge of HIV management. Interaction with Public Health and Family Planning. Day job with no on call.

Cons: Conversationally taxing – it's a lifetime of asking intricately about sexual habits, warts and all.

Skills: Being able to jam a swab halfway up a man's urethra without flinching if you are a man or smiling if you are a woman. Not exactly glamorous.

Risks: Low – plenty of patients available and little competition.

Little known fact: The notorious gangster Al Capone died from the complications of syphilis.

Contact: British Association for Sexual Health and HIV: www.bashh.org; The Royal College of Physicians: www.rcplondon.ac.uk/specialty/GUM.asp

Geriatric medicine, including stroke medicine

Pros: One of the few remaining 'general' subspecialties, thus a wide range of pathology seen. Rewarding investment of time with slow rehab patients – you'll know what I mean after you've done geriatrics. The chance to reverse a TACS with thrombolysis can give you your adrenaline kicks if needed.

Cons: Can be used as a 'dumping ground' by other specialties. Lots of delayed discharges and waiting for social services which is not in the patients' best interests.

Skills: Being able to generate a problem list with over ten points and still feel motivated.

Risks: Low as more jobs will be created as the numbers of elderly increase.

Little known facts: What is the secret to longevity? Sprightly 111-year old Lucy D'Abreu, from Stirling, thought to be the oldest Briton on record, claimed it was the 'grace of God' (thescotsman.scotsman.com/uk.cfm?id=584272003). The oldest man in the world, thought to be over 120 years old, was Chinese, and he was a smoker (www.bbc.co.uk/dna/actionnetwork/A6521933).

Contact: British Geriatrics Society: www.bgs.org.uk; Royal College of Physicians: www.rcplondon.ac.uk/specialty/Geriatric.asp

Haematology

Pros: Complex range of pathologies, from assessing someone with anaemia ? cause, to interpreting cytogenetic results from a bone marrow aspirate, to managing genetic haematological disorders. Grateful patients, with whom you tend to form a lasting relationship.

Cons: Can get bogged down with lab management. Other doctors are often ignorant of haematology – a dim and distant memory from med school (see Dermatology). Long career path (currently MRCP and MRCPath), but the new career structure should shorten this.

Skills: Knowing the many causes of a raised APTT. Ability to perform a sternal bone marrow biopsy without fear of piercing the heart/lungs/mediastinum.

Risks: Low as the complex relationship between the lab and clinical medicine does not suit many.

Little known fact: March haemoglobinuria, a condition seen in soldiers who march a lot, has also been described in bongo players.

Contact: The British Society for Haematology: www.b-s-h.org.uk

Histopathology, including cytopathology, forensic pathology, neuropathology and paediatric pathology

Pros: Diagnostically challenging. Your findings are often the final piece in the diagnostic puzzle, so can be heavily relied upon. Lots of sub-subspecialties to delve into. Good hours – mostly 9–5. Few, if any, on-call commitments. New training structure with excellent supervision and early assessment of aptitude. Three schools of pathology were created in 2001, in Leicester, Southampton and Leeds.

Cons: Can be isolated from patients, and other doctors sometimes. You will invariably do postmortems, so avoid if squeamish. May have to relocate to get a training post in one of the new schools.

Skills: Being able to tell tissue type, diagnosis and prognosis from a glass slide with a smattering of pink and blue dots on it.

Risks: Low, many vacant posts but marketization in the NHS may see pathology jobs hived off to the private sector.

Little known fact: You may have heard that hair and nails continue to grow after death. Sadly, this is a myth. They just appear to do that as the skin around them dehydrates and shrinks back (http://dying.about.com).

Contact: Royal College of Pathologists: 020 7451 6700; www.rcpath.org

Immunology

Pros: Near the top of the intellectual food chain – everyone forgets the details of immunology after medical school. Good opportunity for research. Dealing with anaphylaxis is challenging and rewarding. Private practice opportunities.

Cons: Can get quite a few inappropriate referrals, thus the skill is differentiating true allergy from a bit of a sniffle.

Skills: Insider's knowledge of the hundreds of cytokines. Ideal dinner party conversation if you want an early night.

Risks: Probably plenty of jobs available in the future.

Contact: Royal College of Pathologists: www.rcpath.org; The British Society for Immunology: www.immunology.org

Infectious diseases

Pros: One of the more fascinating specialties. A 'Ripley's believe it or not' caseload with regard to tropical medicine, along with the commoner diseases (pneumonia, cellulitis, gastroenteritis). Good research opportunities.

Cons: Few jobs available. Lots of on call for that reason.

Skills: Consultants give the best lectures – purely on graphic merit.

Risks: Old-style national training numbers were thin on the ground. The Foundation programme should create more opportunities.

Little known fact: Hydrophobia, present in about 50% of rabies sufferers, is due to pharyngeal spasm on attempting to eat or drink (www.gpnotebook. co.uk/simplepage.cfm?ID=1147535352).

Contact: Royal Society of Tropical Medicine & Hygiene: www.rstmh.org; British Infection Society: www.britishinfectionsociety.org; see also the RCP and RCPath websites.

Intensive care medicine

Pros: All the best bits of medicine, without the social side – or so they say. Combines physiology with major practical procedures and regular contact with other specialties. Definitely for adrenaline junkies.

Cons: Not much patient follow-up or patient interaction, as most of the time they are sedated. Long working hours and on-call commitments.

Skills: Technically demanding procedures, including intubation.

Risks: An ever-popular and ever-competitive specialty. No shortage anticipated as the specialism is increasingly recognised.

Contact: Intercollegiate Board for Training in Intensive Care Medicine: www.ibticm.org; Intensive Care Society: www.ics.ac.uk

Medical microbiology and virology

Pros: Mix of lab and clinical work (including ITU). Diagnostically challenging in terms of correctly identifying a pathogen, ensuring it is not a contaminant and choosing appropriate treatment. Health promotion opportunities (handwashing) and experience in infection control (MRSA, *C. diff*).

Cons: Little opportunity for patient follow-up, unless ITU case or prolonged stay. Often relying on other clinicians for the facts (e.g. with regard to blood cultures).

Skills: Noses of steel. The smell of fermenting anaerobes just missed out on the top five worst smells in medicine (see above). They are also good at reminding us that we are the victims of our own demise in terms of handwashing.

Risks: Increasing workload. The Foundation programme is striving to produce more microbiologists.

Little known fact: Alcohol gel kills MRSA, but not *C. diff*. So wash those hands with soap.

Contact: The Royal College of Pathologists: www.rcpath.org

Medical oncology

You may have read clinical oncology above. These two subspecialties are slightly different but share common ground. In 1993 the Joint Committee on Clinical Oncology was set up to look into combining the two aspects of training into one subspecialty. See address below for details.

Pros: More holistic, and more prolonged patient contact, than clinical oncology. Has its roots in chemotherapy, and is a relatively new subspecialty from the Royal College of Physicians. Liaison with most specialties, in particular haematology (leukaemia, lymphoma, myeloma).

Cons: See clinical oncology. Rationing of healthcare resources can be frustrating for you and the patient (e.g. the media spotlight on Herceptin (transtuzamab) in metastatic breast cancer).

Risks: Low – increasing demand from patients for specialist care means that you are likely to be needed.

Contact: The Association of Cancer Physicians: www.cancerphysicians. org.uk; Royal College of Physicians: www.rcplondon.ac.uk/specialty/ MedicalOncology.asp; Joint Committee on Clinical Oncology, Royal College of Physicians, 11 St Andrews Place, London NW1 4LE

Medical ophthalmology and ophthalmology

Pros: One of the trendier specialties, probably due to better training. Rewarding job, appreciative patients. Opportunity for surgical or medical ophthalmology work. Another specialty near the top of the intellectual food chain. Private practice possible.

Cons: Under-resourced, highly competitive, and as the number of elderly people grows, so will the number of eye consultations.

Skills: The ophthalmological surgeons take the plaudits for being able to work through a 3 mm incision for cataract surgery and are the only doctors who know how the slit lamp microscope works.

Risks: Highly competitive – currently about 30 consultant vacancies a year (careerfocus.bmjjournals.com).

Little known fact: The green light on an ophthalmoscope is actually the 'red-free filter' and is used to highlight blood vessels and any haemorrhages on the fundus (they show up as black).

Contact: Royal College of Ophthalmologists: www.rcophth.ac.uk; 020 7935 0702

Neurology

Pros: Theoretical, challenging and rewarding once the diagnosis is made. Mix of acute presentations (e.g. Guillain-Barré syndrome) and chronic (e.g. multiple sclerosis).

Cons: Can be frustrating – once you've made the diagnosis, there is a perception that there's very little you can do about it. Competitive.

Skills: Able to complete a full neurological examination without collapsing from exhaustion halfway through.

Risks: Very competitive but the new training scheme for all 'neurosciences' is likely to lead to more opportunities.

Little known fact: The Argyll-Robertson pupil, commonly caused by neurosyphilis, is also known as the 'prostitute's pupil', because it accommodates but doesn't react.

Contact: Association of British Neurologists: 020 7405 4060; www.theabn. org

Neurosurgery

Pros: Technically demanding, very hands-on and lots of exciting emergency surgery. You get to say 'I'm a brain surgeon' at dinner parties.

Cons: Lots of telephone referrals, so you need to have patience and accept that you may get a lot of chaff, and only a bit of wheat. On-call commitments are demanding. Depressing dealing with the head-injured young.

Skills: Stimulating patients' brains while they are awake during surgery.

Little known fact: Harvey Cushing, the American neurosurgeon, was one of the first doctors to use gloves in theatre. The glove manufacturers? Goodyear (en.wikipedia.org).

Contact: Society of British Neurological Surgeons: 020 7869 6892; www.sbns. org.uk; European Association of Neurosurgical Societies; www.eans.org

Nuclear medicine

Pros: Diagnostically important – positron emission tomography imaging really does get to the parts of the body other techniques don't reach (e.g. pulmonary embolism in certain cases, labelled white cell scan in inflammatory bowel disease, bone scans). Opportunities for research.

Cons: As it is a service, the system is open to dubious referrals, which is frustrating for nuclear medicine team. (You will find out when you start work and begin requesting V/Q scans.)

Contact: The British Nuclear Medicine Society: 020 8676 7864; www.bnms. org.uk

Obstetrics and gynaecology, including the subspecialties gynaecological oncology, maternal and foetal medicine, reproductive medicine, urogynaecology and sexual and reproductive health

Pros: Vast specialty, with *Modernizing Medical Careers* creating more subspecialties. Maternal medicine, for example, deals mainly with antenatal care and requires a general medical background. Reproductive medicine ranges from sexual health and well women's clinics to psychosexual counselling, to rape crisis centres. The specialty is undergoing a facelift to make it more accessible to Foundation programme trainees.

Cons: Obstetrics can be stressful when things don't go to plan. Litigation is rife. Telling pregnant patients that smoking really is bad for them and their unborn child, then seeing them light up outside clinic.

Skills: Delivering difficult presentations and keeping a cool head when needed.

Risks: Low in terms of career. High chance of public naming and shaming by the media before the full facts are known and with no right of reply.

Contact: Faculty of Family Planning and Reproductive Health Care: 020 7724 5524; www.ffprhc.org.uk; Royal College of Obstetricians and Gynaecologists: 020 7772 6200; www.rcog.org.uk

Occupational medicine

Pros: Working with people from all walks of life and industry. Not just confined to the Occupational Health department in your hospital. Opportunity for travel, depending on how far the company you are working with stretches. Your position involves assessing someone's fitness to return to work, or begin work, and advice to employers about how to minimise injury in the workplace – a lot of responsibility. No on-call work.

Cons: Due to the low-profile nature of the job and the fact that most of it is away from hospital you may be undervalued by your colleagues. Currently consultant posts are few and far between.

Skills: Spotting malingerers a mile off.

Risks: With the Foundation programme it is hoped more Specialty Training posts will become available. There is currently only one SHO post (careerfocus.bmjjournals.com).

Contact: Faculty of Occupational Medicine of the Royal College of Physicians: 020 7317 5890; www.facoccmed.ac.uk; Society of Occupational Medicine: www.som.org.uk

Old age psychiatry

Pros: Rewarding specialty. Able to restore quality of life, whether improving someone's mood after the death of their spouse, or arranging 24-hour care for someone with dementia. Pleasantly confused patients can be fun to work with.

Cons: Because it's a relatively new specialty and fairly low profile, funding hasn't been good, so some aspects are under-resourced. Patient assessment is labour-intensive if cognitive problems are apparent.

Skills: Knowing what different bits of the MMSE actually mean in terms of brain functioning.

Risks: Low. With a growing elderly population, it is likely to expand.

Contact: Royal College of Psychiatrists: 020 7235 2351; www.rcpsych.ac.uk

Ophthalmology

See Medical ophthalmology and ophthalmology.

Oral and maxillo-facial surgery

Pros: Unique, self-sufficient specialty, highly respected (once people know what your job entails) and highly sought. Varied and rewarding caseload, from complex dental surgery to facial reconstruction following trauma.

Cons: Probably one of the most competitive specialties. Research needed. It's a long career pathway – you need to be dual-qualified in medicine and dentistry.

Skills: Anyone who has studied for that long must be pretty good at making a mangled face look beautiful again.

Risks: Highly competitive and not that many consultant posts – so spice up your application form if you're thinking about max-fax.

Contact: British Association of Oral and Maxillofacial Surgeons: www.baoms. org.uk

Otolaryngology, also known as Ear, Nose and Throat

Pros: Varied specialty with lots of subspecialties on offer. Close liaison with allergists, immunologists, speech and language therapists. Wide range of patient age. Rewarding. Scope for private practice.

Cons: Competitive and with an SHO-to-registrar bottleneck, though that promises to be widened with the advent of the Foundation programme. Research is more or less mandatory, but this is likely to change.

Skills: Being able to tinker with the smallest bones in the human body without losing them.

Risks: Currently not a great outlook to get on Higher Specialty training.

Contact: The British Association of Otorhinolaryngologists – Head and Neck Surgeons (ENT-UK): www.entuk.org

Paediatric cardiology

Pros: Complex, challenging, glamorous, rigorous but rewarding. Opportunity for interventional procedures. A 'pure' form of adult cardiology, as not many neonates smoke. Fascinating congenital cardiac pathology.

Cons: Intensely competitive, requiring research to get ahead in the pre-MMC era.

Skills: Ability to interpret paediatric ECHOs.

Risk: An SHO-to-registrar bottleneck, as a legacy of the old career structure. The career structure can be approached from different angles depending on whether your background is MRCPCH (Member of the Royal College of Paediatrics and Child Health) or MRCP (Member of the Royal College of Physicians).

Contact: Royal College of Paediatrics and Child Health: www.rcpch.ac.uk; Royal College of Physicians: www.rcplondon.ac.uk

Paediatric surgery

Pros: Technically demanding, but highly rewarding. High level of clinical acumen required, particularly in young patients whose parents provide the history. Fascinating variety of general surgery, from gastroschisis in premature babies to lung transplants in cystic fibrosis patients.

Cons: Competitive. Research is desirable.

Skills: Adult surgery is complicated enough. Doing all that on a body a third the size – that's impressive.

Risk: Competitive. Registrar posts are difficult to come by, so make sure your application form is ready when the opportunity arises.

Contact: British Association of Paediatric Surgeons: 020 7869 6915; www.baps. org.uk

Paediatrics, including community child health, neonatal medicine, paediatric pharmacology and therapeutics, paediatric subspecialties of endocrinology, gastroenterology, infectious diseases and immunology, intensive care, nephrology, neuro-disability, neurology, oncology, respiratory medicine and rheumatology

Pros: A vast area of medicine. Diagnostically challenging. Kids are generally fun to work with. Long-lasting relationships formed with patients who have chronic illness and their families. Opportunity to sub-specialise as in adult medicine, but paediatrics still remains one of the few generalist areas left. Flexible working is widely accepted.

Cons: Angry or aggressive parents. Harrowing cases of child abuse. Likely to be resident on call in many hospitals. Workload variable – quiet in the summer, overrun in the winter. May have to decide on applying for paediatrics without ever having worked in it as there are few Foundation programme posts.

Skills: Putting a venflon in a screaming kid is like jousting with a blind man on a galloping horse – and that's from the kid's perspective. Paediatricians also have free access to those stickers that say 'I've been brave today'.

Risks: Low if you get on to the Specialty Training programme, but this is likely to be competitive.

Little known fact: The piercing scream of a child comes in at a hefty 110 dB – that's between a chainsaw and a rock concert (www.ata.org).

Contact: Royal College of Paediatrics and Child Health: 020 7307 5600; www.rcpch.ac.uk

Palliative care

Pros: Rewarding, comprising a wide range of diseases, from metastatic cancer to advanced COPD, heart failure or HIV infection. Close patient relationships formed.

Cons: Perhaps evolving too quickly – some areas are under-resourced. Need to get used to dealing with death on a daily basis.

Skills: Making a good death happen. Too many 'bad' deaths happen in hospital, due to poor organization or lack of communication.

Risks: Favourable prospects for consultant posts. Palliative care posts in the Foundation programme will make it more accessible.

Little known fact: Macmillan Cancer Support was started in 1911 by Douglas Macmillan. After watching his father die a painful death from cancer, Douglas created the Society for the Prevention and Relief of Cancer. His aims were to help patients and their relatives. One hundred years on and they are still an invaluable resource (www.macmillan.org.uk).

Contact: The Association for Palliative Medicine of Great Britain and Ireland: www.palliative-medicine.org; Royal College of Physicians: www.rcplondon.ac.uk/specialty/Palliative.asp

Pharmaceutical medicine

Pros: A different take on a medical degree. Focus is still on patient health, but from the perspective of a drug company. Lots of opportunities at different levels of drug production. Attractive salary. National or international travel may be involved.

Cons: Tricky to return to the NHS once you've left. As you are now working for a business, lots of paperwork and bureaucracy.

Skills: Being responsible for endorsing the safety of a drug. One wrong decision and it could be millions of pounds down the drain, and the 'Employee of the Month' sign ripped from your door.

Risks: Lots of opportunity to go into this specialty but companies frequently merge or consolidate so long-term job security is not like working in the NHS.

Contact: The Faculty of Pharmaceutical Medicine of the Royal Colleges of Physicians of the United Kingdom: 020 7224 0343; www.fpm.org.uk; British Association of Pharmaceutical Physicians: 0118 934 1943; www.brapp.org.uk; The Association of the British Pharmaceutical Industry: 0870 890 4333; www.abpi.org.uk

Plastic surgery

Pros: Technically challenging. Varied caseload – the majority of emergency work will be dealing with burns victims. Elective work involves reconstruction of congenital defects, which can be rewarding. Private practice opportunities and the glamour aspect.

Cons: Very competitive. Research desirable. Unfortunately, litigation is creeping in.

Skills: Extreme hand–eye coordination needed as much operating done through magnifying devices. Need to be able to deal with acutely ill patients and long-term psychological issues.

Risks: As with any other surgical specialty, competitive and limited number of SpR posts. NHS plastics seems to be in a mini-crisis.

Little known fact: The first attempted breast augmentation was performed in 1895, using a lipoma on the patient's back as fatty tissue.

Contact: British Association of Plastic Reconstructive and Aesthetic Surgeons: www.bapras.org.uk; British Association of Aesthetic Plastic Surgeons: www.baaps.org.uk; British Society for Surgery of the Hand: 020 7831 5162; www.bssh.ac.uk

Psychiatry of learning disability

Pros: Opportunity to develop a niche in a fascinating, challenging specialty, requiring excellent communication skills. Very little on-call work.

Cons: Under-resourced. A lot of time needed to invest in your patients due to the interaction of psychiatric illness and learning disability. Emotionally draining.

Skills: Among the most patient doctors, with the best communication skills.

Risks: Low. Consultant posts pre-Foundation programme were never given much press, so it is hoped it will become more popular.

Contact: Royal College of Psychiatrists: 020 7235 2351; www.rcpsych.ac.uk

Psychotherapy

Pros: Opportunity to interact with a wide variety of patients and their problems, with rewarding outcomes.

Cons: Lack of evidence base to support results of therapy. Poorly resourced.

Skills: Being able to listen. Ability to suspend disbelief when listening to disagreements between Freudians and Jungians.

Risks: Generally funded at SHA level. With the lack of evidence base and changes to the structure of the NHS, resources are likely to shrink, not increase. Private work may be available.

Contacts: UK Council of Psychotherapists: www.psychotherapy.org.uk; British Association of Psychotherapists: www.bap-psychotherapy.org

Public health medicine

Pros: The 'bigger picture' specialty, focusing on prevention rather than cure. Rewarding and challenging work, using clinical and epidemiological skills to formulate a solution to problems. Appears to yield ultimate power with control of NHS finances. Little on-call commitment.

Cons: Career structure needs a facelift. Recent shift to recruitment of non-medically trained people may undermine status and pay.

Skills: Good with stats and able to understand what the ethical principle of 'justice' means.

Risks: Public health is in a state of flux. Has been reorganised several times. May become more important with its role in management of national risks such as pandemic flu and bio-terrorism.

Contact: Faculty of Public Health: 020 7935 0243; www.fph.org.uk

Rehabilitation medicine

Pros: Rewarding and very much focused on teamwork. Few on-call commitments.

Cons: Under-resourced somewhat due to low-profile nature. May take months to notice an appreciable difference in a patient. Can be difficult to manage patient expectations (Christopher Reeve being a prime example)

Skills: Patience and working in a multidisciplinary team.

Risks: Increasingly popular with recent investment in service provision. Keep your application form polished.

Little known fact: Botox injections were first used to help with flexion contractures and can cause botulism. (If only Hollywood knew.)

Contact: British Society for Rehabilitation Medicine: www.bsrm.co.uk

Renal medicine

Pros: Nice mix of esoteric rare stuff, such as the vasculitides, and the chronic disease management skills required for caring for people on renal replacement therapy waiting for a renal transplant. Intellectual interest from the basic physiology.

Cons: Lots of hypertension that does not respond to treatment.

Skills: Invaluable knowledge of renal physiology. Renal biopsy.

Risks: Few. Renal failure is increasing with an ageing population and defining stages of renal impairment that must be referred to a renal physician (see the NSF) ensures that the workload will stay high.

Point of interest: Tread carefully when asked to re-site a venflon on the renal unit.

Respiratory medicine

Pros: Lots of diagnostic conundrums with only a few symptoms to differentiate them. Mix of practical skills (e.g. bronchoscopy and transthoracic procedures) and levels of care, from acute illness to palliative care.

Cons: The eternal battle involved in trying to get patients to stop smoking! Dealing with shortness of breath and cough.

Skills: Able to understand what a lagger does and remember the anatomy of the lung.

Risks: None, smokers will continue to keep you occupied until your retirement.

Little known fact: There is a database dedicated to patients with rare ('orphan') lung diseases on the British Thoracic Society website called BOLD (British Orphan Lung Disease).

Contact: British Thoracic Society: 020 7831 8778; www.brit-thoracic.org.uk

Rheumatology

Pros: Vast range of presentations, from life-threatening acute systemic vasculitis, to the challenges of connective tissue disease refractory to treatment in young patients, to the long-lasting relationships formed with the rheumatoid and osteoarthritis patients. Lots of practical skills, including musculoskeletal ultrasound. Grateful patients. Few on-call commitments.

Cons: Mostly out-patient work. Time-consuming – patients need a lot of investment in their ideas, concerns and expectations due to the social and psychological effects of the disease and treatments.

Skills: Ability to stick a needle in someone's knee joint without cringing, and with aseptic technique. Insider's knowledge of auto-antibodies.

Risks: Rheumatology is popular. You will need to go to rheumatology clinics and think about audits if you want to stand out from the crowd.

Contact: British Society for Rheumatology: 020 7842 0900; www.rheumatology.org.uk

Trauma and orthopaedic surgery

Pros: Probably the most practical of all the specialties. Rewarding in terms of seeing someone regain independence after joint replacement. Double your NHS income in private practice.

Cons: Fierce competition. Male-dominated at present but this could change. Not well known for a holistic approach to the patient ('That's what ortho-geriatrics is for').

Skills: Wielding a power saw without causing injury. Knowing the definition of a Colles' fracture, including the fact that Abraham Colles was Irish, and first described this in 1814. (Next time you refer the old lady who's fallen onto an outstretched hand and broken her wrist, say 'distal radius fracture' to avoid being shot down.)

Risks: Private practice could run dry if New Labour gets rid of waiting lists. At least you will have legal reports to fall back on. Getting colonised with MRSA – look forward to a career in 'office orthopaedics'!

Little known fact: Orthopaedic means 'straight child' in Greek, stemming from the specialty's origin in treating children with disabilities.

Contact: British Orthopaedic Association: 020 7405 6507; www.boa.ac.uk

Urology

Pros: Dynamic specialty spearheading the new run-through specialty training programmes via *Modernizing Medical Careers*, so quite trendy. Interaction between medical and surgical management of urological disease. Good mix of acute presentations (e.g. urinary retention, pyonephrosis), renal transplant and out-patient management of prostate cancer. Also, have the right to wear wellies in theatre.

Cons: Competitive. The proposed run-through programme may make the specialty two-tiered, so initially you will be performing fairly benign proce-dures and may have to wait before you get on to the major surgery.

Skills: All-seeing index finger that can tell you the volume of a prostate.

Risks: Low. The run-through programme will help get rid of any bottlenecks, but as it is a competitive specialty you will still need to be looking for audits and research to get ahead.

Contact: British Association of Urological Surgeons: www.baus.org.uk

Working abroad

If the travel bug bites you, here is a list of organizations that help doctors find work abroad, in the developed or developing world. If you do decide to do this, communication is vital. Your employers will want to know if you intend to come back to work for them so they can reap the benefits of investing in you. Make sure everyone knows what you are doing though. The next few years are going to see dynamic changes to the career structure in the UK, and the last thing you want is to be left out on a limb.

Contact: BMA International Activities: 020 7383 6793; www.bma.org.uk/ international; Medics Travel: www.medicstravel.co.uk (contains everything you need to organise your time abroad); RedR – Engineers for Disaster Relief: www.redr.org (recruits and trains people to be able to work in areas where humanitarian relief work is provided); Medical Emergency Relief International: 020 7014 1600; www.merlin.org.uk (humanitarian relief work); Médecins Sans Frontières: www.msf.org (it requires fairly experienced doctors, but the website is useful for getting a look at what they do); Voluntary Services Overseas: 020 8780 7500; www.vso.org.uk (well-established organisation that caters for all types of people, not just doctors).

Index

Index

Index